Stem Cell and Tissue Engineering

This book covers conventional clinical treatment methods for handling bone, cartilage, and related disorders along with their limitations and highlights the current state of the art of tissue engineering as an alternative for regenerating such defective tissue. Potential biomimetic scaffolding materials and their development, desired properties, modifications, and optimizations are described. The design and advancement in fabrication, characterization, properties, and biological functions of scaffolds, their integration with stem cells and various bioreactor systems for tissue regeneration are presented. It further reviews *in vitro* and *in vivo (pre-clinical)* assessments of tissue constructs, involved translational challenges, and strategies in various stages of neotissue production.

Features:

- Discusses the key aspects of generating engineered bone, cartilage, and associated tissues through tissue engineering approach.
- Describes multiple engineering principles, and processes involved in the various stages of developing biomaterials and scaffolds.
- Covers integration of stem cells with scaffolds, including assessment of tissue grafts, and translational strategy.
- Explores key factors influencing tissue graft generation in bioreactors and challenges involved in various stages.
- Includes several exercises including review questions and numerical problems, for better understanding of the subject.

This book is aimed at researchers, students, and professionals in biomedical engineering, tissue engineering, stem cells, biomaterials, and orthopaedics.

Stem Cell and Tissue Engineering

Bone, Cartilage, and Associated Joint Tissue Defects

Krishna Pramanik

CRC Press
Taylor & Francis Group
Boca Raton London New York

CRC Press is an imprint of the
Taylor & Francis Group, an **informa** business

First edition published 2024
by CRC Press
2385 NW Executive Center Drive, Suite 320, Boca Raton FL 33431

and by CRC Press
4 Park Square, Milton Park, Abingdon, Oxon, OX14 4RN

CRC Press is an imprint of Taylor & Francis Group, LLC

© 2024 Krishna Pramanik

ISBN: 9781032156880 (hbk)
ISBN: 9781032156897 (pbk)
ISBN: 9781003245353 (ebk)

DOI: 10.1201/9781003245353

Typeset in Times
by Newgen Publishing UK

Contents

About the Author

Krishna Pramanik obtained her PhD in chemical technology from the University of Calcutta, India, in 1995. She has 30 years of experience in industry, research, and teaching in the field of Chemical Engineering, Biotechnology and Biomedical Engineering. She is presently Professor in the Department of Biotechnology and Medical Engineering and heads the Centre of Excellence in Tissue Engineering, National Institute of Technology Rourkela, India. Her current major research activity includes the field of tissue engineering, with main focus on the development of biopolymeric and polymer-composite-based tissue scaffold with nano-features, integration of scaffold with stem cells to generate tissue constructs, and tissue grafts for bone, cartilage, skin, and corneal tissue defects. She has published nearly 150 papers and 16 book chapters in international publications and edited three books. She has supervised 20 doctoral and five post-doctoral fellows, most of which in the area of Biomaterial and Tissue Engineering. She has been serving as the Editor and Editorial Board Member of international journals, including the Associate Editor of *Biocell* and currently Associate Editor of *Biomaterials* (specialty section of *Frontiers in Materials, Frontiers in Bioengineering and Biotechnology,* and *Frontiers in Molecular Biosciences*).

1 Basic Biology of Bone, Cartilage, and Surrounding Tissues

INTRODUCTION

Bone and cartilage, the specialized connective tissues comprising different types of cells embedded within the extracellular matrix, constitute the vital element of the human skeletal system. Both these tissues have important functions in protecting other tissues and organs of our body by providing structural support and surfaces for necessary muscle attachment. However, bone, cartilage, and their associated joint tissues are prone to damage because of trauma or accidental injury, ageing or degeneration, developmental abnormalities, etc., the consequences of which lead to severe pain and loss of mobility (Kock et al. 2012). Typically surgical repair or replacement is needed for relieving pain and restoring respective tissue functions by removing or restoring the defective skeletal part (Demirkiran 2013). In the United States, 6.3 million bone fracture cases arise and 2 million people suffer from osteoporosis coupled with bone fracture, which costs an approximate worth of 20 billion dollars per year (Kim et al. 2017). Tissue engineering, an emerging field in engineering and regenerative medicine, has been considered to offer ideal medical treatment for sustainable improvement in the quality of human life, resulting in an improved clinical outcome for the patient. The tissue engineering approach providing engineered biological substitute can overcome the limitations of the conventional grafting methods. However, to understand the concept and the development of tissue engineering strategy, the fundamental knowledge of the bone, cartilage, and their derivatives like the complex joint tissue, the various issues pertaining to their damage or diseases, and the current scenario of their treatment are of utmost importance to deal with. Therefore, in this chapter, an overview of the basic biology of bone, cartilage, and other associated tissues including their types, composition, structure, and function has been described. The common diseases and damages that affect the cartilage, bone, and joint tissues as well as the various issues related to their defects have been discussed. Furthermore, the presently used treatment methods including the non-surgical treatment or conservative medications focusing on pain management, prevention of inflammation, etc., and the surgical treatment emphasizing the more complex and critical joint defects have been highlighted.

BONE: ITS COMPOSITION, TYPES, STRUCTURE, AND FUNCTION

COMPOSITION OF BONE

Bone is a specialized connective tissue that functions both as a tissue and an organ system (Downey and Siegel 2006b). Bone consists of heterogeneous composite materials such as mineral phase (70–90%) of hydroxyapatite ($Ca_{10}(PO_4)_6(OH)_2$), an organic phase of type I collagen, noncollagenous proteins, and water (Dalén and Olsson 2009). Of the organic material, 90% is collagen (Marie 1992) and the rest is a noncollagenous protein matrix mostly consisting of proteoglycans and glycoproteins with mineral salts comprising calcium phosphate (85%), calcium carbonate (10%), and a small amount of calcium fluoride and magnesium fluoride. These complexes of bone are responsible for the maintenance of the bone structure (Dalén and Olsson 2009). Fifteen per cent weight of the bone consists of cellular content (Downey and Siegel 2006b). The major constituent of bone extracellular matrix is type I collagen which is fibrous in nature (Raouf et al. 2015) and it provides a three-dimensional structure, in which the carbonate apatite mineral crystals are developed (Abdelmagid 2006). The organic component of the bone matrix includes different types of proteins, namely, proteoglycans, glycoproteins, sialoproteins, bone "gla" proteins, etc. Some more proteins are found in the organic phase of bone matrix which play an important role in the development of healthy bone, such as osteocalcin, osteonectin, thrombospondin, fibronectin, byglican, decorin, osteopontin, bone sialoprotein, etc. These proteins have their own specific functions to make healthy and stable bone.

TYPES AND STRUCTURE OF BONE

The bone is a highly vascularized tissue that has the unique capability of remodelling and self-healing. Two major sections of bone consist of cortical bone which is compact in nature and trabecular bone which is spongy in nature (Downey and Siegel 2006b; Raouf et al. 2015).

Cortical or compact bone is the outer hard layer comprising 90% of calcified region of the bone, whereas the spongy cancellous or trabecular bone is the inner part with 25% calcified region encircling numerous large spaces with a honeycomb appearance (Gibson 1985). The compact bone is developed from closely packed osteons which are made up of haversian canals surrounded by circumferential bone lamellae. Cancellous bone is formed from randomly arranged trabeculae (Abdelmagid 2006). The haversian canal of compact bone is the central canal of the bone, which is connected to Volkmann's or perforating canals, and the primary function of these two canals is the supply of nutrients and blood to bone tissue (Kim et al. 2015). Osteocytes, the mature bone cells, are located in tiny cavities between the lamellae known as lacunae (Reilly 2000). Canaliculi is a system of linking tunnels that interconnect the lacunae. Cortical bone bears a significant portion of the skeleton's total load (Augat and Schorlemmer 2006).

In spongy bone, lacunae are found in random matrix network form known as trabeculae instead of concentric circles. Spaces in spongy bone contain red bone marrow that is saved by trabeculae, where hematopoiesis takes place. This porous bone and middle cavity get nutrients from arteries that pass through the outer hard bone. The spongy cancellous bone provides balance to the dense compact bone by making bones lighter, thereby making the movement of muscles easier. It also acts as a shock absorber during joint movement (Safadi et al. 2009).

According to the structure, bones are of four different types, namely, long bone, short bone, flat bone, and irregular bone (Clarke 2008). A long bone is long and thin in shape (Onar and Belli 2005). It has three regions, including the two broader terminals (epiphyses), a cylindrical pipe in the middle (diaphysis), and a growing zone among them (metaphysis) (Abdelmagid 2006). Long bones serve as levers, allowing movement with the support of muscles (Lieberman, Polk, and Demes 2004). Some examples of long bones include clavicles, humeri, radii, ulnae, metacarpals, femur, tibia, fibula, metatarsals, and phalanges (Clarke 2008). The short bone is a cube-shaped bone. The carpal and tarsal bones of the hand and foot are examples of short bones. The centre of this bone is spongy in nature and is covered by a thin layer of compact bone. Flat bone has a flattened and broad surface. The skull bone is an example of flat bone that is made up of the inner and outer layers of compact bone with spongy bone between them (Safadi et al. 2009). Some other examples of flat bones are mandible, scapulae, sternum, and ribs (Clarke 2008). Irregular bone does not have any regular shape like the other three bone types (Zhang et al. 2018) and has a thin sheet of compact bone on the outside and a spongy bone on the inside (Safadi et al. 2009). Some of the examples of irregular bones are vertebrae, maxillofacial bone, etc. (Bogduk 2016).

TYPES OF BONE CELLS

The major types of bone cells include osteoblast and osteoclast, bone lining cells, and osteocytes (Mohamed 2008; Buckwalter et al. 1996; Downey and Siegel 2006a).

Osteoblasts

These types of bone cells exist along the bone surface and are responsible for the formation of new bone by producing a unique protein called osteoid. Osteoblasts synthesize bone matrix mainly in two main steps including the deposition of organic matrix by secreting collagen proteins, non-collagen proteins, and proteoglycans, and further mineralization by two phases such as vesicular and the fibrillar phases (Anderson 2003; Yoshiko et al. 2007). Osteoblast cells can be obtained from mesenchymal stem cells (MSCs) and they help in repairing old bones.

Osteocytes

These cells, which comprise 90–95% of the total bone cells, are basically entrapped osteoblast cells and exist within the bone itself. Osteocytes represent the most mature differentiation state of osteoblast lineage. These inactive osteoblast cells help in communication within bone tissue and also maintain the mineral concentration of the bone by secretion of enzymes (Franz-Odendaal, Hall, and Witten 2006).

Osteoclast

These cells, formed usually by monocyte fusion, are large specialized multinucleate cells having 2–12 nucleus per cell. The nuclei break down the bone cells and digest them by releasing specific enzymes (e.g. lytic enzyme) and acids. They also help in remodelling damaged bone through its degradation or resorbtion and create pathways for blood vessels and nerves. Osteoclasts and their precursors can regulate the differentiation of osteoblast precursors (Boyce, Yao, and Xing 2009).

FUNCTION OF BONE

Bone contributes towards good health and imparts significant functions to the body (Marie 1992). Bone protects internal organs from external impacts like the skull safeguards brain, ribs protect lungs, heart, etc.; provides structural support, movement, and stabilization of other vital organs; helps in blood supply and mineral reserves like calcium, phosphorous, growth factors, and homeostasis; and assists in blood pH control by releasing and absorbing basic salts, multiple progenitor cell housing and others (Kim et al. 2015). Bone marrow also produces blood cells. Cancellous bones help in producing red blood cells (RBC), white blood cells (WBC), and platelets. Bones release hormone that helps in controlling blood sugar levels. It can also absorb heavy metals and other toxic elements from the blood. Muscles, cartilage, ligaments, and tendons are attached to bone and help in movement.

CARTILAGE: ITS COMPOSITION, TYPES, STRUCTURE, AND FUNCTION

Cartilage is a shiny, white, flexible connective tissue found throughout the body. It is comprised of chondroblast or perichondral cells that are differentiated into the chondrocytes, thereby forming the extracellular matrix (ECM). The later is generally composed of water, collagen and proteoglycans, and other non-collagenous proteins and glycoproteins. Chondrocytes lie in lacunae and collagen fibres. This tissue covers the bone ends at the joint as a cushion and provides support (Figure 1.1) and exists in different parts of the human body. Cartilage is a unique tissue type without any blood vessels or nerves (avascular). Its unique structure makes it strong and flexible. In spite of having such properties, it can be damaged easily, thereby imparting joint pain, stiffness, restriction in movement, and inflammation or swelling. The injured, inflamed, or damaged cartilage also causes joint damage and deformity. Cartilage damage may occur due to tears and injuries for example, accidental or sports-related injury, genetic defect, and other disorders like arthritis. Tissues like bone, skin, muscle, etc., can regenerate tissue on their own, whereas cartilage has poor regeneration ability. Therefore, cartilage performs a very specific function.

It consists of different layers that are articular surface, superficial tangential zone (STZ), middle zone, deep zone, calcified zone, and subchondral bone. The STZ region is 10–20% and 40–60% middle zone of the total cartilage. The deep zone is 30–40% that is composed of chondrocytes and ends with tidemark near the calcified zone that is 30–40%. The deepest layer is the subchondral bone layer which is made up of cancellous bone. Cartilage in our body is of three types, namely, hyaline cartilage, fibro cartilage, and elastic cartilage, which are discussed next.

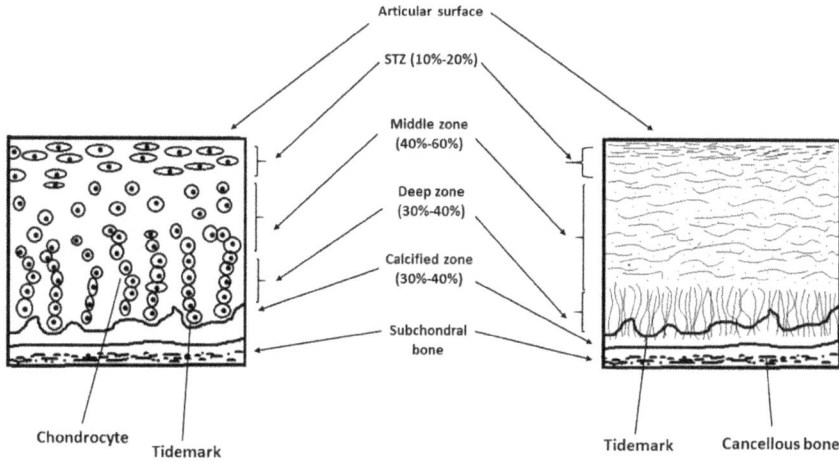

FIGURE 1.1 Structure of cartilage.

Hyaline Cartilage

The term "hyaline" means glassy and it is originated from the Greek word *hyalos*. The hyaline cartilage is the most common type of cartilage in our body and is shiny, semi-transparent in appearance, strong, and elastic in nature. It is found in the nose, larynx, trachea, bronchi, and joints (known as articular cartilage AC). It is a precursor of bone. This cartilage consists of many thin collagen fibres that help to provide strength. However, hyaline cartilage is considered as the weakest among all the three types of cartilage.

Fibro Cartilage

This is the strongest cartilage tissue among the three types of cartilage and is able to hold heavy weights. Fibro cartilage has thick layers of collagen fibres comprising type I collagen and running linearly through the tissue separated by cartilage matrix having chondrocytes. Fibro cartilage is predominantly present in special pads which is known as menisci, in the invertebral discs, vertebrae of the spine, at the interface of tendon and ligament, between the bones in hip and pelvis, joint capsules, etc. These pads play a vital role in reducing the friction in joints, such as the knee.

Elastic Cartilage

Elastic cartilage, also referred to as yellow cartilage, is another form of cartilaginous tissue. They are arranged into elastic fibres consisting of abundant chondrocytes, thereby making a network of matrix that is composed of glycosaminoglycans (GAGs), proteoglycans, and glycoproteins. They are found in the external ears, epiglottis (in throat), and some parts of the nose, trachea, and larynx. This type of cartilage provides strength and flexibility or elasticity to the organs and can maintain the shape of some body structures, like the outer ear.

FUNCTION OF CARTILAGE

Cartilage has different functions in the human body that include the following: it acts as a cushion at the surface of the joints, thereby reducing friction and preventing abrasion and damage; provides shape to certain parts of the body, *viz.*, ears, nose, etc.; acts as a template for the fast growth and development of musculoskeletal system; enhances bone resilience; and holds bones together, for example, bones in the rib-cage. Cartilage can also serve as a lubricating surface and shock absorber that protects the joint against weight-bearing stresses. Cartilage also has a role in bone repair, and in the embryo, it acts as a template for ossification.

OTHER TISSUES

Tendon

Tendons are the linkers between muscles and bones, deliver force from the muscle to the bone, and allow joint movement. Tendons are whitish in colour with elastic nature, thereby showing excellent resistance to mechanical loads. Tendons are comprised of type I collagen and elastin. The outer structures of tendons are divided into five categories: fibrous and synovial sheath, reflection pulleys, peritendinous sheet, and tendon bursae. Normally at each end of the muscle, tendons are present: at the prox-imal end proximal tendon and at the distal end distal tendon. The point of fusion with a muscle and the point of junction with a bone is called myotendinous junction and osteotendinous junction, respectively (Kannus 2000).

Ligament

Ligaments, also known as articular ligaments, are dense bands of connective tissue usually consisting of tough collagenous fibres and they remain intact even during elastic movement. They are viscoelastic and are of different shapes and sizes, such as string, arch-shaped, narrow or wide bands, etc. However, their shapes are changed when strain is applied for a prolonged period of time. They also act as linkers between bone joints and bone. Ligaments play an important role in stabilizing and controlling joints through their normal range of motion when subjected to a tensile load (Frank 2004). Ligaments exist in different locations of the joints, such as in knees, ankles, elbows, shoulders, etc. So, the joint becomes unstable upon stretching or tearing of the ligament.

BONE, CARTILAGE, AND JOINT DAMAGES AND DISEASES

CARTILAGE DISORDERS

Although cartilage is beneficial to our body, it has some limitations, including its inability to heal itself, unlike most other tissues. Damaged cartilage requires much longer period than other tissues to heal due to non-supply of blood in it. Furthermore, the cartilaginous cells which are known as chondrocytes do not easily replicate or repair themselves, which does not permit the damaged cartilage to heal well without medical intervention. Cartilage damage may occur due to various other reasons including the direct impact, progressive wear and tear, lack of movement, poor joint alignment, etc. Direct or forced impact occurs when joints are subjected to a heavy impact, which may be because of a bad fall or an accident. Sports people like footballer, wrester, athletics, and others are more prone to high risk of cartilage damage, particularly AC damage. Joints may also be damaged due to wear and tear when they experience stress for a long period of time. People with obesity easily get their knee joint damage more than a normal person due to experiencing extensive physical stress. Cartilage is often naturally degraded with age and stiffness, especially after long periods of inactivity or immobility which lead to severe pain, inflammation, and even disability. One of the most common examples of such cartilage deterioration is osteoarthritis (OA). One-third of Americans aged over 45 years have been reported to suffer from knee pain. Although AC damage most often occurs in the knees, joints in hips, elbows, wrists, ankles, and shoulder also may be affected. When cartilage damages severely, the joint may be locked that leads to bleeding in the joint, the condition of which is known as haemarthrosis (Uttarilli et al. 2019). Some of the common conditions that lead to cartilage degeneration are the followings.

Costochondritis

Costochondritis is a condition of inflammation of the cartilage that connects the ribs attached to the rib cage (sternum), which is known as the costosternal joint. Although the condition is normally temporary, it may also become chronic. The condition causes uncomfortable chest pain. Although the exact cause of costochondritis may not be known in most of the patients, some conditions like trauma to the chest arising due to an accident or fall, strainful or high-impact activities like weight lifting, strenuous exercise, people having allergies and arthritis, spondylitis, etc., may be responsible. Women and middle-aged people mostly suffer from costochondritis.

Herniated Disk/Herniation

The soft gel-like material in the cartilage disk sticks out due to the rupture of outer cartilage present between two vertebrae, thereby pressing against soft tissue and nerves causing severe pain which is known as a herniated or slipped disk. This type of situation usually happens when degenerative changes occur as a side effect of ageing. People with a major accident or back injury can have herniated disk causing severe pain often in the back and down the legs. Disc herniation usually occurs when hyaline cartilage pulls out from the vertebral endplates. The fragments of cartilage may increase the risk of persisting sciatica and the lost cartilage may increase the permeability of endplate, leading to endplate inflammation and disc infection.

Joint Defects

Cartilage acting as a cushion allows bones for free and easy movement against each other. The synovium, also known as synovial membrane, is a soft connective tissue surrounding the joints that secrets and renews a fluid, thereby lubricating and protecting the cartilage from damage due to friction; thus, the healthy cartilage in turn protects the bones in the joints (Redondo, Christian, and Yanke 2019). When the synovial membrane becomes inflamed and thickened caused by joint overuse, it leads to wear and tear of the cartilage and builds up of extra fluid within joints causing swelling. Most of the joints in knees, hips, hands, feet, and spine are commonly affected by OA. If cartilage further deteriorates, it loses its ability to provide adequate cushioning to the underlying bones because of which bone surfaces are exposed and come in direct contact with each other that results in additional pain and inflammation in joints and its surrounding tissues. If this condition continues, bones grow osteophytes or bone spurs which are the most common phenomena in joints with OA (Nicol et al. 2019).

Chondromalacia Patellae

In this condition, the cartilage of the femur or thigh bone deteriorates due to sliding of backside of kneecap or patella in the knee joint. This condition arises due to several factors such as injury, poor alignment, or muscle weakness, and is most common in younger and sports people like athletic. Aged people with knee arthritis also suffer from this disorder. Different factors are responsible for the high risk of chondromalacia patellae, such as age (particularly in juveniles and young adults), sex (females are more vulnerable than males as they typically possess less weight of muscle), flat feet (which creates much stress on the knee joints), previous injury or dislocation, and high activity like frequent exercise that creates pressure and thereby augments the risk of knee problems. Cartilage may also be damaged by several diseases which are usually characterized by changes and abnormalities in growth, causing devastating consequences. Some of the common cartilage diseases and disorders are discussed here.

Articular Cartilage Injury

Articular cartilage (AC), the smooth cushion covering the bony surface of joints, is composed of chondrocyte cells with a matrix made up of protein collagen. AC consists of different distinct layers with different structural and biochemical features and provides low friction surface, thereby enabling the joint to withstand high load or weight and easy movement. But once damaged, this cartilage cannot heal on its own and cause significant pain and weakness. Cartilage disorder happens as a consequence of traumatic mechanical destruction (e.g. sports injury) which most often occurs in young adults, progressive mechanical degeneration like wear and tear, obesity, OA, and inflammatory arthritis in adults. When cartilage is worn or torn away, it exposes the underlying bone known as subchondral bone. Since AC lies inside joints, there is no direct blood supply within this cartilage and this avascular nature makes it limited ability to self-regenerate, thereby requiring more time for repairing damaged AC. In knee injury, AC may rupture (Forlino et al. 2011).

Growth Plate Cartilage Damage

Growth plates are the areas of cartilage found in the long bones like the femur or thigh bone. The fracture of growth plate mostly occurs from falling or twisting, thereby affecting the layer of growing tissue of the kid's bones and thus disrupting their normal cartilage growth. Growth plates are very soft and even weaker than surrounding ligaments and tendons, so any injury may tear the ligament causing joint sprain in adults and growth plate fracture in children. About 15% of all juvenile fractures and 1–30% of sports-related injuries belong to this category (on Osteoporosis Prevention Diagnosis and Therapy 2001). Besides external injury, the damage of growth plate cartilage may be caused by genetic mutations, a condition known as chondrodysplasias, which disturbs normal skeletal growth.

Osteochondritis Dissecans (OCD)

This is a type of bone and cartilage disorder that forms loose bodies in the joints without any injury or trauma. OCD occurs when a small section of bone starts to dissociate from the surrounding tissue due to inadequate blood supply, causing the risk of instability and damage of the adjacent AC, thereby developing premature OA (Cantarini et al. 2014). The OCD lesion commonly occurs in the articular cartilage at the end of the femur bone in the knee joint (Figure 1.2). Although the reason is not known, this joint disorder most often affects the knee joint, ankle, and elbow, due to repetitive trauma or stresses on the joints over time, lack of vitamin D, and genetic predisposition. The disorder may also occur in other joints such as shoulder and hip joints. Although people of any age may develop OCD, it mostly affects children and adolescents aged between 10 and 20 years, especially young athletes.

Relapsing Polychondritis (RP)

RP is a rare multisystemic situation which results in recurrent inflammation and breakdown of the cartilage. This immune-mediated condition results in progressive anatomical deformation and functionally impairs the involved structures. People suffering from RP are often associated with other conditions like autoimmune diseases,

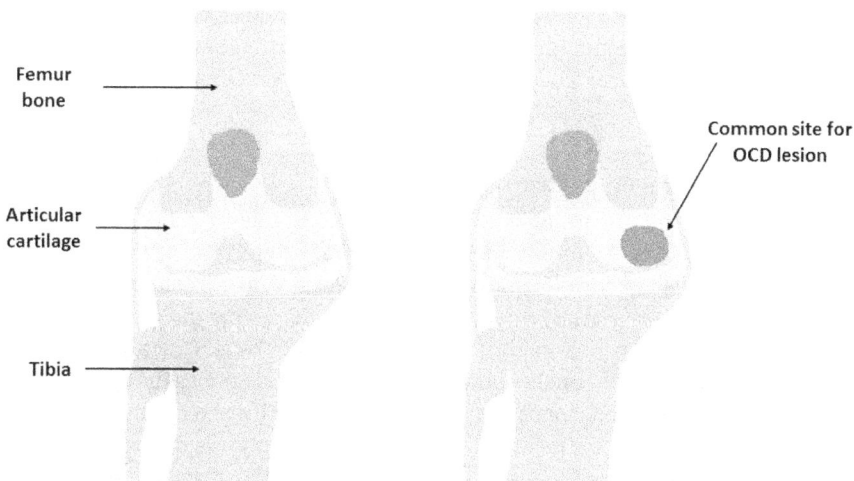

FIGURE 1.2 Osteochondritis dissecans disorder.

vasculitis, and hematologic disorders. RP can affect people of all ages; however, the median age of onset has been reported to be between the fourth and fifth decades of life (Borgia et al. 2018). Symptoms of RP usually commence with sudden onset of pain, which is followed by tenderness and swelling of the cartilage. Although the exact cause of RP is not well known, it is thought to be an autoimmune disorder. It is also not considered to be a familial disease. Chondritis and polyarthritis are the most common clinical features of RP. However, bilateral auricular chondritis can be seen in a majority of patients. The major parts affected by RP are ears, joints, nose, ribs, spine, and windpipe. However, any cartilage in the body can be affected by RP. Mild forms of RP can be treated with nonsteroidal anti-inflammatory drugs (NSAIDs), dapsone, colchicine, and low-dose corticosteroids. Life-threatening complications require corticosteroids and immunosuppressants (De Filippi, Diderich, and Wouters 1992). The disease may follow a progressive course leading to complete damage of the affected tissue, the damage of nasal cartilage, the so called "saddle nose" is one of the examples. Respiratory failure followed by the occurrence of cardiovascular condition is the most common cause of death in RP patients.

Chondrocalcinosis

Chondrocalcinosis refers to calcification (deposition of calcium salts) in hyaline cartilage and/or fibrocartilage present in the joints. The deposited calcium salts are comprised of either calcium pyrophosphate dehydrate (CPPD) or calcium phosphate like carbonate-substituted hydroxyapatite, tricalcium phosphate, octacalcium phosphate, and dicalcium phosphate dihydrate, with CPPD crystal deposition. In some cases, magnesium deficiency has been found to be linked to chondrocalcinosis (Hubert et al. 2018). Chondrocalcinosis in weight-bearing joints such as the knee is associated with OA (Seeman and Delmas 2006). Chondrocalcinosis caused due to CPPD is often asymptomatic. Inflammatory and cartilage damaging responses are seen in the case of deposition of basic calcium phosphate crystals. CPPD crystal deposition occurs predominantly in the pericellular spaces surrounding the chondrocytes in cartilage tissue, the release of which into the joint space causes acute inflammatory reaction leading to pseudo gout condition.

Benign or Non-Cancerous Tumours

This tumour is made of cartilaginous tissues and constitutes a major class of bone tumours, the so-called chondroma, and is unlikely to spread. They can occur in any bone, but usually in big ones like the femur, tibia, upper arm bone, and pelvis. Some types of these tumours are more common like in spine or near the growth plates of the long bones, thereby weakening the bone, leading to break (fracture), and even causing disability or death. Enchondroma is a stage of cartilaginous tumour involving hyaline cartilage and osteochondroma, an overgrowth of cartilage and bone occurring near the growth plate, are the most common non-cancerous cartilaginous tumours that account for about 34% and 30% of all types of benign cartilaginous tumours, respectively. These types of tumours rarely become malignant and are normally treated by excision (curettage) along with a bone graft (Chesney 2001).

Malignant cartilaginous tumours, the so-called chondrosarcomas (CHS), primarily affect the cartilage cells which are present in femur, knee, spine, pelvis, etc., and can also spread to other parts of the body. It is the second most common type of primary bone cancer and these cartilage tumours are usually treated with intralesional surgery combined with an adjuvant like cryosurgery. The severe chondrosarcoma and CHS of axial skeleton are surgically resected in wide margins with an intermediate risk of local recurrence (Pettifor 2005).

Inflammatory Arthropathy

The cartilage tissue may be severely damaged by the inflammatory rheumatic diseases causing many arthritis including the rheumatoid arthritis, gout, infantile idiopathic arthritis, systemic lupus erythematosus, seronegative spondyloarthropathies, etc.; some of which are discussed in later section.

BONE DISORDERS

There are many bone disorders that lead to health complications. Some common bone diseases or disorders include the following:

Metabolic Bone Diseases

These are the conditions of bone strength that cause an abnormal bone mass or bone structure due to deficiency of minerals like calcium, phosphorus, etc., or vitamins (e.g. vitamin D). Osteoporosis, one of the metabolic bone diseases, is caused by bone loss and deterioration of bone structure. This disease usually occurs in aged people. The other metabolic bone diseases include osteomalacia caused due to bone softening, hyperparathyroidism caused due to overactive gland causing loss of bone calcium, and Paget's disease (abnormally large, but weak bone involving cellular remodelling and deformity) (Lips and Van Schoor 2011; Martin et al. 2004).

Bone Cancer

Bone cancer may occur in any type of bone, but it mostly affects the pelvis or long bones in the arms and legs. Bone cancer is rare, and the benign bone tumour is much more common compared to the malignant ones. This type of cancer can spread to bones of the other parts of the body; for example, metastatic tumour, "multiple myeloma", is a type of blood cancer that affects the function of bone marrow and also new bone formation in the hips, ribs, pelvis, shoulders, spine, etc., thereby enhancing the risk of fracture.

Scoliosis

Scoliosis is a medical condition that involves the deformation of spine or backbone leading to an abnormal sideways curvature of the vertebrae. Infants or early adolescents mostly suffer from this disorder. The causes of this disease are mostly unknown in about 80% of patients, although birth defects, neurological abnormalities, and genetic conditions have been reported as the possible reasons.

Osteoporosis

Osteoporosis is the most frequent systemic skeletal disease that develops when bone mass and mineral density diminish, and the bone quality and structure may also change. This reduces bone strength and makes the bones more susceptible to failure when subjected to mild stress. It is characterized by symptoms such as back pain (because of a collapsing vertebra), stooped posture, gradual loss of height with time and age, and weakening of bone. The wrist, hip, forearm, and spine vertebrae are the most often afflicted bones by osteoporosis. Osteoporosis could be caused by abnormally high bone loss and less-than-normal maximum bone mass. This condition may also be caused by glucocorticoid steroids, anorexia, alcoholism, surgical ovary removal, hyperthyroidism, renal disease, selective serotonin reuptake inhibitors, proton pump inhibitors, chemotherapies, and antiseizure medicines. Physical variables like gender, age, family history, race, and body size essentially contribute to the development of osteoporosis. Although postmenopausal women and older men are more vulnerable, certain teenagers and toddlers may acquire an unusual idiopathic juvenile osteoporosis. Osteoporosis may be avoided by following a healthy diet from infancy and avoiding drugs that accelerate bone loss. Calcium consumption, vitamin D exposure, exercise, and osteoporosis medications reduce bone loss and, in the long run, may prevent the disease. Biophosphate medicines may assist in preventing future bone fractures if bones have already been damaged. If there have been no past fractured bones, this drug is less effective (Wells et al. 2008, 2022; Golob and Laya 2015).

Bone Fracture

Bone fracture refers to a broken bone that occurs when the bone is subjected to a sudden strong pressure or force, for example, accidental injury. Bone fracture can happen completely or partially as well as in different ways, *viz.,* crosswise, lengthwise, in pieces, etc. The severity of bone fracture depends on the force applied. Bones may crack when their breaking point slightly exceeds. Older people are at a high risk of bone fractures compared to children because bones of the later are more flexible and resilient, making rapid healing of fractures.

Bone fractures are usually of two types, namely, closed or open, and completely or partially.

Closed or Open Fractures

Closed fractures are simple bone fractures that occur without affecting the skin, whereas an open bone fracture, which is also known as compound fracture, may occur when the ends of the fractured bone tear through the skin. The open fracture exposes the bone and its surrounding tissues, thereby causing a higher risk of infection.

Total or Partial Fractures

Partial or incomplete fracture is the diverse set of fractures that occur when bones crack without complete breaking down and it most commonly affects long bones in young patients. On the other hand, total or complete fracture occurs when the force applied to the bone exceeds the structural integrity of the bone, resulting in the crushing of the bone into multiple pieces. Both types of fractures have a slew of variations, depending on the pattern and the status after breakage. The majority of forearm and lower leg fractures result from an indirect injury, for example, a fall on an outstretched arm or a leap from a great height, rather than a direct injury (e.g. strike with a bat). The force applied and the angle of the force cause a variety of injuries in various instances (Giustina, Mazziotti, and Canalis 2008; Dupree and Dobs 2004).

Hip Fracture

Hip fracture occurs when the upper half of the thighbone (femur) breaks; a fall and a car collision are the most common causes of this fracture. Because bones weaken and become more brittle with age, therefore, hip fractures more likely occur in elderly people. The majority of hip fractures produce excruciating pain and necessitate emergency treatment. After a hip fracture, some people require a total hip replacement. Hip fractures usually occur in the femoral neck fracture and intertrochanteric fracture, a specific hip fracture that causes the breaking of the femur between the greater and the lesser trochanters, that is, femoral neck and long straight part of the femur. Figure 1.3 depicts a typical hip joint defect, in which a narrowed joint space is caused by the bone spurs and destroyed cartilage.

Stress Fracture

Stress fracture is the result of an overuse injury that occurs when muscles become exhausted and lose the ability to withstand additional trauma, and ultimately transfers the stress to the bone, thereby causing fracture. These types of conditions are usually

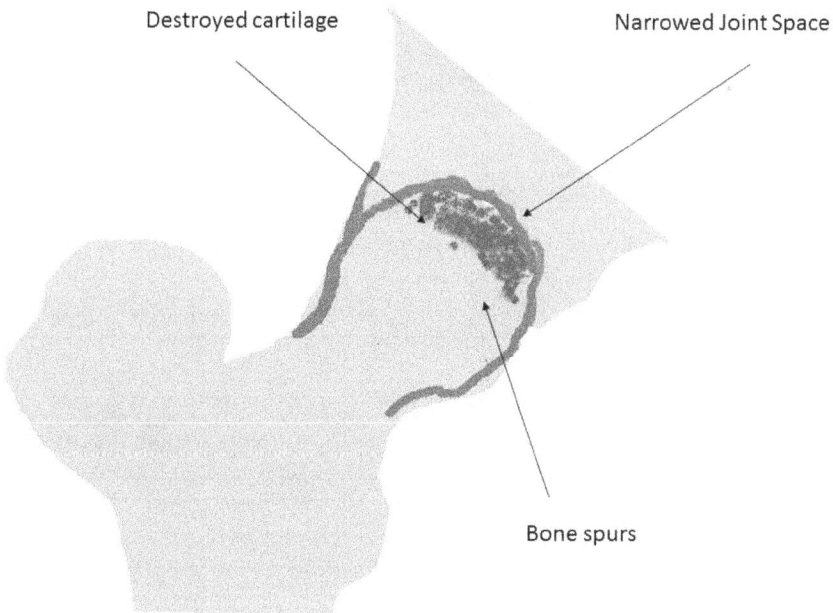

FIGURE 1.3 Hip joint defect.

caused by a sudden increase in an activity, but they may also happen by the impact of an unaccustomed surface (e.g. switching from a soft clay court to a hard one by a tennis player); inappropriate sports goods (e.g. wearing worn or less flexible shoes by a runner); and excessive physical stress (e.g. increase in playing time for a basketball player).

Knee Fracture

It is another form of injury that breaks the patella, or the kneecap, the bone that covers the knee joint. The fracture may happen in many ways; it can be a minor or partial crack or can be severe by a complete break into pieces. Kneecap fracture sometimes may lead to the ligaments or tendons attached to sprain or tear. Knee fractures are usually traumatic injuries such as a fall onto concrete or a high-speed collision like a car accident, causing immediate severe pain, swelling and bruising, restriction in movement, feeling of scraping or grinding during movement, muscle spasms, etc. (Lawrence et al. 2008).

Paget's Disease

This disease, also known as the osteitis deformans, is a chronic bone disorder that can affect both single (monostotic) and multiple bones (polyostotic), *viz.*, femer, tibia, pelvis, skull, and lumbar vertebrae. However, Paget's disease does not affect the whole skeleton and cannot spread from one bone to another. This disease also causes bones to grow misshapen and more prone to fracture. Older people aged more than 55 years and male mostly get this disease. The affected bones exhibit dysregulated bone remodelling at the microscopic level, secondary arthritis, bone fracture, and disorganized new bone formation. Paget's disease often leads to bone pain, fracture, bone deformities (e.g. spine curvature), joint cartilage damage, and neurological problems. Genetic factors or acquired factors such as viral infections are responsible for this disorder (Shaker 2009; Tuck et al. 2017; Ralston 2013).

Osteopetrosis Disease

Osteopetrosis is one of the rare disorders that happen due to abnormal bone growth leading to the bone rupture. Osteogenesis imperfecta diseases are the consequences of genetic disease. This condition is also known as brittle bone disease, which makes bones weak and breaks easily (Davel et al. 1956). Malignant infantile osteopetrosis and adult osteopetrosis are the types of fosteopetrosis conditions.

Osteonecrosis Disease

Osteonecrosis or avascular necrosis is a disease that occurs usually due to lack of blood supply to the bone, causing the bone cells and bone tissue death, and often affects the age group between 30 and 50 years irrespective of gender. Globally about 10,000–20,000 people are affected annually by this disease. This type of disease may occur to any one or multiple bones at a time or at different times and more frequently happens in the femur, balls of the hip and shoulder joints (upper humerus), ankle joints, etc. Besides, the lack of blood supply may also occur due to accidental injuries, consumption of excess alcohol, high doses of steroids, etc., for a prolonged period of time. This type of necrosis can make joint surface collapse that gradually increases the pain and joint stiffness, thereby resisting its movement, and it may also cause arthritis. Osteonecrosis may make patients without any risk factor so-called idiopathic; however, if the disease is left untreated, bones may crack and eventually collapse (Lombard et al. 2016; Dieppe 2011).

Sprains and Strains

Sprain refers to an injury to ligament tissue resulting from wrenching or twisting of a joint, whereas strains are injuries affecting the muscle or tendons. Both sprains and strains are associated with sports injuries and are usually caused by minor trauma. Ankle injury is the most common sprained or strained joint.

Tendinitis

Tendinitis, also called tendonitis, refers to joint pain and swelling that usually occurs due to repeated injuries of the tendon, a joint that connects muscles to bones. In this condition, the connective tissues between muscles and tendons become inflamed. Although this condition can occur in any tendon, it most often affects the shoulders, elbows, knees, heels, hip, Achilles tendon, and base of the thumb. Various risk factors include age and participation in sports associated with repetitive motions like golf, running, swimming, tennis, etc. If the inflammation or irritation of the tendon persists for a long time (e.g. a month or more), a condition like tendinosis may be resulted due to degenerative changes and abnormal growth of new blood vessels in the tendon. Calcific tendinitis is a frequent condition that primarily affects people between the ages of 40 and 60 years. Women appear to be more vulnerable than men. Various factors, such as aberrant thyroid gland activity, metabolic illnesses (e.g. diabetes), and hereditary susceptibility, have been suggested to have a role in this syndrome (Abate et al. 2013).

Sports Injury

These are the most common types of injuries found in developed countries and their treatments are not only difficult but also often expensive, and time-consuming. So, preventive strategies and activities are promoted on both medical and economic grounds. These types of situations arise from the consequence of overtraining, poor conditioning, or poor form or technique. The most common sports injuries include bruises, sprains, strains, rips, and shattered bones. However, tissues like muscles, ligaments, tendons, fascia, and bursae can also be affected. Among these, sprains, strains, knee injuries, Achilles tendon rupture, joint dislocations, and brain injury are the most common types of sports injuries.

Torn Anterior Cruciate Ligament (ACL) and Medial Collateral Ligament (MCL)

The ligament is a connective tissue that joins two bones. Ligaments such as the ACL and MCL connect the femur to the tibia bone, thereby making knee joint stable. Ligaments are tight, non-stretchable fibres that hold bones together. The ACL, together with the posterior cruciate ligament (PCL), MCL, lateral collateral ligament (LCL), and menisci (cartilage pads), keeps the knee stable when running, jumping, and landing by preventing it from slipping, turning, and hyperextending. It resists over-rotation by preventing the bones from stretching beyond a normal angle. ACL may be torn by both contact and noncontact manoeuvres. More than 70% of all injuries are the result of noncontact injuries, which are mostly related to sports like athletics. A direct impact can cause the knee to hyperextend or bend inward in contact injuries, a condition which is known as valgus stress. Pain, swelling, and loss of movement are the outcome of torn ACL and MCL and these may cause joint instability causing difficulty to walk.

Dislocation is a condition that results from the displacement of bones of any joint, leading to the disruption of adjoining tissues. Various causes of dislocation include high-impact stresses resulting from trauma (accident or fall) or the weakening of muscles and tendons that make resistance to the ligaments, muscles, etc., to hold the joint intact.

Osteomyelitis

Osteomyelitis is a bone infection caused by bacteria or fungi. Haematogenous or contiguous microbial seeding of the bone can cause osteomyelitis. The most prevalent infecting bacterium is *Staphylococcus aureus* that reaches the bone through the bloodstream or by extension from a local injury followed by inflammation and thereby destructs the porous or cancellous bone and marrow (Urish and Cassat 2020). Although osteomyelitis can affect any bone, long-bone, vertebral, and foot osteomyelitis accounting for the vast majority of occurrences, the results of a bone sample and bone cultures are frequently used to confirm an osteomyelitis diagnosis.

Avascular Necrosis

Avascular Necrosis also called osteonecrosis, is a bone disease condition that leads to small breaks in the bone and cause the bone to collapse. Avascular necrosis involves the death of the bone tissue due to inadequate blood supply to the defect area and it normally affects the femur (thigh bone); but other bones such as bones of the upper arm, shoulder, knee, and ankle are also affected.

Carpal Tunnel Syndrome (CTS)

The carpal tunnel is a narrow passage encircled by bones and ligaments in the wrist that encompasses and protects the median nerve and the nine flexor tendons. CTS is a condition that is caused by excessive pressure on the median nerve present in the carpal tunnel of the wrist and controls the movement of the hand and the fingers. It is a case of compression neuropathy, where the median nerve gets compressed, leading to nerve damage and worsening conditions. Bones in the carpal form the floor and sides, whereas transverse carpal ligament forms the roof of the tunnel forming a rigid surrounding. The median nerve provides feelings in the thumb, and fingers, as well as controls the muscles around the base of the thumb (Dorwart 1984). The pressure exerted on the median nerve can be due to interstitial fluid pressure within the carpal canal or when the tunnel becomes narrow due to direct contact pressure on the nerve from adjacent tissues called synovium that lubricates the tendons. Synovial thickening in limited space may emerge as a result of the increase of the fluid pressure over time (Werner and Armstrong 1997).

The condition worsens and thereby damages the nerve over time. It mostly affects middle-aged individuals, with females being at a greater risk compared to males. A number of factors can be responsible for causing CTS, such as heredity, physical stress due to excessive hand use, pregnancy, and other health issues.

JOINT DEFECTS AND DISEASES

Besides bone and cartilage as discussed in the previous section, healthy joints such as shoulder joints, knee joints, ankle, and finger joints allow us for easy movement, provide support to bear the body weight, as well as to perform work. Joint disorder may occur due to joint diseases or trauma, the consequences of which lead to great suffering to human beings. The common joint disorders are described in the next section.

Arthritis

Arthritis is a leading cause of joint disorder that affects people with severe pain and inflammation worldwide. According to the Centers for Disease Control and Prevention, about 80 million US adults will have some form of arthritis by 2040. The ageing global population has caused a consistent rise in the disease burden of various types of arthritis and it poses a considerable public health challenge globally (Dalal, Bull, and Stanley 2007; Desai, Steiger, and Anders 2017; Gibofsky 2014; Felson 2006). It causes impairment of mobility of an individual by causing inflammation and pain in the hip, shoulder, knee, and other joints, affecting their activities in daily life such as opening locks and doors, causing immense economic burden on the individual as well as society (Kardos et al. 2019; Morrey 2008). Various types of arthritis exist, with the most common being the non-inflammatory OA that is caused by the degeneration of AC, hypertrophy of bone-ends, subchondral sclerosis, and a range of alterations to the biochemical composition of the synovial membrane and joint capsule (Morrey 2008). Gout is also a common form of inflammatory arthritis which is the result of the monosodium urate crystals deposition in the joints. Rheumatoid arthritis (RA) is an autoimmune condition that leads to destruction of articulating cartilage and juxta-articular bone. Inflammation of joints is also caused by various other diseases such as lupus and fibromyalgia and psoriatic arthritis. OA and RA are the two basic categories of joint disorders which are discussed in detail in the following section.

Rheumatoid Arthritis

It is an autoimmune disease condition in which the body's immune cells interact with the local joint cells, resulting in ever-increasing inflammation or painful swelling that causes destruction of the cartilage and bone (Figure 1.4). It affects multiple joints such as hands, wrists, knees, etc., producing chronic pain, lack of balance, distortions, and stiffness together with soreness and swelling that occur symmetrically on both sides of the body, for example, in both wrists and both knees. Although the primary

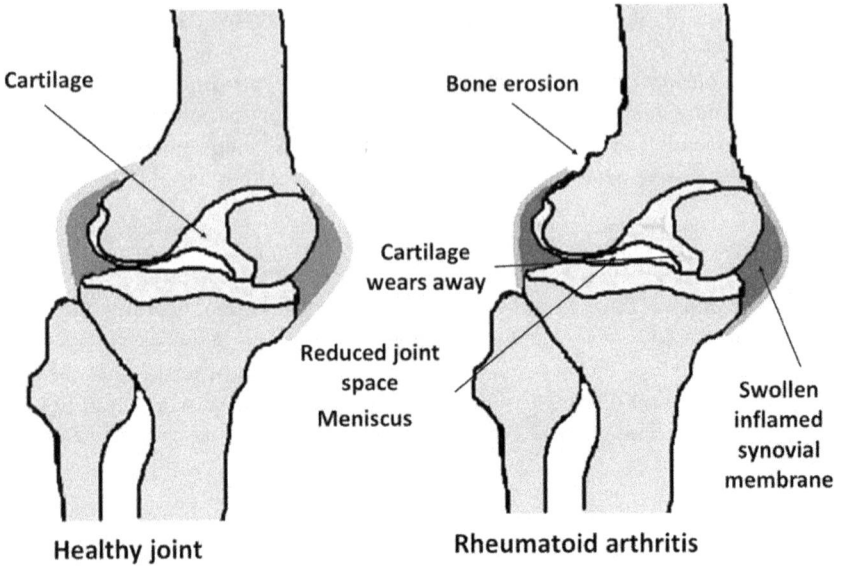

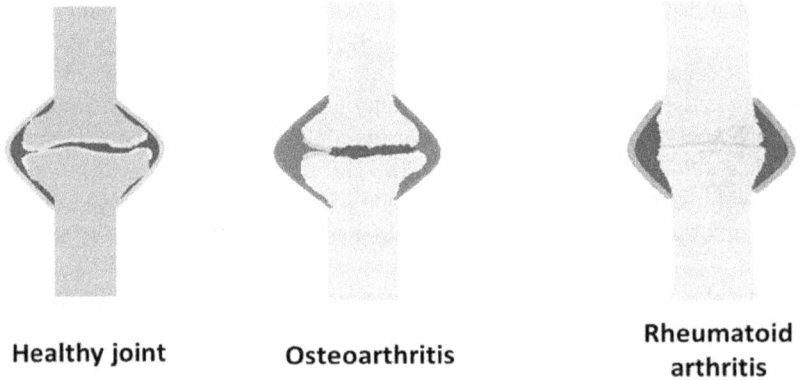

FIGURE 1.4 Rheumatoid arthritis.

cause of this condition is not known well, factors like gender, age, genetics, smoking particularly at an early age, obesity, etc., are associated with this arthritis.

Swelling of joints in RA is the result of complex autoimmune process and inflammatory reactions involving innate as well as adaptive immunity. Triggered by genetic susceptibility, environmental factors, or even chance, the individual loses tolerance to self-proteins that contain a citrulline residue. Hence, these proteins are not recognized as "self" and are targeted by the immune system which develops anti-citrullinated protein/peptide antibodies. Disease progression involves the interaction between innate and adaptive immunity (Tekaya et al. 2018; Murata et al. 2020).

In this type of arthritis, the inflammation of synovial membrane occurs due to the infiltration of peripheral blood cells and proliferation of fibroblast-like synoviocytes leading to pannus development. These cells release pro-inflammatory mediators and autoantibodies in the joint that sustain the inflammatory process along with cartilage damage and osteoclast-mediated bone erosion that cause invasion of the pannus tissue and irreversible joint deformation.

Osteoarthritis

OA is one of the most common joint disorders and occurs when cartilage in the joints is in "wear-and-tear" form or breaks down, leading to stiffness, pain, resistance to movement, etc. This disorder produces joint friction causing swelling and stiffness in the affected area. Figure 1.5 shows a typical osteoarthritis condition of elbow.

The various risk factors associated with this disorder are ageing, weight, intensity of joint activity, sports-related injuries, family history, etc. The situation becomes more critical with patients having hip and knee arthritis (Figure 1.6). Although it is more likely to develop in adults with 50 years of age and older, women are more vulnerable.

The cartilage is in a state of dynamic remodelling, where the rate of regeneration of cartilage matches the rate of degradation. In OA, degradation enzymes are overexpressed, causing a net loss in the mass of cartilage. This can be caused by ageing due to a reduction in growth factors and an increase in oxidative stress. The AC offers a smooth surface for sliding for movement, as well as acts as a "shock absorber", thereby reducing the pressure on the bone. The degradation of cartilage causes the surface to get rough, as well as reduces the thickness of the cartilage.

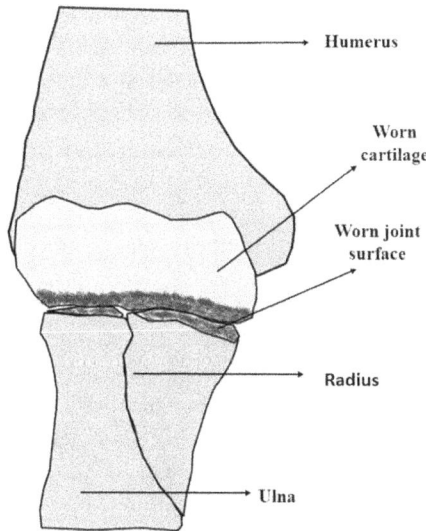

FIGURE 1.5 Osteoarthritis of elbow.

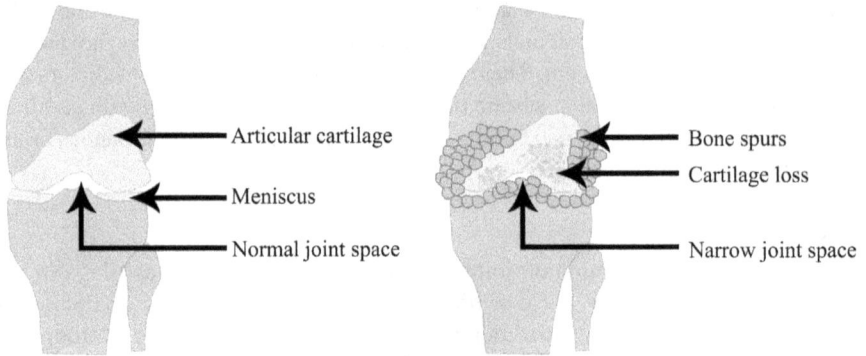

FIGURE 1.6   A typical knee joint defect.

Roughness causes problems in joint movement and the thinning of the cartilage exposes the bones to destruction as they are more susceptible to forces.

Spondyloarthritis

Spondyloarthritis is also known as spondylitis that includes some other rheumatoid diseases, namely, enteropathic arthritis, ankylosing spondylitis, psoriatic arthritis, reactive arthritis, undifferentiated spondyloarthritis, and a subtype of juvenile idiopathic arthritis. Enteropathic arthritis is a condition of inflammatory bowel disease that causes inflammatory back and/or joint pain, inflammation in the intestine, etc. Ankylosing spondylitis causes fusion of parts of the spine in a fixed position, inflammation, pain, and stiffness in joints in shoulders, hips, ribs, etc. Juvenile idiopathic arthritis, a chronic joint condition, is mostly found in kids and it is inflammatory, affecting the muscles, joints, ligaments, internal organs, and others. Reactive arthritis is an infection in the intestine or urinary tract that causes inflammation and pain in the joints. Psoriatic arthritis often causes pain and swelling in the joints in finger and toe. It also causes pain and stiffness in the spine. Undifferentiated spondyloarthritis causes heel pain and knee swelling.

Gout

This is another common inflammatory arthritis that occurs due to the deposition of uric acid crystal, which is a waste product of blood, in and around the joints, and surrounding tissues in the body (Figure 1.7). The most affected areas include the joint connecting the big toe, small toe joints, knees, and ankle. Acute gouty arthritis, a severe form of arthritis that happens due to repeated occurrence of gout in the early phase. Figure 1.8 illustrates the necroinflammation in acute gouty arthritis caused by the deposition of uric acid and the release of cytokines and chemokines, thereby recruiting the neutrophil that causes necrosis, some of which are mediated by factors like IL and NF-κβ and inflammation in joints. Gout tends to resolve after a few days through suppression mechanism to reduce inflammation and clear dead cells. Chronic gout is the consequence of tophus formation by the monosodium urate (MSU) crystals

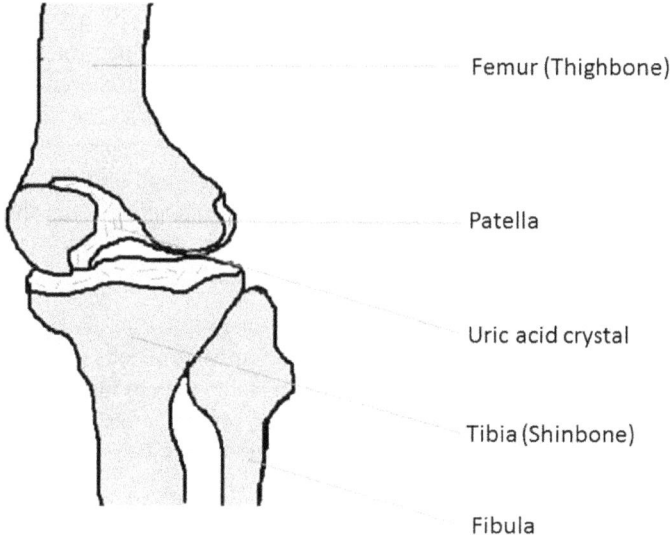

FIGURE 1.7 Deposition of uric acid crystals causing gout arthritis.

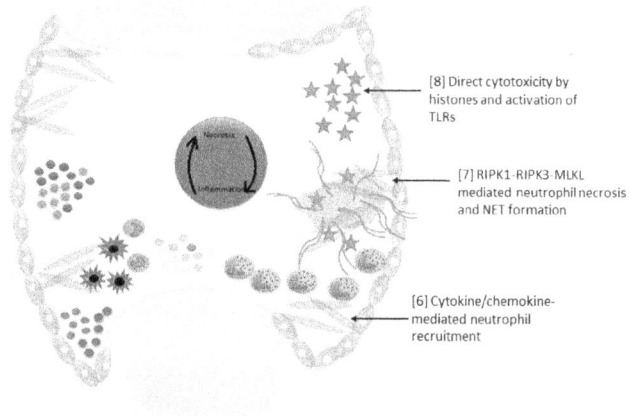

FIGURE 1.8 Necroinflammation in acute gouty arthritis.

and neutrophil extracellular traps (NETs) that damages the surrounding tissues. Some of the risk factors associated with this disease include gender, obesity, consumption of alcohol, some medications like diuretics, high-fructose food and drink, a purine-rich diet, etc.

Bursitis

Bursitis is a common condition that involves swelling and pain in joints because of inflammation of fluid-filled sacs, the so-called bursae that act as a cushion and lubricant between bones, muscles, and tendons near the joints. The common causes of bursitis include injury or overuse of joints near bursae, repetitive motion, bacterial infection, trauma or RA, gout, tendonitis, diabetes, and thyroid, and the cause also may be unknown. Bursitis causes pain, stiffness, and aches in the afflicted joint, swelling, and redness over the joint itself.

Lupus

Lupus is an autoimmune disease that occurs when healthy cells and tissues of our body are attacked by the immune system by mistake, thereby damaging the joints, bones, and other organs such as the skin, internal organs, brain, etc. It may prompt arthritis in hands, elbows, kidneys, shoulders, knees, and feet. Pain or swelling in joints, muscles, and chest is caused by this disease.

CURRENT TREATMENT OPTIONS

Most of the treatments of bone- and cartilage-related disorders focus on pain management, prevention of inflammation, and surgery. The later is particularly used for joint disorders. The various methods are categorized in the following section.

NON-SURGICAL TREATMENT OR CONSERVATIVE MEDICATIONS

A variety of conservative medications including NSAIDs like ibuprofen (Advil), naproxen (Aleve), and celecoxib (Celebrex) are used to treat OA. Duloxetine is used to treat anxiety and depression. This medicine can also be used as a pain reliever for many conditions and OA patients when NSAID does not work to relieve pain. The early-stage OA can be treated without surgery with physical and occupational therapy and the use of NSAIDs may delay surgery in some cases. Platelet-rich plasma injections may also be benefitted. This anti-inflammatory medication may be beneficial in relieving some symptoms shown with AC disorders. However, for severe damage surgery is a must. In some cases, there is no option but to go for a total knee replacement.

The effects of early-stage knee arthritis may be reduced by strengthening thigh muscles through appropriate physical therapy or exercise to provide better support to the joint together with maintaining good nutrition and healthy weight. These reduce pressure on the knee joints, thereby decreasing the knee pain and improving function. Although exercise is useful in many cases, it is most unlikely to help or take part in tissue regeneration activity.

Other non-operative treatments such as hyperbaric oxygen and shock wave therapies, electrical stimulation, physiotherapy, and muscle strengthening exercises, and their combinations, are sometimes used, but the effectiveness and conflicting results of some of these treatments are to be determined for confirmation. Non-surgical treatment cannot be used as conservative treatment, as they do not normally slow the advancement of the disease and most of them provide simply pain relief. Other non-pharmaceutical means include losing weight, use of heat or cold packs in affected area, cognitive behavioural therapy, use of medical devices (e.g. walking cane) to prevent falls or a sleeve or brace to support the knee, etc.

SURGICAL TREATMENT

As already mentioned, surgical treatment is needed when conservative treatments fail to respond and in the case of severe damage. It is a clinical procedure involving an incision performed to investigate or repair the damage or disease in living tissue. There are different types of surgical treatments available and a specific surgical method is selected depending on various factors including the age and activity level of the patient, size, and age of injury and damage.

Some of the common surgical treatments for bone-related disorders are described here.

Core Decompression

This surgical procedure typically involves the drilling into the area of damaged bone at the joint. This procedure reduces pressure within the bone and allows increased blood flow, thereby decreasing or even stopping the progression of the bone and joint destruction. Core decompression is usually applied for the treatment of osteonecrosis.

Osteotomy

This surgical method used to treat orthopaedic disorders involves the cutting and reshaping of the bones to reduce pressure on the defect area, thereby preventing or lessening the damage. This type of procedure can be used to repair a damaged joint and also used to shorten or lengthen or realign the defect bone. This treatment is most effective for advanced osteonecrosis and bone with a small area of defect or damage. It is also used to correct a hallux valgus (toe deformity) or straighten a fractured bone and relieve pain of arthritis related to the hip and knee. Currently, it is being replaced by joint replacement in older patients.

Bone Grafting

Bone grafting is a medical procedure that involves the removal of tissues from one place and putting in a damaged area for repairing and rebuilding the diseased or damaged bones that are extremely complex in nature posing a significant health risk. Common donor sites are the skull, hips, ribs, and knee of the patient (the so-called autograft) or donor (allograft), with hip being the most common harvesting place for a graft. Defects that require major bone grafting include traumatic injury involving multiple fractures, tumour surgery, or congenital defects. The bone graft also helps in bone healing surrounding the surgically implanted devices used for joint replacements, such as plates, screws, etc.

Arthroplasty/Joint Replacement

The term "arthroplasty" refers to a surgical reconstruction or replacement of a joint for restoring the joint function. It is also known as joint replacement surgery that is eventually needed when the disease has progressed to the stage of collapse of the bone. A prosthesis or artificial joint may be used in this procedure, especially in the case of total joint replacement. In the total hip replacement, the so-called total hip arthroplasty, the damaged bone and cartilage are replaced with prosthetics which are made from metal, plastic, or ceramic materials that mimic the shape and movement of a natural joint. In total joint replacement, for example, in the treatment of late-stage osteonecrosis, the damaged joint is replaced with artificial parts. The joint replacement surgery can restore the normal activity of the patient. Hip and knee replacement surgeries have become the most trusted treatments to restore mobility and relieve pain in patients. This surgery may also be an option for people with arthritis in shoulder, elbow, wrist, ankle, etc.

Arthroscopic Debridement

Arthroscopic debridement is an orthopaedic surgery that involves a "clean-up" procedure to remove the cartilage or bone debris and inflammatory substances by flushing fluid through the joint. Arthroscopy procedure in the knee and wrist is commonly used to reduce pain, achieve fast recovery, and improve movement.

Marrow Stimulation

In this technique, tiny holes are created by drilling to remove the damaged cartilage debris and calcified cartilage layers followed by penetrating subchondral bone plate, enabling the entry of blood and bone marrow containing MSCs to the defect site that initiates a biologic repair response resulting in fibrocartilage formation. This procedure can be successfully used to treat young age people usually under the age of 40 years with small chondral defects (Herrington and Al-Sherhi 2007).

Mosaicplasty

Mosaicplasty is also called osteochondral grafting. This surgical procedure removes healthy cartilage from unaffected site and harvests them in the damaged area. Mosaicplasty is mostly used for isolated and small size (10–20 mm) cartilage damage and is limited to use in patients under the age of 50 who suffer from accidental injury.

Autologous Chondrocyte Implantation (ACI)

The poor capability of self-repairing characteristic leads to permanent damage of AC and hence its repair is a great challenge. ACI is a surgical procedure in which chondrocytes are harvested from the joint, cultured *in vitro*, and implanted in the defect site for repairing AC through regeneration process. Besides pain relief, this treatment slows down the progression or delays partial or total joint replacement surgery, and therefore patients may regain mobility and relieve pain. This procedure is usually applied for accidental injury.

This treatment method suffers from several risk factors including infection, bleeding and blood clotting during the process or post-surgery fracture, nerve damage, continued pain, stiffness, allergy, excess bone formation at the artificial knee joint, and excess scar tissue restricting knee movement, kneecap instability, resulting in painful dislocation of the knee surface, etc.

Microfracture

This surgical method is used to treat damaged cartilage. The procedure uses the combined effects of surgery and rehabilitation for cartilage repair by stimulating the neo-cartilage tissue growth in a small area of the damaged cartilage. The method creates small holes by drilling the rigid interface that exists between cartilage and the subchondral bone forming a blood clot rich in bone marrow stem cells that grow and form strong, dense, and elastic fibrocartilage, thereby filling the defect or lesion. It is most commonly used in the chondral defects like knee joint, specifically in patients with full thickness damage, but can also be used to repair other joint defects like hip, ankle, shoulder, etc.

Osteochondral Autograft Transplantation

Osteochondral autograft transfer involves the harvesting of a "plug" of healthy bone and AC tissue from the non-load-bearing area of the joint to repair defects in the high load-bearing space. This is done arthroscopically. When multiples of such tissue "plugs" are used, it results in a mosaic pattern which is called "mosaicplasty".

COMPLEX JOINT DISORDERS

OSTEOARTHRITIS

So far there is no solution for OA to make it reverse as repairing or replacement of damaged cartilage is too difficult. However, depending on the severity of symptoms and their location, some non-surgical treatments or conservative medications, or their combination, are used to reduce the pain and stiffness and make the patient's movement better. Some of the medications that can be used to relieve OA pain are NSAIDs and duloxetine (Cymbalta). Besides exercise, physiotherapy and occupational therapy sometimes may be useful. The medications pose severe side effects like cardiovascular problems, liver damage, kidney damage, etc. Although some steroid injections reduce inflammation in the affected area, they can also cause additional joint damage upon repeated use. Glucocorticoids and hyaluronic acid injections are also used for knee or hip OA. Platelet-rich plasma and stem cell injections are recently being explored on experimental basis. Devices like walking cane to prevent falls or a sleeve or brace to support the knee are used for temporary relief of pain. There is no option but one has to go for surgery for the treatment of severe and critical OA. Osteotomy procedure can be used around the knee joint to relief OA pain. Sometimes, arthrodesis, a bone fusion technique, is beneficial to treat the severely damaged joints like those in fingers, wrists, ankles, etc.; but, it is rarely applied in hip or knee joints. However, arthroplasty involving a total joint replacement providing long-lasting pain relief is performed for severely arthritic hip and knee joints.

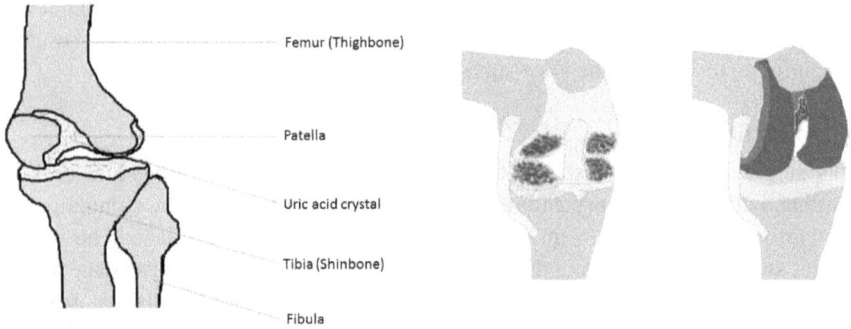

FIGURE 1.9 Damaged knee joint, and its replacement.

KNEE JOINT REPLACEMENT

As discussed above, arthroplasty surgery involving the replacement of damaged or injured knee joint with an artificial joint or prosthesis decreases pain and allows the knee to move properly (Figure 1.9). There are three common reasons for knee replacement: OA (age-related wear and tear of knee joint), RA (membrane surrounding the knee joint becomes inflamed), and post-traumatic arthritis (critical knee injury, bones at the knee break or ligament tear, affecting cartilage).

Knee replacement can be total or partial. The different types of knee replacement surgery are discussed next.

Partial Knee Replacement

This type of surgical method is performed to replace only one part, either the inside or outside or kneecap part of the damaged knee with an artificial implant, called a prosthetic, without involving much bone removal and with a smaller incision requiring less recovery time. Although it can relieve pain and stiffness and post-operative rehabilitation is often associated with less risk of infection, blood loss, and blood clotting, unlike total replacement, however, it does not last long.

Kneecap Replacement

This is an alternative surgical technique that is used in place of total knee replacement. This type of surgery is a short surgical procedure but a speedy recovery is performed when only the kneecap is deteriorated.

Mini-Incision Surgery

This technique creates a small incision in front of the knee, through which a specialized instrument is introduced to manoeuver around the tissue. This method offers several advantages, such as less harmful, faster recovery of patient's mobility, less pain, less blood loss, aesthetic impact, minimum health resources required, and less aggressive when dealing with soft tissues.

Image-Guided Surgery

In this procedure computerized images and infrared beacons are used in surgery, allowing the surgeon to work from the different operating theatres. Image-guided surgery offers surgeons to perform the operation safer and make it less invasive. This procedure has now become a recognized standard of care in managing joint disorders. Other methods like arthroscopic washout and debridement and osteotomy can also be used.

Chondromalacia Patellae Treatment

Chondromalacia Patellae disorder It is an anterior knee pain which is caused due to physical and biomechanical changes and mostly happens in young population. In this condition, the AC of the posterior surface of the patella undergoes degenerative changes that cause softening, swelling, and erosion of the hyaline cartilage underlying the patella and sclerosis of the underlying bone (Gagliardi et al. 2013).

Fire needling and acupuncture may be used to get relief from chondromalacia patellae and recovering the biodynamical structure of patellae. The first line of treatment aims to reduce pressure on the kneecap and joint. This can be done by resting (damaged cartilage due to the runner's knee), stabilizing, and icing the joint. Anti-inflammatory medication, like ibuprofen, may work in reducing inflammation around the joint. Physical therapy or exercise, specifically non-weight-bearing exercises (e.g. swimming), focusing on stretching and strengthening may be helpful to improve muscle strength and balance, thereby preventing knee misalignment. Isometric exercises that involve muscle contraction can help to maintain muscle strength and mass. When the conservative medication does not work, various surgical operations can be performed. Anthroscopic surgery is most commonly performed for diagnosis of the affected area and to determine the misalignment of the knee. This procedure involves cutting some of the ligaments to reduce tension and make movement ease. Other surgical methods are implantation of cartilage graft, drilling, chondrectomy, and autologous chondrocyte transplantation.

Investigational or Stem Cell Therapy

In recent decades research interest has been directed towards using stem cell therapy. Adult stem cells, specifically MSCs which have the potential to provide different cell types, are under active research. The patient's own MSCs can be cultured *in vitro* and transplanted at the site of the damaged bone, cartilage or joint to stimulate targeted tissue repair and regeneration; this procedure is known as autologous transplantation. MSCs can also be isolated from sources such as bone marrow, fat or adipose tissue, umbilical cord blood, umbilical cord tissue etc., and they have the ability to differentiate into many other tissues like bone, cartilage, muscle, etc. Although human clinical trials have shown promising results in using MSCs for tissue regeneration, long-term studies are needed before its application in the normal clinical setting. Moreover, stem cell therapy has been reported to have low efficacy.

EXERCISE

1. What is the major composition of bone? What are the functions of bone?
2. What is osteoporosis? What happens when osteoporosis occurs?
3. What is osteoarthritis? What causes osteoarthritis? What is the difference between osteoarthritis and rheumatoid arthritis?
4. Which joints are most commonly affected by arthritis? What are the symptoms of osteoarthritis? How is osteoarthritis diagnosed?
5. What are the various strategies for the treatment of osteoarthritis?
6. What are the nonsurgical options for treating osteoarthritis pain?
7. Write short notes on the following: Paget's disease, osteonecrosis, and marrow stimulating.
8. What is cartilage? What are the different types of cartilage?
9. How can cartilage become damaged? Can cartilage repair itself?
10. What is costochondritis? What causes costochondritis? Who are more vulnerable to costochondritis?
11. What are the surgical options that are currently used for the treatment of osteoarthritis pain?
12. What is growth plate? How growth plate damage occurs and what are the treatment methods?
13. What are the strategies that can be adopted for relieving tissue pain in human?
14. Explain the various currently used grafting methods. And advantages and disadvantages.
15. Discuss about stem cell therapy and its impacts on human health care.
16. What is cartilage made of?

REFERENCES

Abate, M., C. Schiavone, V. Salini, & I. Andia. 2013. "Occurrence of tendon pathologies in metabolic disorders." Rheumatology, 52(4): 599–608.

Abdelmagid, S. 2006. "Characterization and regulation of osteoactivin expression in osteoblasts." *Temple University.*

Anderson, H. C. 2003. "Matrix vesicles and calcification." *Current Rheumatology Reports* 5 (3): 222–226. https://doi.org/10.1007/S11926-003-0071-Z

Augat, P., and S. Schorlemmer. 2006. "The role of cortical bone and its microstructure in bone strength." *Age and Ageing* 35 (2): 27–31. https://doi.org/10.1093/AGEING/AFL081

Bogduk, N. 2016. *Functional Anatomy of the Spine. Handbook of Clinical Neurology.* 1st ed. Vol. 136. Elsevier B.V. https://doi.org/10.1016/B978-0-444-53486-6.00032-6

Borgia, F., F. Giuffrida, F. Guarneri, and S. P. Cannavò. 2018. "Relapsing polychondritis: An updated review." *Biomedicines* 6 (3): 84. https://doi.org/10.3390/BIOMEDICINES6030084.

Boyce, B., Z. Yao, and L. Xing. 2009. "Osteoclasts have multiple roles in bone in addition to bone resorption." *Critical Reviews & Trade; in Eukaryotic Gene Expression* 19 (3): 171–180. https://doi.org/10.1615/CRITREVEUKARGENEEXPR.V19.I3.10

Buckwalter, J. A., M. J. Glimcher, R. R. Cooper, and R. Recker. 1996. "Bone biology. I: Structure, blood supply, cells, matrix, and mineralization." Instructional Course Lectures 45 (January): 371–386. https://europepmc.org/article/med/8727757

Cantarini, L., A. Vitale, M. G. Brizi, F. Caso, B. Frediani, L. Punzi, M. Galeazzi, and D. Rigante. 2014. "Diagnosis and classification of relapsing polychondritis." *Journal of Autoimmunity* 48–49 (February): 53–59. https://doi.org/10.1016/J.JAUT.2014.01.026

Chesney, R. W. 2001. "Vitamin D deficiency and rickets." *Reviews in Endocrine & Metabolic Disorders* 2 (2): 145.

Clarke, B. 2008. "Normal bone anatomy and physiology." *Clinical Journal of the American Society of Nephrology: CJASN* 3(3): S131–S139. https://doi.org/10.2215/CJN.04151206

Dalal, S., M. Bull, and D. Stanley. 2007. "Radiographic changes at the elbow in primary osteoarthritis: A comparison with normal aging of the elbow joint." *Journal of Shoulder and Elbow Surgery* 16 (3): 358–361. https://doi.org/10.1016/J.JSE.2006.08.005

Dalén, N, and K. E. Olsson. 2009. "Bone mineral content and physical activity." *Acta Orthopaedica Scandinavica* 45 (1–4): 170–174. https://doi.org/10.3109/1745367740 8989136

Desai, J., S. Steiger, and H. J. Anders. 2017. "Molecular pathophysiology of gout." *Trends in Molecular Medicine* 23 (8): 756–768. https://doi.org/10.1016/J.MOLMED.2017.06.005

Dieppe, P. 2011. "Developments in osteoarthritis." *Rheumatology* 50 (2): 245–247. https://doi.org/10.1093/RHEUMATOLOGY/KEQ373

Dorwart, B. B. 1984. "Carpal tunnel syndrome: A review." *Seminars in Arthritis and Rheumatism* 14 (2): 134–140. https://doi.org/10.1016/0049-0172(84)90003-9

Downey, P. A., and M. I. Siegel. 2006a. "Bone biology and the clinical implications for osteoporosis." *Physical Therapy* 86 (1): 77–91. https://doi.org/10.1093/PTJ/86.1.77

Downey, P. A., and M. I. Siegel. 2006b. "Bone biology and the clinical implications for osteoporosis." *Physical Therapy* 86 (1): 77–91. https://doi.org/10.1093/PTJ/86.1.77

Dupree, K., and A. Dobs. 2004. "Osteopenia and male hypogonadism." *Reviews in Urology* 6 (6): S30. /pmc/articles/PMC1472878/

Felson, D. T. 2006. "Osteoarthritis of the knee." *New England Journal of Medicine.* 354 (8): 841–848. https://doi.org/10.1056/NEJMCP051726.

Filippi, J. P. De, P. P. N. M. Diderich, and J. M. G. W. Wouters. 1992. "Hypomagnesemia and chondrocalcinosis." *Nederlands Tijdschrift Voor Geneeskunde* 136 (3): 139–141. https://europepmc.org/article/med/1732847

Forlino, A., W. A. Cabral, A. M. Barnes, and J. C. Marini. 2011. "New perspectives on osteogenesis imperfecta." *Nature Reviews Endocrinology* 7 (9): 540–557. https://doi.org/10.1038/nrendo.2011.81

Frank, C. B. 2004. "Ligament structure,pPhysiology and function." *Journal of Musculoskeletal & Neuronal Interactions* 4 (2): 199–201. https://europepmc.org/article/med/15615126

Franz-Odendaal, T. A., B. K. Hall, and P. E. Witten. 2006. "Buried alive: How osteoblasts become osteocytes." *Developmental Dynamics* 235 (1): 176–190. https://doi.org/10.1002/DVDY.20603

Gagliardi, J. A., E. M. Chung, V. P. Chandnani, K. L. Kesling, K. P. Christensen, R. N. Null, M. G. Radvany, and M. F. Hansen. 2013. "Detection and staging of chondromalacia patellae: Relative efficacies of conventional MR imaging, MR arthrography, and CT arthrography." *American Journal of Roentgenology* 163 (3): 629–636. https://doi.org/10.2214/AJR.163.3.8079858

Gibofsky, A. 2014. "Epidemiology, pathophysiology, and diagnosis of rheumatoid arthritis: A synopsis." *The American Journal of Managed Care* 20 (7): S128–35. https://europepmc.org/article/med/25180621

Gibson, L. J. 1985. "The mechanical behaviour of cancellous bone." *Journal of Biomechanics* 18 (5): 317–328. https://doi.org/10.1016/0021-9290(85)90287-8

Giustina, A., G. Mazziotti, and E. Canalis. 2008. "Growth hormone, insulin-like growth factors, and the skeleton." *Endocrine Reviews* 29 (5): 535–59. https://doi.org/10.1210/ER.2007-0036

Golob, A. L., and M. B. Laya. 2015. "Osteoporosis: screening, prevention, and management." *Medical Clinics* 99 (3): 587–606. https://doi.org/10.1016/J.MCNA.2015.01.010

Herrington, L., and A. Al-Sherhi. 2007. "A controlled trial of weight-bearing versus non—weight-bearing exercises for patellofemoral pain." *The Journal of Orthopaedic and Sports Physical Therapy* 37 (4): 155–160. https://doi.org/10.2519/JOSPT.2007.2433

Hubert, J., L. Weiser, S. Hischke, A. Uhlig, T. Rolvien, T. Schmidt, S. K. Butscheidt, et al. 2018. "Cartilage calcification of the ankle joint is associated with osteoarthritis in the general population." *BMC Musculoskeletal Disorders* 19 (1): 1–8. https://doi.org/10.1186/S12891-018-2094-7/FIGURES/4

Kannus, P. 2000. "Structure of the tendon connective tissue." *Scandinavian Journal of Medicine & Science in Sports* 10 (6): 312–320. https://doi.org/10.1034/J.1600-0838.2000.010006312.X

Kardos, D., B. Marschall, M. Simon, I Hornyák, A. Hinsenkamp, O. Kuten, Z. Gyevnár, et al. 2019. "Investigation of cytokine changes in osteoarthritic knee joint tissues in response to hyperacute serum treatment." *Cells* 8 (8): 824. https://doi.org/10.3390/CELLS8080824

Kim, J. N., J. Y. Lee, K. J. Shin, Y. C. Gil, K. S. Koh, and W. C. Song. 2015. "Haversian system of compact bone and comparison between endosteal and periosteal sides using three-dimensional reconstruction in rat." *Anatomy & Cell Biology* 48 (4): 258–261. https://doi.org/10.5115/ACB.2015.48.4.258

Kim, D. K., J. I. Kim, T. I. Hwang, B. R. Sim, and G. Khang. 2017. "Bioengineered osteoinductive broussonetia kazinoki/silk fibroin composite scaffolds for bone tissue regeneration," *ACS Applied. Materials and Interfaces* 9 (2), 1384–1394.

Kock, L., C. C. Van Donkelaar, and K. Ito. 2012. "Tissue engineering of functional articular cartilage: The current status." *Cell Tissue Res* 347:613–627.

Lawrence, R. C., D. T. Felson, C. G. Helmick, L. M. Arnold, H. Choi, R. A. Deyo, S. Gabriel, et al. 2008. "Estimates of the prevalence of arthritis and other rheumatic conditions in the United States: Part II." *Arthritis & Rheumatism* 58 (1): 26–35. https://doi.org/10.1002/ART.23176

Lieberman, D. E., J. D. Polk, and B. Demes. 2004. "Predicting long bone loading from cross-sectional geometry" 171: 156–171. https://doi.org/10.1002/ajpa.10316

Lips, P., and N. M. Van Schoor. 2011. "The effect of vitamin D on bone and osteoporosis." *Best Practice & Research Clinical Endocrinology & Metabolism* 25 (4): 585–591. https://doi.org/10.1016/J.BEEM.2011.05.002

Lombard, T., V. Neirinckx, B. Rogister, Y. Gilon, and S. Wislet. 2016. "Medication-related osteonecrosis of the jaw: New insights into molecular mechanisms and cellular therapeutic approaches." *Stem Cells International*, 1–16, 2016. https://doi.org/10.1155/2016/8768162

Mancini, T., M. Doga, G. Mazziotti, and A. Giustina. 2005. "Cushing's syndrome and bone." *Pituitary* 7 (4): 249–252. https://doi.org/10.1007/S11102-005-1051-2

Marie, P. J. 1992. "Physiologie du tissu osseux." *Immuno-Analyse & Biologie Spécialisée* 7 (6): 17–24. https://doi.org/10.1016/S0923-2532(05)80182-6

Martin, K. J., K. Olgaard, J. W. Coburn, G. M. Coen, M. Fukagawa, C. Langman, H. H. Malluche, et al. 2004. "Diagnosis, assessment, and treatment of bone turnover abnormalities in renal osteodystrophy." *American Journal of Kidney Diseases* 43 (3): 558–565. https://doi.org/10.1053/J.AJKD.2003.12.003

Mohamed, A. M. F. S. 2008. "An overview of bone cells and their regulating factors of differentiation." *The Malaysian Journal of Medical Sciences: MJMS* 15 (1): 4. /pmc/articles/PMC3341892/

Morrey, B. F. 2008. "Results of arthroscopic debridement for osteochondritis dissecans of the elbow rahusen FThG, Brinkman JM, Eygendaal D (St Maartenskliniek, Nijmegen, the Netherlands; Amphia Hosp, Breda, the Netherlands) Br J Sports Med 40: 966–969, 2006." *Year Book of Orthopedics* 2008: 195–196.

Murata, K., H. Ito, M. Hashimoto, K. Murakami, R. Watanabe, M. Tanaka, ... & S. Matsuda. 2020. "Fluctuation in anti-cyclic citrullinated protein antibody level predicts relapse from remission in rheumatoid arthritis: KURAMA cohort." *Arthritis Research & Therapy* 22: 1–10.

Nicol, L., P. Morar, Y. Wang, K. Henriksen, S. Sun, M. Karsdal, R. Smith, et al. 2019. "Alterations in non-type I collagen biomarkers in osteogenesis imperfecta." *Bone* 120 (March): 70–74. https://doi.org/10.1016/J.BONE.2018.09.024

On Osteoporosis Prevention Diagnosis, and Therapy. 2001. "Osteoporosis Prevention, Diagnosis, and Therapy." *JAMA* 285 (6): 785–795. https://doi.org/10.1001/jama.285.6.785.

Onar, V., and O. Belli. 2005. "Estimation of shoulder height from long bone measurements on dogs unearthed from the Van-Yoncatepe early iron age necropolis in eastern Anatolia." *Revue de Medecine Veterinaire* 156 (1): 53–60.

Pettifor, J. M. 2005. "Rickets." *The Bone and Mineral Manual*, January, 39–44. https://doi.org/10.1016/B978-012088569-5/50010-3

Ralston, S. H. 2013. "Paget's disease of bone." *New England Journal of Medicine* 368 (7): 644–650. https://doi.org/10.1056/NEJMCP1204713

Raouf, G. A., H. Gashlan, A. Khedr, S. Hamedy, and H. Al-Jabbri. 2015. "In vitro new biopolymer for bone grafting and bone cement." *International Journal of Latest Research in Science and Technology ISSN* 4 (2): 46–55. http://www.mnkjournals.com/ijlrst.htm

Redondo, M. L., D. R. Christian, and A. B. Yanke. 2019. "The role of synovium and synovial fluid in joint Hemostasis." *Joint Preservation of the Knee: A Clinical Casebook*, January, 57–67. https://doi.org/10.1007/978-3-030-01491-9_4/COVER/

Reilly, G. C. 2000. "Observations of microdamage around Osteocyte Lacunae in Bone." *Journal of Biomechanics* 33 (9): 1131–1134. https://doi.org/10.1016/S0021-9290(00)00090-7

Safadi, F. F., M. F. Barbe, S. M. Abdelmagid, M. C. Rico, R. A. Aswad, J Litvin, and S. N. Popoff. 2009. *Bone Structure, Development and Bone Biology. Bone Pathology, 2:1–50.* https://doi.org/10.1007/978-1-59745-347-9

Seeman, E., and P. D. Delmas. 2006. "Bone quality — The material and structural basis of bone strength and fragility." *The New England Journal of Medicine* 354 (21): 2250–2261. https://doi.org/10.1056/NEJMRA053077

Shaker, J. L. 2009. "Paget's disease of bone: A review of epidemiology, pathophysiology and management." *Therapeutic Advances in Musculoskeletal Disease* 1 (2): 107–125. https://doi.org/10.1177/1759720X09351779

Tekaya, R., A. B. Tekaya, O. Saidane, H. B. Said, A. Gaja, H Sahli, I. Mahmoud, and L. Abdelmoula. 2018. "Tophaceous hip gouty arthritis revealing asymptomatic axial gout." *The Egyptian Rheumatologist* 40 (3): 209–212. https://doi.org/10.1016/J.EJR.2017.10.001

Tuck, S. P., R. Layfield, J. Walker, B. Mekkayil, and R. Francis. 2017. "Adult paget's disease of bone: A review." *Rheumatology* 56 (12): 2050–2059. https://doi.org/10.1093/RHEUMATOLOGY/KEW430

Urish, K. L., & Cassat, J. E. (2020). "*Staphylococcus aureus* osteomyelitis: bone, bugs, and surgery." *Infection and Immunity*, 88(7), 10–1128.

Uttarilli, A., H. Shah, G. S. L. Bhavani, P. Upadhyai, A. Shukla, and K. M. Girisha. 2019. "Phenotyping and genotyping of skeletal dysplasias: Evolution of a center and a decade of Eexperience in India." *Bone* 120 (March): 204–211. https://doi.org/10.1016/J.BONE.2018.10.026

Wells, G. A., A. Cranney, J. Peterson, M. Boucher, B. Shea, V. Robinson, D. Coyle, and P. Tugwell. 2008. "Alendronate for the primary and secondary prevention of osteoporotic fractures in postmenopausal women." *Cochrane Database of Systematic Reviews* 1. https://doi.org/10.1002/14651858.CD001155.PUB2/INFORMATION/EN

Wells, G. A., S. Ching Hsieh, C. Zheng, J. Peterson, P. Tugwell, and W. Liu. 2022. "Risedronate for the primary and secondary prevention of osteoporotic fractures in postmenopausal women." *Cochrane Database of Systematic Reviews* 2022 (5). https://doi.org/10.1002/14651858.CD004523.PUB4/INFORMATION/EN

Werner, R. A., and T. J. Armstrong. 1997. "Carpal tunnel syndrome: Ergonomic risk factors and intracarpal." *Physical Medicine and Rehabilitation Clinics of North America* 8 (3): 555–569. https://doi.org/10.1016/S1047-9651(18)30317-6

Yoshiko, Y., G. A. Candeliere, N. Maeda, and J. E. Aubin. 2007. " Osteoblast autonomous P i regulation via Pit1 plays a role in bone mineralization." *Molecular and Cellular Biology* 27 (12): 4465–4474. https://doi.org/10.1128/MCB.00104-07/ASSET/3B4863A7-8E2B-4B9B-9EF7-474FCA6AAD0D/ASSETS/GRAPHIC/ZMB0120768090007.JPEG

Zhang, X., Y. Zhu, L. Cao, X. Wang, A. Zheng, J. Chang, J. Wu, et al. 2018. "Alginate-Aker injectable composite hydrogels promoted irregular bone regeneration through stem cell recruitment and osteogenic differentiation." *Journal of Materials Chemistry B* 6 (13): 1951–1964. https://doi.org/10.1039/c7tb03315j

2 Tissue Engineering as an Alternative Approach

INTRODUCTION

The bone and cartilage tissue damages and disorders due to injuries and congenital and degenerative diseases are quite common issues that have greatly impacted human life. The conventional non-surgical therapeutics, surgical intervention, and their combination suffer from various complications in their procedures as well as adverse after-effects causing the patients to continue with their pain for a longer period of time. The extensive surgical procedure often needed both at the recipient and the donor sites for the conventional grafts to be used for the reconstruction of bone, cartilage, and their complex tissues for their rehabilitation is extremely inconvenient to patients (Hernandez, Ruiz-Magnaz, and Guijarro-Martinez 2012). The use of allogenic and xenogenic grafts has the disadvantages of donor scarcity, donor morbidity, and immunogenic rejection. The lack of potential clinical techniques to reconstruct the damaged bone, cartilage, and other tissues has prompted to search for an efficient alternative method. In recent decades, the advancement in life sciences has made the scientists to discover new ideas, with ultimate goals to fully repair, regenerate, and maintain the functionality of the damaged human tissue. In this context, Tissue engineering (TE), a subfield of biomedical engineering discipline, has been evolved to cure these tissue disorders by avoiding the limitations emanated from the traditional clinical treatment. The TE technique integrates biology with engineering disciplines to produce engineered tissue or cellular products *in vitro* for repairing and preserving the structure as well as the function of tissues and/or organs through the regeneration of lost tissues by appropriate clinical strategies (Langer and Vacanti 1993). This technique has tremendous potential to repair, regenerate, and maintain the functionality of the lost or damaged human tissue; hence, it is under active research (Ghosh and Pal 2016). This is a multidisciplinary field for which inputs from various scientific knowledge, skill, and expertise are needed for its development. Although the field is speedily developing and has the potential to influence significantly the biological system, a lot of challenges prevailed in TE being a comparatively new field. To achieve the success of TE, we should have clear concepts about the vital background information including the basic principles and tissue regeneration processes and challenges. This chapter describes the basic concept of TE technique, its general strategy for tissue regeneration including the bone and associated tissues, various challenges associated with this technique, and future prospect.

BASIC CONCEPT

The loss or failure of organs and/or tissues is the most frequent, traumatic, and expensive ailments in human health care. Millions of people worldwide suffer from various diseases that are associated with bone, cartilage, skin, burn, muscle, tendon, and ligament tissues every year (Sikavitsas, Bancroft, and Mikos 2002; Sittinger et al. 1996). Current treatment methods like tissue or organ transplantation have several drawbacks, including infection and device rejection, and they normally do not let the patients to resume their normal activities completely. A national survey indicates that the waiting list of patients who need organ transplantation far exceeds the number of donors available. Health care survey of India (February 2008) reveals that revenue from the health care sector accounts for 5.2% of the gross domestic product (GDP), making it the third largest growth sector, indicating the suffering of patient population. Studies have further estimated that almost half of the national health care bill is due to the tissue loss or organ failure. This alarming situation in health care can only be effectively solved when a permanent solution towards these losses is discovered. In this context, TE has emerged as a promising strategy to replace damaged tissues or organs. This method not only offers an effective and permanent solution but also reduces the overall cost of treatment.

TE is an interdisciplinary field in engineering and medicine that creates functionalized artificial tissues by applying the principles and methods of engineering and biology (Figure 2.1). The goal of this field is to develop biologically active substitutes by combining living cells, biomaterials, and physicochemical factors that can replace the damaged or diseased tissues including bone, cartilage, joint tissues, etc., and there by to restore, maintain, or improve their functions. The term "regenerative medicine" is frequently used synonymously with TE, although the former gives more emphasis on using stem cells or progenitor cells directly to produce tissues. The origin of "tissue engineering" can be clearly traced to a specific individual. In 1986, Y.C. Fung, a pioneer in biomechanics field, first established an engineering research centre named "Centre for the Engineering of Living Tissues". In 1988, the first scientific meeting on TE held at Lake Tahoe, California (Skalak and Fox 1988; Nerem and Sambanis 1995), recognized its concept and importance.

DEFINITION OF TISSUE ENGINEERING

TE has been defined in various ways by different scientists:

- First time Langer and Vacanti defined TE as follows: "it is an interdisciplinary field that involves the application of different engineering principles and life sciences for the development of biologically functionalized substitutes that are able to restore, maintain, or improve tissue function or a whole organ".
- Y. C. Fung defined TE as "the application of the principles and methods of engineering and life sciences toward the fundamental understanding of

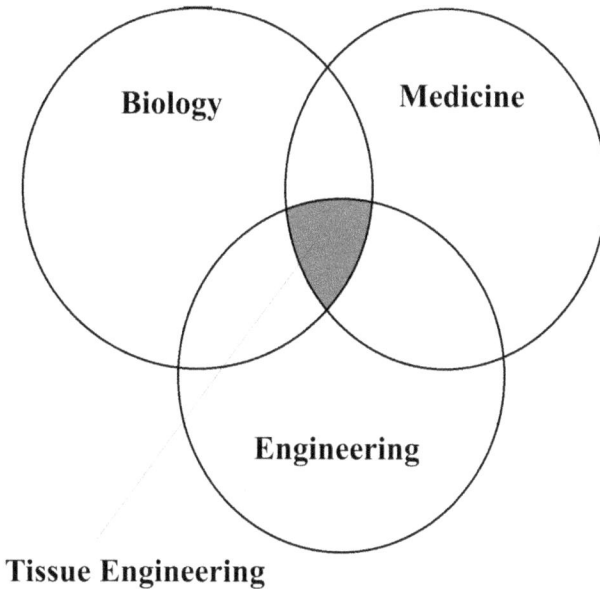

Tissue Engineering

FIGURE 2.1   Different disciplines involved in tissue engineering field.

structure function relationships in normal and pathological mammalian tissue and the development of biological substitutes to restore, maintain, or improve tissue function".

- C. T. Laurencin defined TE as "the application of biological, chemical, and engineering principles toward the repair, restoration, or regeneration of living tissues using biomaterials, cells, and factors alone or in combination".

The concept of TE to create neotissue from a combined effect of cells, and scaffold (an engineered matrix) derived from suitable biomaterial is presented in Figure 2.2. Besides suitable cell source and scaffolds acting as cell recruiter, and guide for cell expansion and differentiation, it requires suitable growth factors and stimulating agents, for example, mechanical stimulation, electrical stimulation depending on targeted tissue to be regenerated.

HISTORY OF TISSUE ENGINEERING

The term "tissue engineering" was evolved long back, about three and half decades earlier. As mentioned earlier, a proposal to establish a "Center for the Engineering of Living Tissues" was first submitted by Y.C. Fung, a scientist in biomechanics and bioengineering, to the National Science Foundation (NSF) in 1985 with a concept to create artificial tissue through engineering approach. Although the proposal was not accepted by NSF, the concept of this engineering approach towards biology relating cells and organs surfaced again at the spring session of NSF in 1987 in Washington, D.C. where a panel meeting was convened to review the proposals under the title

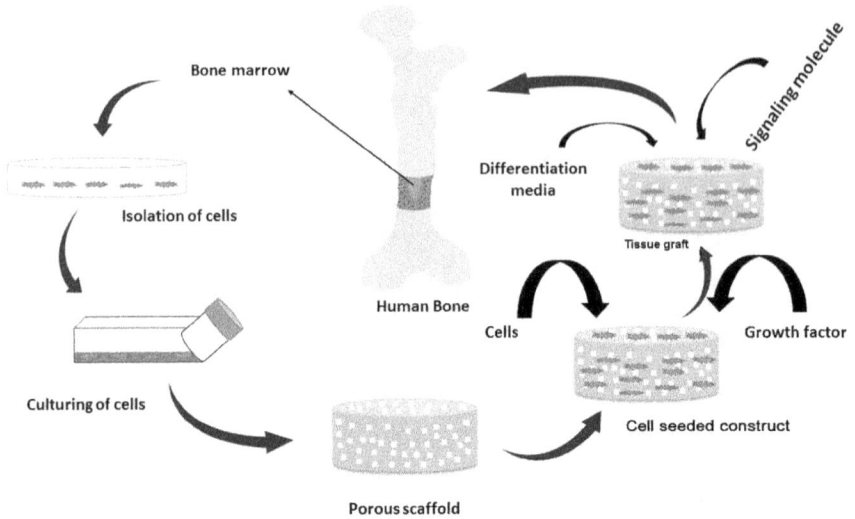

FIGURE 2.2   Concept of tissue engineering technique.

"Bioengineering and Research" including Fung's proposal. In this meeting, the term "tissue engineering" was coined. Following this the first scientific meeting entitled "tissue engineering" conference was held in the beginning of 1988 at Lake Tahoe, California. In the early 1990s, the concept of application of engineering principles for repairing the defect or damaged biological tissue led to the fast growth of TE as an interdisciplinary field having potential to revolutionize the many important areas of medicine (Skalak and Fox 1988; Vacanti 2006; Fung 2001). TE is not new and existing since ancient times, although the term "tissue engineering" was not evolved at that time. Some of the examples of application of this field are noted in the following.

Sushruta, an Indian physician, and regarded as the "Father of Indian Medicine" and "Father of Plastic Surgery", lived sometime between 600 and 1000 BC developed surgical techniques for reconstructing noses, earlobes, and genitalia and performed nose transplants (Champaneria, Workman, and Gupta 2014; Sorta-Bilajac and Muzur 2007). In the 1580s (16th century), Gaspare Tagliacozzi (1545–1599), a professor of surgery and anatomy at the University of Bologna, Italy, did reconstruction of the nose, using forearm flap (Ménard 2019). Similarly, tooth transplantation was happened in the mid-17th century. The corneal transplantation was proposed in the 17th century, and, subsequently, Samuel Bigger published a report on the successful corneal transplantation in a gazettee in 1837 (Crawford, Patel, and McGhee 2013). The skin grafting originated in ancient time for more than 3,500 years ago and this ancient skin graft technique was taking place 1500 BC. However, according to the "Sushruta Samhita, an early text of Ayurveda, in ancient time, the skin grafting was performed by the Hindu more than 3000 years ago" (Reverdin 1909; Kohlhauser et al. 2021).

Aseptic or sterile techniques were first adopted in surgery in the late 19th century following the germ theory of Louis Pasteur in the mid-19th century. And this was an inspiration for Joseph Lister to adopt antiseptic surgery using carbolic acid (e.g. phenol) as a disinfectant or sterilizing agent in the 1860s (2018). During this period, reconstructive surgery was emerged. In the 20th century, the modern-day transplantation surgery using conventional grafting methods and the use of synthetic materials for tissue repair emerged. In the late 20th century, scientific focus was shifted towards the development of cell-based reconstructive therapies through tissue regeneration. This resulted in the kidney, heart, lung, and bone marrow transplantations. After the mid-1980s the concept of applying engineering principle to tissue and organ was evolved and subsequently, the term "tissue engineering" was evolved in 1985 followed by the organization of the First Symposium on Tissue Engineering in 1988.

GENERAL STRATEGIES FOR TISSUE REGENERATION

TE requires a fundamental understanding of the structure and function of tissues, including bone, cartilage, etc., and their replacement and/or repair when they get damaged due to injury or tissue degeneration. This technique can solve the existing problems associated with tissue or organ by developing an artificial extracellular matrix (ECM) with biofunctionalized characteristics that is used as the delivery vehicle for stem cells and bioactive molecules, thereby producing the target tissue. However, in general, tissue regeneration can be achieved using the following approaches.

Cell and Tissue-Based Therapy

In this approach, cells are isolated from a suitable source and expanded using appropriate culture media. The expanded cells are directly injected intravenously or into specific host organs to repair the damaged or diseased tissues thereby restoring the lost tissue or organ function. The cells utilize the blood stream that provides nutrients and required bioactive molecules, whereas the host tissue matrix acts as a cell support system for desired cellular interaction including cell attachment, migration, proliferation, differentiation, and host tissue integration (Holzapfel et al. 2013). Unlike organ transplantation which usually involves a complex surgical procedure, cell therapy is comparatively easier to perform and can also easily be reached to wider population. Cell therapy can be used for the treatment of a wide variety of diseases, *viz.*, diabetes; neurodegenerative diseases, such as Parkinson's, Alzheimer's, and Huntinton's diseases, etc.; and lesions in the cardiovascular diseases, cornea, skeletal muscle, skin, joints, bones, etc. Various cell types like stem cells including embryonic stem cells, multipotent adult progenitor cells, etc., can be used for tissue regeneration in the defect or disease sites. Although, cell therapy is considered as the most promising future technique for therapeutic treatment in restoring tissue or organ function, this injection approach suffers from its low efficacy as the major drawback (Sánchez, Schimmang, and García-Sancho 2012).

Inducing Tissue Regeneration by Soluble Bioactive Factors

The soluble bioactive factors, for example, growth factors, play an important role in different cellular actions, such as cell viability, proliferation, and differentiation

through cell signalling activity. Natural ECM contains numerous adhesive molecules, the so-called ligands, which are able to bind and modulate the bioactivity of signalling molecules (Discher, Janmey, and Wang 2005). The bioactive signalling molecules such as low-molecular-weight drugs, oligonucleotides, and numerous protein compounds like cytokines, chemokines, hormones, and growth factors have the ability to regulate specific cellular metabolism inside the host, resulting in a specific cellular response including the cell survival, proliferation (growth factors-inducing proliferation, mitogens—stimulating cell division), and differentiation (morphogens control cell differentiation) of cells and thereby enabling tissue regeneration by triggering specific activation reaction in metabolic j+46
pathway (Chan and Leong 2008). Therefore, precise control of bioactivity through these signalling molecules at the defect site of the patient can effectively control tissue regeneration process.

Scaffold or Matrix-Based Artificial Support System

Although cell-based therapy is the most promising future approach for tissue regeneration, the low efficacy of this therapy is a major obstacle for its commercial use. To increase the efficacy of the cell therapy, scaffold-based support system has been evolved. This approach primarily targets the development and use of a functionalized artificial extracellular matrix, the so-called scaffold, which are derived from natural or synthetic biomaterials. These scaffolds act as cell career and provide structural support to the cells and guidance for tissue regeneration, thereby producing cell-scaffold construct and subsequently tissue graft by differentiation of the cells on the scaffold (Mayer et al. 2000).

TISSUE ENGINEERING STRATEGIES FOR BONE AND CARTILAGE REGENERATION

Bone, cartilage, and joint defects caused by trauma, infection, and degenerative diseases are frequent phenomena and become critical due to therapeutic limitations. Bone lesions are the most common problems, whose severity increases with time once they become damaged. According to the International Osteoporosis Foundation, in India ~26 million osteoporosis patients were reported in 2010 and this number is expected to reach 36 million in the future. Worldwide, cartilage defects are estimated to be the fourth leading cause of disability. In USA, ~1 million bone injury cases are reported every year and an alarming increase in bone-related defects is expected worldwide in the future. In patients younger than 40 years, osteochondral defects are observed in 34–62% of knee arthroscopies and 4.2–6.2% full-thickness focal lesions (1–2 cm^2). In comparison to general population, there is the highest demand of knee by the athletes who are likely to develop osteoarthritis 12 times more (Amoako and Pujalte 2014). The conventional bone substitutes such as autografts, allograft, and xenografts have their own limitation, including the lack of availability, immunogenic response, and zoonotic disease transfer, whereas most of the metal implants often fail due to corrosion, post-operative loosening or failure to osteo-integrate. Such intrinsic problems associated with currently available clinical strategy led to the introduction of bone and cartilage TE as a clinical alternative. This led to growing demands of engineered tissue grafts to cope with the alarming situation of different types of orthopaedic tissue defects. Like general TE approach, the three major components for the creation of a tissue-engineered bone and cartilage constructs are the cells, scaffolds, and bioactive factors.

Development of biomaterials with biomimetic properties is a prerequisite, which offers a great challenge in TE technique. The design and fabrication of three-dimensional (3D) scaffold structures and subsequently the production of tissue grafts using this scaffold and suitable cells like stem cells for the production of tissue grafts for regeneration of bone and cartilage or their combination, for example, osteochondral, joints, etc., in a clinical manner, are other challenges. Bone tissue extracellular matrix consists of two major components: a biomineral component constituted of hydroxyapatite (65–70%) and an organic component consisting of proteoglycans, glycoproteins, bone sialoproteins, and bone Gla proteins which cover 25–30%. Bone damages are often associated with surrounding tissue damage like cartilage. The strategy in alternative medicine is to develop biomaterials for fabricating scaffolds which can act as artificial extracellular platforms for recruiting cells and guiding cell differentiation as well as reorganization of the ECM. Bone and cartilage TE often is an integrative process which is influenced by important moieties like growth factors to control and regulate this process. Growth factors also influence the physiological function during bone regeneration. Osteogenic and chondrogenic cells along with appropriate growth factors and scaffolds derived from suitable biomaterials form the foundation of cartilage and bone TE strategies which are applied for repairing and restoring damaged tissues (Qasim, Chae, and Lee 2020). Strategically, for bone defects repair, developing matrices with osteogenic (capable of directing or inducing bone tissue formation), osteoconductive (ability to allow cells for bone tissue growth on a surface like scaffold or matrix), and osteoinductive (ability to induce osteogenesis by recruiting and stimulating the cells to form bone-forming cells, e.g. preosteoblasts) properties with 3D nanostructures should be the target.

TE AS A MULTIDISCIPLINARY APPROACH

TE is an interdisciplinary field that requires much input and skills from a range of science including biology, engineering, and medical disciplines. The various disciplines involved in TE field are shown in the schematic diagram (Figure 2.3). The method combines cells, tissue-engineered materials, as well as a variety of biochemical and physico-chemical factors. Besides biology and medicine, the field covers a wide range of engineering principles that are related to chemical engineering, mechanical engineering, material science and engineering, computer engineering, polymer engineering, surface engineering, bioscience and bioengineering, etc. (Pedrero, Llamas-Sillero, and Serrano-López 2021; Stock and Vacanti 2001). Biologists are involved in developing innovative and effective methods for isolating and growing cells from different sources. They also discover new growth factors, useful bioactive molecules that are acted as cell signalling molecules, and characteristics of the stem cells and other cells for better understanding of their function and what causes them to change.

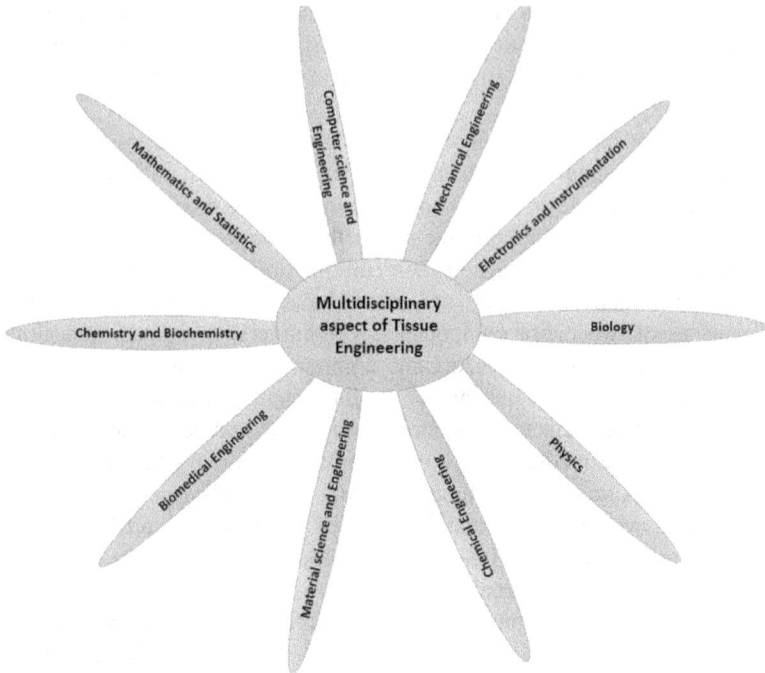

FIGURE 2.3   Multidisciplinary aspects of tissue engineering.

The architecture of TE scaffolds is another important and critical factor. The engineered matrix should possess an interconnected porous structure and high porosity, typically more than 70% for proper cellular penetration within the scaffold and sufficient diffusion of nutrients to the cells located inside the construct and to the newly synthesized extra-cellular matrix by these cells. For this purpose, specially mechanical engineering plays an important role in the design of the scaffolds by devising an appropriate fabrication technique. The knowledge of instrumentation and electronic engineers are important for the operation, control, and maintenance of the bioreactors during the tissue regeneration *in vitro* and developing online monitoring device. Biologists can contribute towards monitoring and maintaining the cell properties of newly seeded cells. Design engineers may also help in 3D printing of tissues and cells on the scaffolds. Computer engineers help to develop artificial programs to monitor and guide mathematically the formation of scaffolds. Development of scaffold biomaterial is of prime importance for which knowledge of material and polymer science including the type, characteristics, and processing technologies is needed. Surface engineering has an important role in modifying the surface properties, thereby making implant or scaffold with better performance for tissue regeneration. For developing tissue construct or engineered tissue grafts, the design of bioreactor is important, which requires mechanical engineers. Long-term preservation of the developed tissue graft or tissue construct with good cell or tissue viability is of immense importance. In this context, appropriate technology can be developed with the help of mechanical engineering or cryogenic engineering. The knowledge of nanotechnology is beneficial in developing scaffolds with nanofeature structures like nanofibre, nanotube, nanocomposite, etc., thereby mimicking the body tissue.

After initial success *at-bench*, the tissue constructs and tissue grafts are needed to be tested *in vivo* to assess their ability for tissue growth. *In vivo* animal models are considered as a proof-of-concept validation for promising *at-bench* tissue growth. The subject of animal biotechnology is needed in this particular stage. Finally, the role of medical professionals and doctors is of utmost importance for application of the engineered tissue grafts in actual clinical use for the treatment of patients. They also contribute to obtaining the detailed statistics of the patient's tissue defect and disability through proper diagnosis using analytical or instrumental techniques as well as observation. Nonetheless, they also conduct *in vivo* clinical trial of the tissue-engineered products in humans before commercialization.

POTENTIAL APPLICATION OF TISSUE ENGINEERING

Although TE research has been extensively carried out targeting a wide spectrum of tissue types in the last two decades, only a very few tissue products have come up in the market. The potential applications of TE are envisioned including skin, cartilage, bone, cardiac/heart, central nervous system, and others like ligaments, tendon, joints, skeletal muscle, neurodegenerative diseases, cancer, liver, kidney, cornea, pancreas, spine, dental, etc. Tissue-engineered skin substitutes can be used for the treatment of patients with severe skin damage due to burn, chronic wound, ulcer, accidental injuries, etc. Damaged musculoskeletal tissues like bone, cartilage, tendon ligaments, and their combination forming more complex joint tissue can be regenerated, thereby restoring their function and structures. Neurodegenerative diseases like Alzheimer's disease, Parkinson's disease, etc., can be treated by tissue regeneration approach. Liver transplantation is the replacement of damaged or diseased liver by surgery. TE offers the potential engineered liver that can treat the patient with acute or chronic liver disorders. The drawbacks associated with corneal transplantation for improving and restoring lost vision can be overcome by the use of corneal substitutes through TE approach (Fagerholm et al. 2014). Similarly, the lost kidney function can be restored by the implantation of engineered grafts generated by renal TE (Montserrat, Garreta, and Izpisua Belmonte 2016; Moon et al. 2016).

There are numerous nontraditional, but important applications of TE strategies, such as drug screening using engineered heart models (Ralphe and de Lange 2013; Nachlas, Li, and Davis 2017), lung (Chen et al. 2017), skin (Danilenko, Phillips, and Diaz 2016), infectious diseases and cancer models (Benam et al. 2017), cartilage (Peck et al. 2018), etc.

CHALLENGES AND FUTURE PROSPECTS OF TE

TE Research and Development

TE is considered as an ultimate ideal clinical treatment option and has tremendous prospect in solving the tissue-related problems, thereby improving the quality of life. However, TE has several challenges that are yet to be addressed. The lack of well-equipped laboratory, research funds, and expertise in this new area provide *in vitro* and *in vivo* experimental results with huge difference and hence it is difficult to assess the actual efficiency of the tissue scaffold in tissue regeneration. Active research and development in multi-directional aspects are needed to overcome many of the challenges persisting in TE. For example, although engineered bone tissue substitutes are considered as the potential alternatives to the conventional bone grafts without displaying any immunogenic reaction, their clinical practices have not progressed much because of numerous issues, including insufficient vascularization at the defect site, inability to self-repair owing to avascular nature of the hyaline cartilage, slow cartilage metabolism compared to other tissues, and hence more difficult for cartilage defect to heal, etc. (Tew et al. 2001). Therefore, a systematic research is necessary to overcome these issues. Cell expansion is important for continuous and fast supply of cells for successful tissue regeneration that requires *in vitro* laboratory-based cell culture system. However, the major concerns involved in this stage are laboratory sterility, ethics, and risks associated with the use of serum-based media which are usually of animal origin (Herberts, Kwa, and Hermsen 2011; Halme and Kessler 2006). The avoidance of *in vitro* laboratory cell culture, and therefore, elimination of these concerns, may be possible by developing a rapid cell isolation technique with higher cell density and their direct or immediate use for tissue regeneration (Francis et al. 2010; Francis et al. 2018). Irrespective of the strategy of rapid isolation and immediate application, methods of culturing of cells without using animal serum-based media may be an appropriate option, although it may be critical in the case of human clinical translation. In this context, developing an animal serum-free medium from the human-derived growth supplements, for example, human platelet lysates (Hemeda, Giebel, and Wagner 2014; Bieback et al. 2009; Crespo-Diaz et al. 2011; Schallmoser and Strunk 2009; Walenda et al. 2012), may be a promising solution for cell culturing. It has also been reported that the development of animal as well as human serum-free media for culturing the most suitable MSCs for neotissue regeneration and their clinical applications is another encouraging strategy (Chase et al. 2010; Lindroos et al. 2009; Patrikoski et al. 2013).

There are numerous scaffolds, some of which are with novel composition developed by the researchers worldwide. Most of these research remain in the published literature, and only a very few are in the stage of clinical trial. Besides composition, further research is needed for appropriate scaffold designs that can optimize its properties, including the biocompatibility, biodegradation, pore size, pore geometry, mechanical strength, stiffness, surface properties, etc. (Stoop 2008; Agrawal et al. 2018; Nava et al. 2016; Arora, Kothari, and Katti 2015). In recent years research has been directed towards matrix development by developing biomaterials with desired functional properties. For example, polymer-composite scaffolds using bioactive ceramic compounds are promising for orthopaedic applications than the simple polymer-blend scaffolds. In later stages, research focus was directed towards the development of composite scaffolds by combining polymer, ceramic materials along with inorganic oxides. Still hardly any scaffold biomaterial that can meet all the desired properties for bone TE is available. There is also concern in the fundamental understanding of the mechanism of differentiation of cells into neotissue that is important for the development of engineered tissue products. Therefore, a systematic research on the development of scaffold biomaterials, cells production and appropriate microenvironment to enhance the bone and bone-related tissue regeneration is of immense importance.

Development of multifunctional scaffold materials with nanostructure hierarchical architecture and biomimetic properties that enable formation of different tissues with varying properties, for example, in the case of more complex situation like joints, is likely to be the focus of future research and/or growth factors. Rapid advances are being made to identify new cell types and their development for tissue regeneration. Stem cells including human mesenchymal stem cells (hMSCs), human embryonic stem cells (hESCs), adult stem cells, and induced pluripotent stem cells (iPSCs) are exciting because of their potency for differentiation, and therefore transformation into various cell or tissue types. Furthermore, there are certain ethical issues involved in various stages of TE that sometimes create barriers for the researchers. Limited research and development funding for a long time is another concern for conducting research in this emerging area. This may become more critical for research in developing countries. Expensive as well as lack of expertise and sophisticated laboratories for conducting *in vivo* experiment become quite difficult. However, there is still growing interest in research and development in this novel field.

TE Clinical Barriers

Over the past three decades, TE has offered ample hope in overcoming the limitations associated with the current clinical treatment methods through active research in this field. Still there are not many clinical trials using the engineered tissues developed through TE technique. Some of the major obstacles in clinical translation of the tissue-engineered products are discussed in the following section.

TE involves the multifactorial nature of the translational process and requires highly complex clinical condition, which are the major obstacles for its translation. TE needs to optimize several intersecting components including the cells, scaffolds, stimulating and signalling factors, and bioreactors to produce tissue products optimally. But the individual component is complex. For example, plenty of scaffolds have been described in the published literature, which can be further modified or improved in many ways. However, there is a need to stop in some stage and proceed to the next stage of development which is difficult to decide as the choice of scaffolds depends on cell type. The expansion of cells with maintained phenotype in large scale and following regulatory issues is another critical factor. Long-term provision for financial support in performing translational research and good manufacturing practices (GMP) facility for getting the Food and Drug Administration (FDA) approval before proceeding for clinical trial are other constraints (Evans 2011; Madry et al. 2014).

INDUSTRIAL CHALLENGES

TE field offers an entirely new paradigm in medical treatment with the potential to make a great change in medical practice. With the progress in TE, the industry has many challenges that are related to quality control of the tissue products, ethical complications, and implant transplantation. The major industrial problems existing in this field include high cost of manufacturing tissue constructs and tissue grafts as well as their maintenance with long self-life, poorly structured agreements with business partners or governments, unrealistic cost–benefit analysis associated with the product produced in the early stage of development, unrealistic sales forecasts leading to excessive fixed costs of sales, lengthy regulatory procedure, the so-called FDA approval, causing financial crisis, and competition with existing recognized drug manufacturing companies such as Johnson & Johnson(J&J), Pfizer, **GlaxoSmithKline (GSK)**, Procter & Gamble(P&G), those produce traditional therapeutic products for various disease treatments. Furthermore, acceptance of new tissue-engineered products is another big concern among the majority of the patients, doctors, and society at large (Sallent et al. 2020). However, in recent decades scientists and researchers have given their utmost effort to make relationship or collaboration with relevant industries to enhance the growth of TE research as well as industrial or large-scale production of engineering tissue, thereby bringing the benefits of this novel technique to improving the quality of life of mass population.

Establishing a consensus quality control programme that ensures the functionality and safety of the tissue-engineered grafts and constructs, as well as the raw materials like cells used for developing these products, is a key challenge for the TE industry. This will have major impact on the application of these tissue substitutes in future health care practice. There is also a need for setting up of industrial-scale production units for the scaffold and cells for producing tissue-engineered products. In addition, the industries should establish GMP facility to ensure FDA standards of the cells and the *in vitro* production of the cell-seeded constructs and tissue grafts. Furthermore, appropriate strategies need to be evolved for preserving the tissue-engineered products for a longer period of time with maintained tissue viability and functionality. Even with massive testing in well-equipped laboratories, industries usually face difficulty for getting FDA approval for commercializing the cellular products. Furthermore, It is observed that most of the investors are from private sectors or small-scale companies which have limited financial abilities (Lynn, Morone, and Paulson 1996; Mendicino et al. 2019).

EXERCISE

1. Which field of study does tissue engineering encompass?
2. What is tissue engineering? State the importance of tissue engineering.
3. Describe the key elements that are required to develop a tissue by tissue engineering approach?
4. Tissue engineering is the frontier area of research in the 21st century—Explain.
5. Tissue engineering is a promising alternative technique for the treatment of defect bone and joints in human body—Justify.
6. Describe the multidisciplinary approach of tissue engineering field with examples..
7. Identify the major challenges involved in tissue engineering technique and explain how to overcome them..

8. Write about the future prospects of tissue engineering in human health care.
9. Discuss about the various industrial challenges involved in tissue-engineered therapiesand suggest appropriate strategy to overcome them.
10. Write a brief history of tissue engineering development.
11. What are the most critical barriers do you feel involved in the application of the tissue-engineered products and suggest some strategy for their remedy. for application of tissue engineering?
12. What are the different applications of tissue engineering?
13. Explain how cell and tissue engineering are important in regenerative medicine.
14. Explain the basic concept of tissue engineering with the help of an appropriate diagram.

REFERENCES

Agrawal, P., K. Pramanik, V. Vishwanath, A. Biswas, A. Bissoyi, and P. K. Patra. 2018. "Enhanced chondrogenesis of mesenchymal stem cells over silk fibroin/chitosan-chondroitin sulfate three dimensional scaffold in dynamic culture condition." *Journal of Biomedical Materials Research Part B Applied Biomaterials* 106 (7): 2576–2587. DOI: 10.1002/jbm.b.34074

Amoako, A. O., and G. G. Pujalte. 2014. "Osteoarthritis in young, active, and athletic individuals." *Clinical Medicine Insights: Arthritis Musculoskelet Disorders* 7: 27–32. DOI: 10.4137/CMAMD.S14386

Arora, A., A. Kothari, and D. S. Katti. 2015. "Pore orientation mediated control of mechanical behavior of scaffolds and its application in cartilage-mimetic scaffold design." *Journal of the Mechanical Behavior of Biomedical Materials* 51: 169–183.

Benam, K. H., M. Mazur, Y. Choe, T. C. Ferrante, R. Novak, and D. E. Ingber. 2017. "Human lung small airway-on-a-chip protocol." In *3D Cell Culture*, edited by Zuzana Koledova. Humana Press, New York, 345–365.

Bieback, K., A. Hecker, A. Kocaömer, H. Lannert, K. Schallmoser, D. Strunk, and H. Klüter. 2009. "Human alternatives to fetal bovine serum for the expansion of mesenchymal stromal cells from bone marrow." *Stem Cells* 27 (9): 2331–2341.

Champaneria, M. C., A. D. Workman, and S. C. Gupta. 2014. "Sushruta: father of plastic surgery." *Annals of Plastic Surgery* 73 (1): 2–7.

Chan, B. P., and K. W. Leong. 2008. "Scaffolding in tissue engineering: General approaches and tissue-specific considerations." *European Spine Journal* 17 (4): 467–479.

Chase, L. G., U. Lakshmipathy, L. A. Solchaga, M. S. Rao, and M. C. Vemuri. 2010. "A novel serum-free medium for the expansion of human mesenchymal stem cells." *Stem Cell Research & Therapy* 1 (1): 1–11.

Chen, Y.-W., S. Xuelian Huang, A. Luisa Rodrigues Toste de Carvalho, S.-H. Ho, M. Naimul Islam, S. Volpi, L. D. Notarangelo, M. Ciancanelli, J.-L. Casanova, and J. Bhattacharya. 2017. "A three-dimensional model of human lung development and disease from pluripotent stem cells." *Nature Cell Biology* 19 (5): 542–549.

Crawford, A. Z., D. V. Patel, and C. N. J. McGhee. 2013. "A brief history of corneal transplantation: From ancient to modern." *Oman Journal of Ophthalmology* 6 (1): S12.

Crespo-Diaz, R., A. Behfar, G. W. Butler, D. J. Padley, M. G. Sarr, J. Bartunek, A. B. Dietz, and A. Terzic. 2011. "Platelet lysate consisting of a natural repair proteome supports human mesenchymal stem cell proliferation and chromosomal stability." *Cell Transplantation* 20 (6): 797–812.

Danilenko, D. M., G. D. Lewis Phillips, and D. Diaz. 2016. "In vitro skin models and their predictability in defining normal and disease biology, pharmacology, and toxicity." *Toxicologic Pathology* 44 (4): 555–563.

Discher, D. E., P. Janmey, and Y.-L. Wang. 2005. "Tissue cells feel and respond to the stiffness of their substrate." *Science* 310 (5751): 1139–1143.

Evans, C. H. 2011. "Barriers to the clinical translation of orthopedic tissue engineering." *Tissue Engineering Part B: Reviews* 17 (6): 437–441.

Fagerholm, P., N. S. Lagali, J. A. Ong, K. Merrett, W. B. J., J. W. Polarek, E. J. Suuronen, Y. Liu, I. Brunette, and M. Griffith. 2014. "Stable corneal regeneration four years after implantation of a cell-free recombinant human collagen scaffold." *Biomaterials* 35 (8): 2420–2427.

Francis, M. P., P. C. Sachs, L. W. Elmore, and S. E. Holt. 2010. "Isolating adipose-derived mesenchymal stem cells from lipoaspirate blood and saline fraction." *Organogenesis* 6 (1): 11–14.

Francis, S. L., S. Duchi, C. Onofrillo, C. Di Bella, and P. F. M. Choong. 2018. "Adipose-derived mesenchymal stem cells in the use of cartilage tissue engineering: The need for a rapid isolation procedure." *Stem Cells International* 2018.

Fung, Y. 2001. "A proposal to the National science foundation for an engineering research centre at USCD." *Center for the Engineering of Living Tissues. UCSD* 865023: 2001.

Ghosh, B., and Imon P. 2016. "Basic ideas and concepts about tissue engineering: A review." *International Journal of Scientific & Engineering Research*, 7 (12): 571–574. ISSN 2229-5518

Halme, D. G., and D. A. Kessler. 2006. "FDA regulation of stem-cell-based therapies." *New England Journal of Medicine* 355 (16): 1730.

Hemeda, H., B. Giebel, and W. Wagner. 2014. "Evaluation of human platelet lysate versus fetal bovine serum for culture of mesenchymal stromal cells." *Cytotherapy* 16 (2): 170–180.

Herberts, C. A., M. S. G. Kwa, and H. P. H. Hermsen. 2011. "Risk factors in the development of stem cell therapy." *Journal of Translational Medicine* 9 (1): 1–14.

Hernandez, F., V. Ruiz-Magnaz, and R. Guijarro-Martinez. 2012. "Mandible reconstruction with tissue engineering in multiple recurrent Ameloblastoma." *The International Journal of Periodontics & Restorative Dentistry* 32: e82–e86.

Holzapfel, B. Michael, J. Christian Reichert, J.-T. Schantz, U. Gbureck, L. Rackwitz, U. Nöth, F. Jakob, M. Rudert, J. Groll, and D. Werner Hutmacher. 2013. "How smart do biomaterials need to be? A translational science and clinical point of view." *Advanced Drug Delivery Reviews* 65 (4): 581–603.

Kohlhauser, M., H. Luze, S. P. Nischwitz, and L. P. Kamolz. 2021. "Historical evolution of skin grafting—a journey through time." *Medicina* 57 (4): 348.

Langer, R., and J. P. Vacanti. 1993. "Tissue engineering." *Science* 260: 920–926.

Lindroos, B., S. Boucher, L. Chase, H. Kuokkanen, H. Huhtala, R. Haataja, M. Vemuri, R. Suuronen, and S. Miettinen. 2009. "Serum-free, xeno-free culture media maintain the proliferation rate and multipotentiality of adipose stem cells in vitro." *Cytotherapy* 11 (7): 958–972.

Lynn, G. S., J. G. Morone, and A. S. Paulson. 1996. "Marketing and discontinuous innovation: The probe and learn process." *California Management Review* 38 (3): 8–37.

Madry, H., M. Alini, M. J. Stoddart, C. Evans, T. Miclau, and Sandra Steiner. 2014. "Barriers and strategies for the clinical translation of advanced orthopaedic tissue engineering protocols." *European Cells and Materials* 27: 17–21.

Mayer, J., E. Karamuk, T. Akaike, and E. Wintermantel. 2000. "Matrices for tissue engineering-scaffold structure for a bioartificial liver support system." *Journal of Controlled Release* 64 (1–3): 81–90.

Ménard, S. 2019. "An unknown renaissance portrait of tagliacozzi (1545–1599), the founder of plastic surgery." *Plastic and Reconstructive Surgery Global Open* 7 (1): 1–6.

Mendicino, M., Y. Fan, D. Griffin, K. C. Gunter, and K. Nichols. 2019. "Current state of US Food and Drug Administration regulation for cellular and gene therapy products: Potential cures on the horizon." *Cytotherapy* 21 (7): 699–724.

Montserrat, N., E. Garreta, and J. C. I. Belmonte. 2016. "Regenerative strategies for kidney engineering." *The FEBS Journal* 283 (18): 3303–3324.

Moon, K. H., I. K. Ko, J. J. Yoo, and A. Atala. 2016. "Kidney diseases and tissue engineering." *Methods* 99: 112–119.

Nachlas, A. L. Y., S. Li, and Michael E D. 2017. "Developing a clinically relevant tissue engineered heart valve—A review of current approaches." *Advanced Healthcare Materials* 6 (24): 1700918.

Nakayama, D. K. 2018. "Antisepsis and asepsis and how they shaped modern surgery." *The American Surgeon* 84 (6): 766–771.

Nava, M. M., L. Draghi, C. Giordano, and R. Pietrabissa. 2016. "The effect of scaffold pore size in cartilage tissue engineering." *Journal of Applied Biomaterials & Functional Materials* 14 (3): e223–e229.

Nerem, R. M., and A. Sambanis. 1995. "Tissue engineering: from biology to biological substitutes." *Tissue Engineering* 1 (1): 3–13.

Patrikoski, M., M. Juntunen, S. Boucher, A. Campbell, M. C. Vemuri, B. Mannerström, and S. Miettinen. 2013. "Development of fully defined xeno-free culture system for the preparation and propagation of cell therapy-compliant human adipose stem cells." *Stem Cell Research & Therapy* 4 (2): 1–15.

Peck, Y., L. T. Leom, P. F. P. Low, and D. Wang. 2018. "Establishment of an in vitro threedimensional model for cartilage damage in rheumatoid arthritis." *Journal of Tissue Engineering and Regenerative Medicine* 12 (1): e237–e249.

Pedrero, S. G., P. Llamas-Sillero, and J. Serrano-López. 2021. "A multidisciplinary journey towards bone tissue engineering." *Materials* 14 (17): 4896–4925.

Qasim, M., D. S. Chae, and N. Y. Lee. 2020. "Bioengineering strategies for bone and cartilage tissue regeneration using growth factors and stem cells." *Journal of Biomedical Materials Research Part A* 108 (3): 394–411.

Ralphe, J. C., and W. J. de Lange. 2013. "3D engineered cardiac tissue models of human heart disease: learning more from our mice." *Trends in Cardiovascular Medicine* 23 (2): 27–32.

Reverdin, E. A. 1909. "Other methods of skin-grafting." *Historical Boston Medical and Surgical Journal* 161: 911–917.

Sallent, I, H. Capella-Monsonís, P. Procter, I. Y. Bozo, R. V. Deev, D. Zubov, R. Vasyliev, G. Perale, G. Pertici, and J. Baker. 2020. "The few who made it: Commercially and clinically successful innovative bone grafts." *Frontiers in Bioengineering and Biotechnology* 8: 952.

Sánchez, A., T. Schimmang, and J. García-Sancho. 2012. "Cell and tissue therapy in regenerative medicine." In *Stem Cell Transplantation*, edited by Carlos Lopez-Larrea, Antonio Lopez-Vazquez, and Beatriz Suarez-Alvarez. Springer, New York, 89–102.

Schallmoser, K., and D. Strunk. 2009. "Preparation of pooled human platelet lysate (pHPL) as an efficient supplement for animal serum-free human stem cell cultures." *JoVE (Journal of Visualized Experiments)* 32: e1523.

Sikavitsas, V. I., G. N. Bancroft, and A. G. Mikos. 2002. "Formation of three-dimensional cell/polymer constructs for bone tissue engineering in a spinner flask and a rotating wall vessel bioreactor." *Journal of Biomedical Materials Research* 62 (1): 136–48. DOI: 10.1002/jbm.10150

Sittinger, M., D. Reitzel, M. Dauner, H. Hierlemann, C. Hammer, E. Kastenbauer, H. Planck, G. R. Burmester, and J. Bujia. 1996. "Resorbable polyesters in cartilage engineering: Affinity and biocompatibility of polymer fiber structures to chondrocytes." *Journal of Biomedical Materials Research: An Official Journal of the Society for Biomaterials and the Japanese Society for Biomaterials* 33 (2): 57–63.

Skalak, R., and C. Fox. 1988. *NSF Workshop, UCLA Symposia on Molecular and Cellular Biology.* New York: Alan R Liss.

Sorta-Bilajac, I., and A. Muzur. 2007. "The nose between ethics and aesthetics: Sushruta's legacy." *Otolaryngology—Head and Neck Surgery* 137 (5): 707–710.

Stock, U. A., and J. P. Vacanti. 2001. "Tissue engineering: Current state." *Annual Review of Medicine* 52: 443–51.

Stoop, R. 2008. "Smart biomaterials for tissue engineering of cartilage." *Injury* 39 (1): 77–87.

Tew, S., S. Redman, A. Kwan, E. Walker, I. Khan, G. Dowthwaite, B. Thomson, and C. W. Archer. 2001. "Differences in repair responses between immature and mature cartilage." *Clinical Orthopaedics and Related Research (1976–2007)* 391: S142–S152.

Vacanti, C. A. 2006. "History of tissue engineering and a glimpse into its future." *Tissue Engineering* 12 (5): 1137–1142.

Walenda, G., H. Hemeda, R. K. Schneider, R. Merkel, B. Hoffmann, and W. Wagner. 2012. "Human platelet lysate gel provides a novel three dimensional-matrix for enhanced culture expansion of mesenchymal stromal cells." *Tissue Engineering Part C: Methods* 18 (12): 924–934.

3 Biomaterials for Repairing Bone, Cartilage, and Associated Joint Tissue Defects

INTRODUCTION

Bone and cartilage tissue engineering is the promising tool that can be used for the purpose of the bone and cartilage-related tissue regeneration, in which biomaterials play a prime role. Biomaterial is used for making scaffold which builds the backbone for the cell and ultimately tissue structure, and provides necessary cues for cellular growth and tissue regeneration. The success of tissue regeneration depends largely on the host response to the implanted scaffold biomaterial components that guides the reconstruction process of the damaged bone and cartilage tissue. Therefore, scaffolding biomaterial is a crucial element in tissue engineering, which not only acts as a carrier for cells and other bioactive molecules like growth factors but also provides the necessary mechanical support to the hosted cells, and regenerated tissue (Wei, Liu et al. 2021). Therefore, the selection of biomaterials with ECM mimicking properties for developing scaffolds is one of the prime factors and also it is a great challenge to achieve for the bone and cartilage tissue engineering.

Keeping this in view, a large number of diverse biomaterials have been explored, researched, and developed with appropriate properties for their use in the purpose of regenerating tissues, thereby repairing of the damaged bone and cartilage.

The biomaterials include natural and synthetic biopolymers, polymer–polymer blends, hydrogels, polymer-ceramic composites, etc. This chapter provides an overview of the ideal biopolymers and advances in the development of biomaterials with biomimicking properties such as polymer blends and polymer composites including the nanocomposite biomaterials for bone, cartilage, and joint defect. The chapter also reviews the recent advances in the methods of processing biomaterials to enhance &/or modify their properties including biochemical, physico-chemical and others, thereby increasing their potentiality to mimic the native extracellular matrix (ECM) tissues and to support the targeted tissue regeneration while demonstrating superior functional performance.

BIOMATERIAL AND ITS HISTORY

Biomaterial can be defined as a substance or material of synthetic or natural origin which can interact with biological systems to support in repairing or regenerating damaged tissue or enhance biological function of a tissue or organ partially or

DOI: 10.1201/9781003245353-3

completely. Thus, biomaterial can play a vital role in medicine in restoring function and healing of the injured or diseased people and other applications in biotechnology field. The biomaterial what is known in the 21st century was used in medicine far back, the date of which is immemorial. However, biomaterials as sutures derived from animal sinew have been used by ancient Egyptians for closing large wounds thousands of years ago, when there was no knowledge of biocompatibility, biodegradability, sterility, etc., which are essential properties of today's biomaterial (Scott 1983).

In the 20th century, the use of biomaterial has become important in many fields including medicine, biology, material science, physics, and chemistry. The field has grown tremendously in the 21st century due to emergence of the tissue engineering and regenerative medicine.

BIOMATERIAL CLASSIFICATION

Biomaterials used for scaffold development are classified based on the following three different generations.

THE FIRST GENERATION OF BIOMATERIALS

The first-generation biomaterials used in biomedical applications were introduced in the 1960s. The main focus at that time was to achieve appropriate biomaterial property that can enhance the performance of the transplanted biomaterial in replacing damaged or diseased tissue with a minimal immunogenic reaction to the host. These biomaterials are mostly biologically inert and can reduce corrosion, release of ions and particles after implantation, thereby minimizing the undesirable immune response and foreign body reaction as well as interact minutely with the surrounding tissues. The examples of these biomaterials are (i) metals like stainless steel and cobalt–chrome-based alloys, (ii) titanium (Ti) and Ti-based alloys, (iii) ceramics like alumina or aluminium oxide (Al_2O_3) and zirconium oxide or zirconia (ZrO2), and (iv) synthetic polymers like silicone rubber, acrylic resins like poly(methyl methaacrylate) (PMMA) and polyetheretherketone (PEEK).

THE SECOND GENERATION OF BIOMATERIALS

The second-generation biomaterials used are bioactive in nature. This class of biomaterials has the ability to interact with the biological systems, thereby enhancing the biological or tissue response through the necessary tissue-surface bonding, and is also biodegradable, thereby facilitating tissue regeneration and healing. Some examples of this class of biomaterials are (i) metals—these are of two types: the first type of metals that are coated with a bioactive ceramic material which makes them bioactive and the second type of metals, the surfaces of which are modified chemically to stimulate protein adsorption or cell adhesion and other tissue–biomaterial interactions, thereby promoting tissue healing; (ii) ceramic materials—these are bioactive glass also known as bioglass, glass-ceramics, calcium sulphate, and calcium phosphates; and (iii) polymers—these are basically biodegradable synthetic polymers e.g. poly(glycolic acid) or polyglycolide (PGA) and polylactic acid or polylactide (PLA) and natural polymers (e.g. collagen).

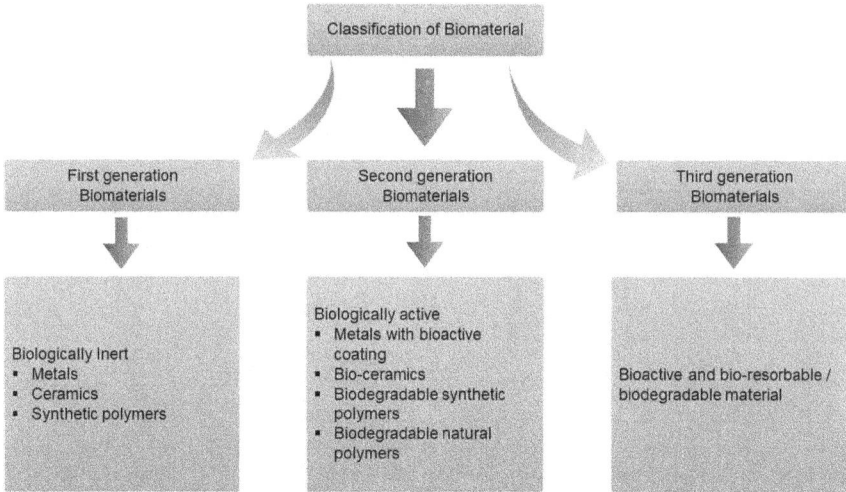

FIGURE 3.1 Classification of biomaterials.

THE THIRD GENERATION OF BIOMATERIALS

These biomaterials are derived from the second-generation biomaterials. These biomaterials are bioactive and biodegradable, and are usually designed as three-dimensional (3D) porous structures with excellent properties, thereby making them capable of stimulating regeneration of living tissue by gene activation. The combining effect of bioactivity and biodegradability in a single platform is the concept of these category of biomaterials. The metals that are used for the development of porous structures were concentrated on Ti and Ti alloys. The biomaterials usually used for tissue engineering application are based on the second and third generations. Figure 3.1 protrays the classification of the biomaterials.

SIMPLE BIOMATERIALS

For the development of scaffold, for tissue engineering applications, the primary interest has been in the use of polymeric materials because they can be easily moulded into different forms like porous, hydrogels, and fibres. Many polymers of natural and synthetic origin have been investigated for bone and cartilage tissue regeneration, which are described in the proceeding section.

NATURAL BIOPOLYMERS

These biomaterials are biocompatible, biodegradable, and have the resemblance with ECM. However, most of these natural polymers possess low mechanical strength. Their physical characteristics can vary from one source to another. Natural polymers have more biological association with cells because of their bioactive features, allowing them to function better in biological systems (Aslan, Şimşek, and Dayi 2006). Potential natural polymers and their characteristics are given in Table 3.1 and are described next.

TABLE 3.1
The List of Potential Natural Polymers and Their Important Characteristics

Name of Natural Bio-polymers	Advantages	Limitations	References
Sodium Alginate	Biocompatible Low cost biodegradable Similarity to GAGs structure Water-soluble Abundant Can be used as gene carriers Low immunogenicity Instant gel forming ability and hence suitable for 3D printing	Low cellular interaction and adhesiveness Low mechanical strength low protein adsorption and cell adhesion	(Tsukuda, Onodera et al. 2015, Choi, Kim et al. 2018, Leslie, Cohen et al. 2018, Bozkurt, Aşık et al. 2019, Khatab, Leijs et al. 2020, Han, Xu et al. 2021), (Chawla, Kaur et al. 2020) Rowley et al. 1999
Chitosan	Resemblance to the structure of GAGs Cheap Biodegradable, Biocompatible Nonantigenicity Adsorption capacity Antimicrobial activity stimulates chondrogenesis hydrophilic	Potential threats from allergens High viscosity and Low solubility in water Low cell-matrix interaction low mechanical strength	(Hunziker 2002, Hoemann, Sun et al. 2005, Chen, Xia et al. 2016, Keller, Regiel-Futyra et al. 2017, Giuliani 2019, Sultankulov, Berillo et al. 2019, Naghizadeh, Karkhaneh et al. 2021) (Soundarya, Menon et al. 2018) (Islam, Rahman et al. 2020)
Gelatin	Encourage cell adhesion Easily adaptable to UV crosslinking Injectable for 3D bioprinting Biocompatible Biodegradable Highly water soluble Cell adhesion	Undesirable mechanical characteristics Unimpressive thermal stability Rapid degradation	(Larsen, Artym et al. 2006, Wang, Du et al. 2014, Han, Xu et al. 2017, Li, Truong et al. 2017, Zhou, Hong et al. 2018, Zhu, Cui et al. 2018, Echave, Hernaez-Moya et al. 2019, Hou, Liu et al. 2020) (Mazaki, Shiozaki et al. 2014)

Material	Advantages	Disadvantages	References
Agarose	Water soluble; Gentle (mild) gelation; Promote ECM secretion ability; High water absorbance capacity	Mechanically weak; Lack of cell adhesion sites; Nondegradability	(Zignego, Jutila et al. 2014, Yin, Stilwell et al. 2015, Zarrintaj, Manouchehri et al. 2018, Salati, Khazai et al. 2020)
Cellulose	Low cost; water soluble; Biodegradable; Biocompatible; Robust mechanical attributes; Non-toxic, Cheap; Natural, Widely available	Lack of mechanical properties	(Isobe, Komamiya et al., O'Sullivan 1997, Hubbe, Tayeb et al. 2017, Tayeb, Amini et al. 2018, Wang, Yuan et al. 2018, Dutta, Patel et al. 2019)
Hyaluronic Acid	Constituent of native cartilage tissue; Encourages the expression of chondrocytes' cartilage marker genes	Low cell adhesion ability; Excessive degradation; Poor mechanical attributes	(Collins and Birkinshaw, Knudson, Casey et al. 2000, Tognana, Padera et al. 2005, Gupta, Lall et al. 2019, Li, Yu et al. 2019, Zheng, Yang et al. 2019)
Fibrin	Tunable reactive species, Stimulates MSC chondrogenesis cell-binding ability, high tensile strength,	Not chondro-permissive; Need to design, develop, and purify peptides properly	(Kuznetsov, Hailu-Lazmi et al. 2019, Yang, Liu et al. 2020)
Fibrin Glue	The elements of the ECM cause fibrin to degrade on their own and into non-toxic terminal components.	Weak mechanical strength limited biodegradability regulation. Its use in humans is restricted to sealing off the periosteal flap in ACI technique.	(Peterson, Brittberg et al. 2002, Fussenegger, Meinhart et al. 2003, Vinatier, Gauthier et al. 2009)
Platelet-rich fibrin	Increased growth factors; Excellent handling and storage characteristics; Low costs; Simple preparation	Weak mechanical features features	(Miron, Fujioka-Kobayashi et al. 2017, Wong, Chen et al. 2017, Wu, Sheu et al. 2017, Barbon, Stocco et al. 2019)

(continued)

TABLE 3.1 (Continued)
The List of Potential Natural Polymers and Their Important Characteristics

Name of Natural Bio-polymers	Advantages	Limitations	References
Collagen	Natural ECM component Immunomodulation Good cell-matrix interaction Biocompatible Low immunogenicity Biodegradable Facilitates cell ingrowth and remodeling Enhanced chondrogenesis & simple processing	Low mechanical properties Rapid degradation High cost Limited number of functional groups for crosslinking Immunoreactivity linked to non-human animals and its bovine origins	(Lee, Singla et al. 2001, Lubiatowski, Kruczynski et al. 2006, Kuroda, Ishida et al. 2007, Türk, Altunsoy et al. 2018, Li, Yu et al. 2019, Marques, Diogo et al. 2019) (Elango, Zhang et al. 2016)
Silk fibroin	Replicates collagen structure of original cartilage sterilizability Excellent mechanical properties Biocompatible Regulated degradation Reduced risk of infection Simple processing Low cost	limited growth factor binding Weak β-sheet crystal biodegradation Low osteogenic potential	(Zhang, Yang et al. 2010, Wang, Hu et al. 2011, Sawatjui, Damrongrungruang et al. 2015, Singh, Bhardwaj et al. 2016, Ratanavaraporn, Soontornvipart et al. 2017, Ma, Wang et al. 2018, Ribeiro, Morais et al. 2018, Zhou, Liang et al. 2018, Bharadwaz and Jayasuriya 2020) (Lee, Tripathy et al. 2017)
Sericin	Nutrition-supplying Low cost	Lack of stability in aqueous solution	(Liu, Qi et al. 2016, Ratanavaraporn, Soontornvipart et al. 2017, Qi, Liu et al. 2018)
Chondroitin sulfate	Nutrition-supplying Control hypertrophy MSC chondrogenesis promotes cartilage ECM production	Rapid degradation	(Wang, Varghese et al. 2007, Chang, Hung et al. 2010, Yu, Cao et al. 2013, Zhou, Zhang et al. 2017, Aisenbrey and Bryant 2019)

Collagen

Collagen is a triple-helix natural protein with a 3D structure and it is the principal constituent of connective tissues, such as bone, tendon, cartilage, skin ligament, etc. Collagen provides structural support to the body. Being a protein, it presents excellent bio- or tissue compatibility, non-toxicity, favourable biodegradation, bioresorbability, and easy availability (Liu et al. 2008), Parenteau-Bareil et al. 2010; Ishida et al. 2007; Elango, Zhang et al. 2016). These properties make collagen an excellent biomaterial for wide use in biomedical field including tissue engineering. Collagen is deteriorated naturally by bacterial collagenase enzymes and serines proteases, and the degradation is usually restricted by the cells present in the tissue (Drury and Mooney 2003). Collagen gel has widely been used as substrates for *articular cartilage and subchondral bone regeneration (*Mueller-Rath et al., 2010; Kon et al., 2011).

Gelatin

Gelatin is a high molecular weight polymer of natural origin. Gelatin comprises of 85–92% of single-stranded protein and has abundant arginine–glycine–aspartate (Arg-Gly-Asp) (RGD) sequences which can enhance integrin-mediated cell adhesion. It is derived from the acid or alkaline hydrolysis of collagen present in bones, tendons, ligament and skin (Echave et al. 2017). It is a low-cost, is biodegradable, bioresorbable, hydrophilic, and biocompatible polymer (Catoira et al. 2019; Echave, Hernaez-Moya et al. 2019; Zhu, Cui et al. 2018; Zhou, Hong et al. 2018) and has the gelling and binding ability thereby promoting cell adhesion, cell proliferation, and differentiation, It also possesses chemically modifiable functional groups and lower antigenicity when compared to parent protein. These unique properties make gelatin a potential material for a wide range of tissue engineering and other biomedical applications. It possesses chemically modifiable functional groups and lower antigenicity when compared to parent protein. However, the low mechanical strength is the major disadvantage of this polymer. Gelatin has been prominently used in tissue engineering field as it is a derivative of collagen, a prominent ECM molecule of cartilage having adhesion sites to chondrocytes (Bello et al. 2020).

Fibrin and Fibrin Glue

Fibrin, a fibrous protein, is a natural biopolymer and is produced by the interaction between fibrinogen and thrombin proteins which are related to blood clotting (Sims et al. 1998). It is also a component of natural ECM. Fibrin finds its wide application in tissue engineering due to its excellent properties like biocompatibility, cell-binding ability, high tensile strength, fast degradability, and easy fabrication. However, poor mechanical properties and unsteady degradation rate are the main drawbacks which limit its application in tissue engineering (Hunziker 2002). Fibrin has been reported to promote the articular cartilage repair. Furthermore, the usage of fibrin glue and chondrocytes is reported to improving cartilage repair *in vivo* (Van Susante et al. 1999; Peretti et al. 2000; Fussenegger et al. 2003). In horses, fibrin glue comprising chondrocytes or MSC aided in the development of new cartilaginous tissue with high type II collagen and proteoglycan contents (Hendrickson et al. 1994; Wilke et al. 2007). Like fibrin, the weak mechanical stability is the main disadvantage that restricts the use of fibrin glue. Fibrin is also an attractive polymer for bone tissue regeneration because of its excellent tissue-compatibility, controllable biodegradability, and ability to provide necessary biochemical cues to the cells (Noori et al. 2017).

Agarose

Agarose is a polysaccharide-based natural polymer having repetitive unit of agarobiose, a disachharide that contains alternating β-D-galactose and 3,6-anhydro-L-galactose units of agarobiose. Agarose is usually extracted from marine algae. This linear polymer can form flexible fibres and web of channels, the diameter of which is at nanometre range. It is non-toxic and acts as a gelling agent, which increases its potentiality for many applications such as in electrophoresis, immunodiffusion techniques, gel plates for cells in tissue culture, chromatographic techniques, etc. The properties of agarose hydrogels can be tuned by blending with other biopolymers. Its structural similarity to ECM, non-immunological feature and high water absorbance capacity promote cell adhesion, cell growth, proliferation and differentiation (Zarrintaj et al. 2018). Agarose, and its derivatives have been widely used in tissue engineering including cartilage and bone regeneration (Roach et al. 2016; Lopez-Heredia et al. 2017). It was used as a scaffolding biomaterial for the *in vitro* 3D culture of chondrocytes. It also supported the differentiation of stem cells into chondrogenic tissue (Awad et al. 2004). However, its slow degradation makes its ability limited in the *in vivo* study.

Sodium Alginate (SA)

Like agarose, SA is also a linear natural polysaccharide. It is basically extracted from brown seaweed or soil bacteria. Alginate is soluble in water and has diverse applications including in food industry as a thickener, drug delivery, wound healing, tissue engineering, and others due to its many advantageous properties like similarity with the extracellular matrix, low cost, non-toxicity, hydrophilicity, biodegradability, and biocompatibility under the usual physiological conditions (Sowjanya et al. 2013, Tsukuda, Onodera et al. 2015; Choi, Kim et al. 2018; Leslie, Cohen et al. 2018; Bozkurt, Aşık et al. 2019; Khatab, Leijs et al. 2020)). Its properties like mechanical, gelation, biodegradability and cell supportive properties can easily be tuned by modification. It can easily form insoluble hydrogel when cross-linked with bivalent cations like Ca^{2+} ions and thus can provide structural support to the cells in *in vivo* and *in vitro* conditions, thereby making it a suitable biomaterial in tissue engineering field (Sun and Tan 2013). Besides hydrogel, alginate can also be transformed into other forms like sponges, fibers, microspheres or microcapsules, foams etc.But the main disadvantage of this polymer is its inferior biomechanical properties and also low protein adsorption and cell adhesion due to its hydrophilic nature (Rowley et al. 1999). Besides hydrogel, alginate can also be transformed into other forms like sponges, fibers, microspheres or microcapsules, foams etc. But the main disadvantage of this polymer is its inferior biomechanical properties and also low protein abdsorption and cell adhesion due to its hydrophilic nature (Rowley et al. 1999).

Hyaluronic Acid (HA)

HA, a non-sulphated Glycosaminoglycans (GAG) component of the cartilaginous ECM, is composed of N-acetylglucosamine and glucuronic acid that are linked together through alternating β-1,4 and β-1,3 glycosidic bonds (Necas et al. 2008). HA plays an essential and important role in cell adhesion, proliferation, migration, differentiation, wound repair, and tissue morphogenesis. It is natively found in adult articular cartilage and involves in cartilage synthesis (Kim, Mauck, and Burdick 2011). A high concentration of this polysaccharide is found in musculoskeletal and dermal tissue matrices (Aslan et al. 2006). HA exhibits various physiological functions including joint lubrication, regulation of vascular permeability, and promotion of defective tissue repair. HA is also known as a natural moisturizing agent because of its water retention capacity that makes its application suitable in cartilage tissue engineering. It is degraded naturally by hyaluronidase enzyme (Drury and Mooney 2003) and the degraded products induce chondrolysis in local area (Knudson et al. 2000). HA can also induce differentiation of MSCs into chondrocytes, thereby maintaining chondrocyte phenotype, and enhances ECM synthesis in cartilage (Bang, Jung, and Noh 2018). HA-based hydrogel has been studied mostly for cartilage tissue engineering (Kim et al. 2011). However, HA shows unsatisfactory cell adhesion ability in *in vivo* study because of its degradation by reactive oxygen, nitrogen, and hyaluronidase and also induces inflammation due to foreign objects (Zhu et al. 2017). It has also been reported that HA enhances formation through increase in mesenchymal stem cell differentiation to osteoblast and hence can be used in bone tissue regeneration (Hanna et al. 2018)..

Chitosan

Chitosan, a natural, semi-crystalline linear polymer, is derived by partial deacetylation of chitin procured mainly from the exoskeleton of crustaceans; crab shells and shrimps being the primary sources. It is comprised of linear polysaccharide of D-glucosamine residues linked by β (1→4) linkage with randomly arranged N-acetyl-glucosamine groups. Similar to native cartilage, this polymer has structural similarity with the proteoglycan components such as GAG and HA of cartilage ECM that interacts with collagen fibres playing an important role in cell–cell adhesion, thereby making it a preferred biomaterial for cartilage tissue engineering. Chitosan is non-toxic, biodegradable, and biocompatible and it has anti-microbial properties that can prevent bacterial infection at the defect site which is very useful in tissue engineering enabling CH as an antibiotic carrier (Hoemann, Sun et al. 2005; Chen, Xia et al. 2016; Keller, Regiel-Futyra et al. 2017).. This polymer can be easily blended with other polymers to form hydrogels and easily modifiable in various forms such as porous sponge, film, microcapsule, beads, fibers and other complex structures. It has the capability to provide necessary microenvironment for cartilage tissue regeneration. Furthermore, it can inspire cell proliferation and also promote tissue regeneration. Chitosan has the ability to entrap or chemically conjugate growth factors through the amine and hydroxyl groups present in it. It has shown to enhance wound healing through the activation and modulation of the role of inflammatory cells like fibroblasts, endothelial cells, etc., and by boosting the formation and organization of granulation tissue (Levengood and Zhang 2014). The poor mechanical strength of pure chitosan limits its application in bone tissue engineering. However, its combination with other polymers and ceramic materials resulting composite biomaterials can promote adhesion and proliferation of osteoblast-related cells, and thus serve as potential substrates for bone-tissue regeneration (Fourie et al. 2022).

Cellulose

Cellulose is the low cost and most widely spread polysaccharide natural biopolymer in the earth consisting of anhydro-D-glucopyranose units. It is derived from plants and some bacteria. It is unresolvable in many solvents like water and other solvents due to its robust intramolecular and intermolecular hydrogen bonding among individual chains. To increase its solubility, cellulose is modified by esterification and etherification at the hydroxyl groups (Kamel et al. 2008). It has excellent biocompatible and biodegradable characteristics which enable it for use in biomedical applications. However, its poor mechanical strength and rapid degradation limited its solo use in medical field (Ao et al. 2017). Cellulose is degraded by cellulase enzymes (Müller et al. 2006). So, composites of cellulose with other biomaterials have been used for bone tissue engineering. Electrospun nanofibrous scaffold of cellulose and hydroxyapatite enhanced the mechanical strength, thermal stability, and cell proliferating activity of scaffold for bone tissue growth (Ao et al. 2017); Isobe, Komamiya et al., O'Sullivan 1997; Hubbe, Tayeb et al. 2017; Tayeb, Amini et al. 2018. Cellulose derived from bacteria is crystalline, fibrous, non-toxic, and biodegradable and possesses significant mechanical properties. In spite of these properties bacterial cellulose is mostly used in artificial blood vessel, artificial skin, wound dressings, and specialty membranes. The composites based on bacterial cellulose are cellulose/collagen, cellulose/agarose, cellulose/poly(3-hydroxybutyrate), cellulose/chitosan, and cellulose /hydroxyapatite which have been used for tissue engineering (Torgbo and Sukyai 2018). Cellulose polymer promoted chondrocytes and exhibited good biocompatibility *in vitro* (Müller et al. 2006). Injectable hydroxypropylmethylcellulose hydrogel was able to promote articular cartilage repair (Vinatier, Gauthier, Fatimi et al. 2009). However, only a few *in vivo* studies have been reported so far for its tissue engineering application.

Silk Fibroin (SF)

SF is a natural biopolymer obtained from silkworm cocoon by degumming method. The common variety of silks are mulberry silk produced by *Bombyx mori* silkworm and non-mulberry silks produced by *Antheraea mylitta* and *Antheraea pernyi* silkworms belonging to the Saturniidae family. SF is biocompatible, biodegradable, soluble in aqueous or organic solvent, easily processable to make different forms of structures like film, fibre, and porous, and has excellent mechanical strength, which make it a potential biopolymer for various tissue engineering applications (Zhang, Yang et al. 2010; Wang, Hu et al. 2011; Ma, Wang et al. 2018; Ribeiro, Morais et al. 2018; Zhou, Liang et al. 2018; Bharadwaz and Jayasuriya

2020; Lee, Tripathy et al. 2017). The inherent tripeptide arginine–glycine–aspartate (RGD) sequence present in non-mulberry silk provides recognition site for integrin serving as the cell surface receptor, thereby promoting cell attachment, cell proliferation, and differentiation (Acharya, Ghosh, and Kundu 2009). SF is considered for biomedical applications as it contains a repetitive glycine–alanine–serine sequence, which forms anti-parallel β-sheet structure. This secondary structure is cross-linked through strong inter- and intra-molecular hydrogen bonds, which provide elasticity and mechanical strength to SF, making it an adequate choice for cartilage tissue engineering applications (Kundu et al. 2013).

In 1959, the property of silk for use as a suture in surgery was reported (Goldenberg 1959), whereas the suitability of extracted silk proteins with mammalian fibroblast cells was first reported over sericin to use as a matrix material. Besides the presence of RGD sequences, electrostatic interactions between cells and substrate promote cell attachment (Kundu et al. 2013) and ease of processing into various forms that led to extensive research on silk fibroin for tissue engineering application. It has also been widely investigated as the most promising biomaterial for BTE application because of its tunable mechanical properties, controllable biodegradability, and biocompatibility (Li et al. 2023).

Carboxymethyl Cellulose (CMC)

CMC is a hydrophilic biocompatible polymer derived from chemical modification of cellulose. Carboxymethyl groups bind to the hydroxyl groups of glucopyranose of cellulose to form CMC. It is a carboxymethyl derivative of cellulose. CMC is mostly used in drug delivery and wound dressing application. It has antimicrobial property. It is mostly used in wound dressing as it is capable of absorbing exudate as well as promoting angiogenesis and autolytic debridement (Kanikireddy et al. 2020). CMC is usually combined with other polymers and ceramic materials for tissue engineering applications. CMC and polyvinyl alcohol blend was used for cartilage tissue engineering. Incorporation of CMC into this polymer modifies the scaffold architecture with swelling ability in positive manner (Namkaew, Sawaddee, and Yodmuang 2019). Its biocompatibility, negligible inflammatory reactions, chelating ability, eliciting homogeneous Ca/P crystal nucleation which is a vital osteogenic property make it an attractive scaffolding biomaterial for bone regeneration. CMC/hydroxyapatite composite has been used in bone tissue engineering (Pasqui et al. 2014; Singh et al. 2016)

Glucosamine Sulphate (GS)

GS, an amino-monosaccharide, is a natural sugar usually present in cartilage tissue. It is a key component of GAG disaccharide units, which create functional proteoglycans found in cartilage matrix (Dodge and Jimenez 2003; Derfoul et al. 2007), and also serves as a cushion in joints. It is also a major component of drugs used for the treatment of OA. Oral intake of GS relieves OA pain and effectively stops joint space loss, therefore altering disease development (Pavelka et al. 2002; Chan, Ng et al. 2011).

The use of GS in clinical therapeutics was first reported in 1980, when its oral administration reduced the symptoms of disease by twofolds and helped in rebuilding the damaged cartilage. Besides symptomatic relief, it provides structural modifications of the cartilage defect areas (Theodosakis, Adderly, and Fox 1997), which has made GS to be applied as a therapeutic agent (nutraceutical) for osteoarthritis treatment. At physiological pH, it remains in non-ionized form of which 90% is absorbed by the body upon oral administration. The orally administered GS takes 4 hours to reach cartilage tissue, whereas only 8–12% is retained by cartilage tissue. A pharmacokinetics study in dogs showed that the concentration of drug reaching cartilage tissue is five times lower in oral administration than that administered by intramuscular or intravenous injection, which may be due to the first-pass effect by the liver that metabolizes the majority of ingested GS to water, CO_2, and urea (Deal and Moskowitz 1999).

When glucosamine sulphate used for the long-term treatment, a delayed disease progression was seen in human knee OA patients, demonstrating the possibility of its role in disease modification (Gatterová et al. 2002). It is also capable of stimulating proteoglycan synthesis as well as modulating aggrecan (Acan) levels, resulting in decreased degradation of proteoglycans that makes GS a potential candidate for cartilage damage treatments (Dodge and Jimenez 2003). It is reported that 10–20% of the orally administered drug reaches articular cartilage; however, when an emulsion was applied locally, the transdermal delivery was about 20% to the joints in human patients (Hammad, Magid, and Sobhy 2015) signifying the important role of the administration method in determining the availability and action of the drug.

Chondroitin Sulphate (CS)

CS is a polysaccharide comprising disaccharide units of D-glucuronic acid and sulphated N-acetylgalactosamine. It is the most abundant GAG component accounting for about 80% of GAG components in adult articular cartilage (Kuiper and Sharma 2015; Alinejad et al. 2018). It has anti-inflammatory activity, ability to control the metabolism of cartilage tissue by synthesizing proteoglycans and inhibiting proteolytic enzymes (Deal and Moskowitz 1999; Muzzarelli, Boudrant et al. 2012) and exhibits an anti-inflammatory response (Wang et al. 2007). CS is usually dispensed orally or by injecting intramuscularly. It is present in Acan molecules that bind to hyaluronan and link proteins to form huge aggregates and provides compressive strength to the tissue (Poole et al. 2002). Depending on the location of sulphate group, usually, two types of CS are found in articular cartilage. Chondroitin 6-sulphate is mostly found in high amount in adults and serves to maintain the integrity of the tissue, whereas chondroitin 4-sulphate content is rich in infant cartilage and plays a crucial role in calcification process (Yokoyama, Somervaille et al. 2005). Because of ageing or degeneration, the amount of CS within cartilage drops (Collin et al. 2017).

SYNTHETIC POLYMERS

Synthetic polymeric materials have the advantages of being modified easily, and therefore their microstructure and degradation are improved. Synthetic polymers have favourable mechanical properties including the stiffness, porosity, and elasticity.

However, the major disadvantages of most of these polymers are their cytotoxicity effects (Lanao et al. 2013; Gentile et al. 2014; Stevens et al. 2015), cost and weak cell supportive property. The list of potential synthetic polymers and their characteristics are given in Table 3.2. and are described next.

TABLE 3.2
The List of Potential Synthetic Polymers and Their Characteristics

Name of Synthetic Polymers	Advantages	Limitations	References
Poly Lactic-co-Glycolic Acid (PLGA)	Good biocompatibility Ease of functionalization Biodegradable	Low bioactivity Expensive, inadequate cell adhesion.	(Morille, Toupet et al. 2016, Wang, Yang et al. 2016, Gui, Li et al. 2017, Sun, Zhang et al. 2018, Zhang, Shi et al. 2018)
Polycaprolactone (PCL)	Biodegradability Good processing ability and compatibility Mechanical stability. Can support chondrocyte proliferation while maintaining phenotype. possesses high drug permeability and slow rate of degradation	Low bioactivity Hydrophobicity Acidic degradation of products and low hydrophilicity may lead to inflammation	(Aydin, Korkusuz et al. 2015, Du, Liu et al. 2017, Filová, Tonar et al. 2020, Lam, Reuveny et al. 2020)
Polylactic acid (PLA)	Biocompatibility biodegradability Low immunogenicity High mechanical strength	Acidic degradation Low bioactivity	(Liu, Chen et al. 2018, Li, Liu et al. 2020, Zeng, Li et al. 2021)
Poly (glycolic acid) (PGA)	High tensile strength and Young's modulus	cytotoxic and partially boosts immune responses.	(Mozumder, Mairpady et al. 2017, Samantaray, Little et al. 2020)

(*continued*)

TABLE 3.2 (Continued)
The List of Potential Synthetic Polymers and Their Characteristics

Name of Synthetic Polymers	Advantages	Limitations	References
Polyethylene glycol (PEG)	Biocompatible Easy to be functionalized Biologically inert Non-immunogenicity good biocompatibility. Low toxicity Excellent hydrophilicity and inorganic solvent solubility Anti-fouling characteristics.	Non-biodegradable	(Gaharwar, Dammu et al. 2011, Skaalure, Dimson et al. 2014, Skaalure, Chu et al. 2015, Sridhar, Brock et al. 2015, Mehrali, Thakur et al. 2017, Armiento, Stoddart et al. 2018)
Poly (N-vinylcaprolactam) (PVCL)	Thermosensitive Cytocompatible to chondrocytes	Weak anti-biofouling, poor mechanical characteristics, modest wettability	(Sala, Kwon et al., Yang, Wang et al. 2015)
Polyvinyl alcohol (PVA)	Mechanically strong Promotes MSCs for chondrogenic differentiation	Biologically inert	(Dashtdar, Murali et al. 2015, Qi, Hu et al. 2015, Li, Gao et al. 2018, Oliveira, Seidi et al. 2019)
Poly(N-isopropylacrylamide) (PNIPAM)	thermo-responsive due to its clearly defined structure and characteristics, particularly its temperature response, is near to that of the human body and is also adjustable.	Low biodegradability, its monomer and cross-linker may have poisonous, teratogenic, and carcinogenic consequences.	(Haq, Su et al. 2017)
Polyurethane (PU)	Remarkable mechanical characteristics	Lacks in biological activity	(Wendels and Avérous 2021)

Polylactic Acid

Lactic acid is the unit of PLA and it is converted to PLA by three polymerization processes, such as, polycondensation, azeotopic dehydration condensation, and ring-opening polymerization (ROP). It is a semi-crystalline polymer with glass transition and melting temperatures of 55°C and 180°C, respectively. It has good mechanical strength (stiffness) but poor toughness which limits its use in requiring plastic deformation (Liu, Chen et al. 2018; Li, Liu et al. 2020; Zeng, Li et al. 2021). PLA is commonly used in food packaging, drug delivery, wound healing and orthopaedic devices. This synthetic polymer is also used to produce biodegradable screws, pins, plates and suture anchors. Pins and screw of PLA are gaining more interest in clinical use where high mechanical strength is not required (Hamad, Kaseem, and Deri 2012). PLA composites with many polymers like PCL (Guarino et al. 2008), chitosan (Jiang et al. 2006), and cellulose were used for bone tissue engineering because of its biocompatibility, biodegradability, nontoxicity, and high mechanical strength (Patil et al. 2020). Similarly, several composites based on PLA polymer were used for cartilage tissue engineering, *for example* PLA/PGA composite (Moran et al. 2003). The major disadvantage of this polymer is its high cost and inadequate cell adhesive ability.

Poly (Lactic-co-Glycolic Acid) (PLGA)

PLGA, a synthetic aliphatic polyester is a biodegradable and biocompatible polymer. PLGAs with low (below 10 kDa) and high molecular weight are synthesized. The former is synthesized by the ring-opening co-polymerization resction between lactic and glycolic acid, whereas high molecular weight PLGA is synthesized following the same process but using some catalysts like 2-ethylhexanoate, tin (II) alkoxides, and aluminium isopropoxide. Here the monomers, glycolic acid and lactic acid, bind together through ester linkages, thereby forming PLGA with a linear and an amorphous structure. Its degradation is a heterogeneous erosion in body fluid environment (Lanao et al. 2013). Like its monomer, PLGA has a poor solubility. PLGA was widely used in bone tissue engineering in different forms including hydrogels (PLGA/polyethyl glycol PEG), films, microspheres (PLGA/hydroxyapatite) and porous scaffolds (PLGA/hydroxyapatite). The nanofibrous structure of PLGA is shown to be similar to ECM which can stimulate bone tissue growth (Gentile et al. 2014).

Poly-L-Lactic Acid (PLLA)

PLLA is a FDA approved synthetic biopolymer which belongs to the family of PLA. It possesses several important properties such as tunable mechanical properties, crystallinity, chemical stability, controlled biodegradability and biocompatibility that make it an excellent biomaterial for developing porous scaffolds with micro and nanostructures for various tissue engineering applications. However, the hydrophobic nature limits its application due to lack of biological signaling and protein adsorption ability. To overcome this limitation, PLLA was combined with other biopolymers and bioceramics. PLLA-based scaffolds have been extensively investigated for bone and cartilage tissue engineering application (Mallick, Pal et al. 2016, Ju, Peng et al. 2019)

Polyethylene Glycol (PEG)

PEG is the linear polymer of ethylene oxide and is formed by the ROP of ethylene oxide. PEG is a biocompatible, hydrophilic, biodegradable, non-immunogenic, and non-toxic polymer (Skaalure, Dimson et al. 2014; Skaalure, Chu et al. 2015; Sridhar, Brock et al. 2015). It can also inhibit nonspecific protein adsorption and has a neutral charge and superior mechanical properties (Stevens et al. 2015). It is soluble in both organic and aqueous solvents and has good mechanical strength (Obermeier et al. 2011). PEG is a popular synthetic hydrogel for tissue engineering purposes (Spicer 2020). PEG has been added to electrospun polylactide to improve swelling, stability, and mechanical strength behaviour of the scaffolds. It also increased the differentiation of MSCs to osteoblasts and upregulated many bone marker genes such as osteopontin, osteocalcin, and collagen-I (Ni et al. 2011). Due to its conductive nature it can be associated with cellulose nanocrystals to form an electrospun mat for bone tissue engineering (Zhang et al. 2015).

Polyvinyl Alcohol (PVA)

PVA, a polar synthetic polymer, was discovered through saponifying poly(vinyl ester) with caustic soda solution. It is a hydrophilic polymer and is widely used in biomedical application due to its hydrogel-forming ability. Its low mechanical strength limits its application. It can easily be cross-linked with many chemicals like boric acid, glutaraldehyde, formaldehyde, and sodium nitrate, thereby increasing its strength (Halima 2016). PVA can also be easily moulded into many architectures which is essential for biomedical applications. The conductive nature of PVA makes it a suitable candidate for electrospinning (Enayati et al. 2018). A 3D bioprinting scaffold made up of alginate/PVA/hydroxyapatite was developed as a implant for bone tissue growth (Bendtsen et al. 2017). Incorporation of PVA hydrogel in a PEG modified macroscopic and degradation profiles of scaffold which are important for bone tissue engineering (Martens, Bryant, and Anseth 2003). PVA-based hydrogel with collagen mimicked the ECM for the growth of chondrocyte and cartilage tissue development (Lan et al. 2020).

Polycaprolactone (PCL)

PCL is a synthetic aliphatic polyester. Caprolactone and 6-hydroxycaproic acid are the monomers of PCL. These monomers are polymerized by two different methods: (i) by condensation of 6-hydroxycaproic acid and (ii) by the ROP of caprolactone. It is a slow degrading polymer but with high mechanical strength. PCL can easily be mixed with other polymers. It was blended with many polymers like poly(vinyl chloride), poly(bisphenol-A), poly(styrene–acrylonitrile), nitrocellulose, cellulose butyrate, poly(acrylonitrile butadiene styrene), etc. (Labet and Thielemans 2009). Composites of PCL/PLA/hydroxyapatite (Hassanajili et al. 2019), PCL/hydroxyapatite (Yao 2015), PCL/octacalcium phosphate (Heydari, Mohebbi-Kalhori, and Afarani 2017), etc., have been used in bone tissue engineering as scaffold for bone regeneration. PCL is also able to maintain phenotype and promote proliferation of chondrocytes. PCL with chondrocyte-encapsulated alginate gel was engineered as an implant for cartilage tissue regeneration, where PCL enhanced the durability and mechanical strength of the scaffold (Leferink et al. 2016; Aydin, Korkusuz et al. 2015; Du, Liu et al. 2017; Filová, Tonar et al. 2020). The major disadvantages of this polymer include the lack of hydrophilicity and production of toxic degradation products that may cause inflammation (Baker et al. 2012).

POLYMER BLENDS AND COMPOSITES

CARTILAGE/OSTEOCHONDRAL DISORDER

In the past two decades a lot of research has been progressed towards scaffold biomaterial development for cartilage tissue engineering (Ngadimin et al. 2021). Scaffolds or hydrogels with desired properties to regenerate cartilage by improving cellular function are yet to succeed. An overview of scaffold biomaterials, which has been developed for cartilage tissue regeneration is described in the proceeding section.

COLLAGEN-BASED BIOMATERIAL

Collagen-based biomaterials have demonstrated outstanding biological processes in a number of investigations. These include biocompatibility, regulated biodegradation, minimal immunogenic response and antigenicity, host cell adhesion and migration, and so forth. Various forms of collagen-based biomaterials have been reported to repair cartilage defects, like sponges, hydrogels, films, fibre including nanofibre mats, nanofibrous membranes, etc., depending on the defect area, preparation methods, and functions (Yu et al. 2022). Collagen-based matrices are one of the most often utilized matrices in cartilage tissue engineering. Collagen-hyaluronic acid (HA) biomaterial was shown to promote cartilage tissue repair. Numerous researches have shown that combining collagen with chondrocytes and stem cells aided *in vitro* and *in vivo* cartilage tissue development. MSC-seeded type II collagen scaffolds produced from bone marrow successfully healed rabbit cartilage defects. In another study, core-shell collagen and poly(L-lactic acid-co-epsilon-caprolactone) nanofibrous scaffold encapsulated rhTGF-β3 and bovine serum albumin into the nanofibres core exhibited potentiality for cartilage regeneration of trachea (Djouad et al. 2007).

These biomaterial matrices improved the repair process of osteochondral defects in the rabbit (Lubiatowski et al. 2006), which are generally associated with chondrocytes (Wakitani et al. 1998) or MSCs (Lee et al. 2003). MSCs-seeded collagen gels of types I and III when implanted in osteochondral defects formed cartilage and subchondral bone (Wakitani et al. 1994). Collagen gels are favourable for chondrocyte culture and ECM synthesis and act as 3D support for culturing autologous human chondrocytes exhibiting hyaline cartilage that consists of type II collagen (Ochi et al. 2002). These gels promoted MSCs transformation into hyaline-like tissue in cartilaginous defects, thereby enabling patients to recover their normal activity (Kuroda et al. 2007). These studies ultimately supported collagen gels as suitable matrices for cartilage tissue regeneration.

A number of bioinspired and biomimetic hydrogels have been reported recently for use in cartilage regeneration including mussel-inspired polydopamine-incorporated hydrogels, with the addition of sugar additives like manuka honey for antibacterial properties and improving mechanical characteristics, to increase mechanical and biological efficiency by mimicking biological structures and networks in terms of cell adhesion and tissue integration (Yu et al. 2022). In both *in vitro* and *in vivo* (cartilage defects in rat), enzymatically cross-linked collagen-HA injectable hydrogels promoted chondrogenic differentiation of bone marrow MSCs, thereby repairing hyaline cartilage (Zhang et al. 2020).

GELATIN-BASED BIOMATERIAL

Gelatin biomaterials has been widely investigated for tissue regeneration purposes, because of their favourable biological and tunable physical properties. At varied doses of ethyl lysine diisocyanate, promising findings for *in vitro* MSC proliferation were obtained in a gelatin-based hydrogel with minimal adjustable mechanical characteristics. When compared to porcine-derived gelatin methacrylated GEL-MA, GEL-MA hydrogels derived from bovines and cross-linked with UV polymerization demonstrated the most identical environment to the native cartilage following 28 days of culture (Pahoff et al. 2019). Furthermore, adding gelatin to other polymers, like alginate, has been proven to improve the cell survival and chondrogenesis when compared to alginate only (Xu et al. 2019). Biomimetic gelatin hydrogels cross-linked with enzymes and loaded with cartilage ECM exhibited excellent outcomes in rabbit knee joint models for hyaline cartilage development and GAG content (Tsai et al. 2020).

ALGINATE-BASED BIOMATERIAL

Alginate-based biomaterial matrices have been widely studied as cartilage replacement matrices, as sodium alginate interacts with cells through particular surface receptors, encouraging cell proliferation and migration (Poole et al. 2001; Dominici et al. 2006). It also enables for the production of ECM proteins and preservation of the chondrocytic phenotype (Bonaventure et al. 1994; Almqvist et al. 2001; Carossino et al. 2007). The subcutaneous implantation of alginate beads combined with MSCs that had been *in vitro* differentiated to a chondrocytic phenotype supported the production of cartilaginous protein in the nude mice (Erickson et al. 2002). The results of *in vivo* study were unsatisfactory since alginate alone limits spontaneous healing (Fragonas et al. 2000). Moreover, when combined with chondrocytes, it failed to heal osteochondral lesions, owing to significant immunological responses (Paige et al. 1996; Mierisch et al. 2003). However, a hybrid agarose–alginate hydrogel, Cartipatch® (Tissue Bank of France, Lyon, France), was investigated for its application *in vivo* as implants containing autologous chondrocytes in humans. After 2 years, 8 of the13 patients exhibited hyaline cartilage in neotissue biopsies (Selmi et al. 2008).

HYALURONIC ACID-BASED BIOMATERIAL

HA-based matrices stimulate chondrocyte ECM production *in vitro* and *in vivo* (Tognana et al. 2005). However, unmodified HA is ineffective for cartilage healing (Goa and Benfield 1994) and requires cross-linking to improve biocompatibility

(Bulpitt and Aeschlimann 1999). HA can also be blended with other polymeric materials, for example, a prepared polymer blend comprising gelatine, chondroitin sulphate, and HA was able to maintain the chondrocytic phenotype and promoted type II collagen synthesis *in vitro* (Chang et al. 2003). In 91.5% of patients, the function of cartilage was improved by Hyalograft (Fidia Advanced Biopolymers, Abano Terme, Italy) and HYAFF 11 (Fidia Advanced Biopolymers, Abano Terme, Italy), which are engineered tissue grafts made from HA-based scaffold and the autologous chondrocytes (Marcacci et al. 2005).

CHITOSAN-BASED BIOMATERIALS

Chitosan (Ch) has been mixed with natural polymers like collagen, agarose, and gelatin to fabricate porous scaffold for cartilage tissue engineering applications (Whu, Hung et al. 2013, Chicatun, Griffanti et al. 2017, Garakani, Khanmohammadi et al. 2020). Polymeric matrices of pure Ch or Ch in combination with other polymers, like alginate or HA, promoted cartilage repair, chondrogenic activity of human chondrocytes, and ECM proteins synthesis as demonstrated by several *in vitro* studies (Torgbo and Sukyai 2018). In an *in vivo* study, Ch-based matrices induced the hyaline-like tissue formation in articular cartilage defects. Ch being cationic in nature facilitates strong ionic interactions with the anionic ECM components and helps in their retention. Since a large number of matrix components found in cartilage tissue are anionic, Ch-based scaffolds are believed to help in colonization of chondrocytes *in vitro* and also upon implantation (Chen, Yu et al. 2016). In an *in vitro* study, a silk fibroin–Ch blend porous scaffold supported the umbilical cord blood-derived hMSCs for cartilage construct generation in a dynamic culture condition (Agrawal, Pramanik, Vishwanath et al. 2018). Porcine knee chondrocytes were encapsulated in microspheres of Ch loaded with TGF-β and that demonstrated the regeneration capacity of damaged articular cartilage. Ch–HA fibrous scaffolds supported the rabbit articular chondrocytes adhesion, proliferation, and ECM production because of the strong interaction between the cationic Ch and anionic HA and ECM components, thereby increasing the mechanical strength of the scaffold as well as facilitating cell adhesion and proliferation (Chen, Yu et al. 2016). The physicochemical properties of Ch-based hydrogels were studied and successful encapsulation of bovine chondrocytes was demonstrated (Hwang et al. 2007). Gelatin–Ch–HA integrated with PLGA microspheres shows its tremendous potential in cartilage tissue regeneration upon culturing chondrocytes derived from rabbit ear. Cross-linking Ch with genipin, glutaraldehyde, and formaldehyde improved its degradation rate, mechanical strength, and biomaterial–cell interaction. However, the cytotoxic effect of cross-linking agents limits their use as a primary component of a scaffold biomaterial.

CELLULOSE-BASED BIOMATERIAL

Cellulose-based scaffold biomaterials have been found to be promising for cartilage tissue engineering (Frank et al. 2006). In an *in vitro* study, the usage of a cellulose polymer permitted chondrocyte growth and demonstrated high biocompatibility

(Müller et al. 2006). In addition, injectable hydroxypropylmethylcellulose hydrogel could be utilized to heal articular cartilage (Vinatier, Gauthier, Fatimi et al. 2009). However, only few *in vivo* investigations in the field of tissue engineering have been conducted till date.

SILK FIBROIN-BASED BIOMATERIAL

SF based biomaterials have been widely investigated for cartilage regeneration and have shown great potential for the treatment of osteoarthritis (Su et al. 2023). Silk fibroin was blended with other proteins, polymers, and inorganic materials to develop biomaterials with desired properties for different tissue engineering applications. RGD-coupled freeze-dried silk scaffolds by culturing and differentiating MSCs to chondrocytes were reported. 3D porous SF matrices developed by salt leaching method demonstrated successful chondrogenesis upon culturing bone marrow-derived hMSCs (Wang, Kim et al. 2005). SF was an important component that regulated cellular activities such as cell proliferation, differentiation, and migration for osteochondral tissue regeneration (Xiao et al. 2019).

GLUCOSAMINE SULFATE-BASED BIOMATERIALS

GS has been combined with few other polymers as one of the tissue-engineered scaffold constituents. For example, the prepared GS–PEG hydrogel was able to differentiate embryonic stem cells to cartilage formation (Hwang, Varghese et al. 2007). GS-incorporated gelatin/HA cryogels demonstrated neocartilage formation in defect cartilage of rabbits (Chen, Kuo et al. 2016). The developed SF/CS–glucosamine composite scaffold promoted chondrogenic differentiation of hMSCs (Agrawal, Pramanik, and Biswas 2018).

CHONDROITIN SULPHATE-BASED BIOMATERIALS

Because of poor mechanical strength, CS is usually combined or cross-linked with other polymers with high mechanical strength to improve its mechanical strength (Alinejad et al. 2018; Bai et al. 2017). CS has been combined as a key component with other polymers such as collagen, hyaluronic acid, poly(l-lactide), etc., for culturing chondrogenic cells (Gong, Zhu et al. 2007, Zhang, Li et al. 2011). CS was first combined with PLA to develop scaffold by salt leaching and solvent casting methods for cartilage tissue engineering applications (Lee, Huang et al. 2006). Hydrogel prepared from CS and PEG demonstrated MSCs aggregation and chondrogenic differentiation (Varghese, Hwang et al. 2008). In an *in vitro* study, collagen–CS–HA freeze-dried scaffolds cross-linked with genipin showed cartilage regeneration ability. In another study, compressive strength, swelling, and degradation of the collagen–CS–HA hydrogels were enhanced by cross-linking (Zhang, Li et al. 2011). CS–CShydrogels prevented collagen degradation, thereby indicating their prospective role in maintaining cell phenotype (Muzzarelli, Boudrant et al. 2012). In 2013, nano-Ch-incorporated freeze-dried CS/HA sponge showed suitability for wound dressings (Anisha, Sankar et al. 2013). Later, highly porous structure of SF–CS and sodium alginate scaffolds were prepared by lyophilization and an improvement in compressive strength was achieved by cross-linking with 1-ethyl-3-(3-dimethylaminopropyl) carbodiimide-ethanol. The cell supportive property studied using rabbit chondrocytes showed improvement in cell attachment and gene expression in the composite scaffold as compared to pure CS scaffold, thereby demonstrating the advantage of this scaffold in tissue engineering (Naeimi, Fathi et al. 2014). An enhanced chondrogenic differentiation of human BM-MSCs in freeze-dried SF/gelatin/CS/HA composite scaffold as compared to SF scaffold or pellet culture was reported (Sawatjui et al. 2015). CS–carboxymethylated pullulan injectable hydrogel supported the growth of porcine auricular chondrocytes and has shown tissue compatibility (Chen et al. 2016). A 3D freeze-dried SF/Ch–CS porous scaffold showed an enhanced chondrogenesis of umbilical cord blood derived hMSCs in a dynamic culture system (Agrawal et al. 2018). CS in conjunction with pullulan hydrogels demonstrated excellent vitality of encapsulated chondrocytes and improved chondrogenesis in enzymatically cross-linked and self-cross-linked hydrogels (Chen, Yu et al. 2016, Karaman et al. 2018). CS-based hydrogels showed higher cartilage matrix deposition throughout in comparison to type I collagen and HA-based hydrogels (Hwang et al. 2007)

COMBINED GLUCOSAMINE / CHONDROITIN SULPHATE BIOMATERIAL

The severity of cartilage tissue defect is directly proportional to GAG loss (Mankin, Dorfman et al. 1971), which causes difficulty in joint movement and this further causes wear and tear in the cartilage tissue. To avoid this, chondroprotective agents have a great role in augmenting synthesis of macromolecules existing in cartilage ECM. The chondroprotective agent should be able to inhibit enzymatic degradation of cartilage ECM components and stimulate synoviocytes for the synthesis of HA, as well as control the deposition of components that may accumulate and block synovial space and blood vessels in joints. To meet all these functions, a combination of GS and CS is beneficial to achieve chondroprotection and chondroregeneration (Hanson, Smalley et al. 1997). For example, an increased *in vitro* GAG synthesis and a decrease in OA progression in rabbits were demonstrated by using combined GS and CS rather than using the single component (Lippiello, Woodward et al. 2000). The effect of oral administration of GS, CS, and manganese ascorbate in combination on the metabolism of articular cartilage in cranial cruciate ligament-deficient dogs showed an elevated concentration of CS epitopes and GAG that resulted in structural improvements in articular cartilage during a 3–5-month period (Johnson, Hulse et al. 2001). An *in vitro* culture of chondrocytes on GS–CS–manganese ascorbate was demonstrated to be beneficial in combating chronic stress in cells obtained from aged joints (Lippiello, Woodward ct al. 2000). A randomized study performed on 35 dogs suffering from OA of hips and elbows depicted an overall improvement in pain, weight-bearing capacity, and other clinical conditions. Furthermore, studies performed on human OA patients also demonstrated beneficial results in the treatment of joint space loss (Sawitzke, Shi et al. 2008, Vangsness Jr, Spiker et al. 2009). In an *in vitro* study, SF/CS scaffold combined with both GS and CS promoted and enhanced chondrogenic differentiation of hMSCs and thereby cartilage-specific ECM production in a dynamic culture system (Agrawal et al. 2018).

POLYLACTIC ACID / POLYGLYCOLIC ACID-BASED BIOMATERIALS

Due to their biocompatible properties, PLGA/PLA are widely used in cartilage tissue engineering alone or in combination with other biomaterial matrices (Hu et al. 2011; Levett et al. 2014) and in various forms like fibrous to sponge. PGA polymers produce the best *in vitro* findings, with cellular density similar to that reported *in vivo* and continuous type II collagen synthesis (Freed, Vunjak-Novakovic, and Langer 1993). The rabbit model was used mostly for *in vivo* research (Freed et al. 1994). BioSeed® (BioTissue Technologies, Freiburg, Germany) comprising autologous articular chondrocytes was used in humans that induced the synthesis of a hyaline cartilage with significant clinical improvement (Ossendorf et al. 2007).

POLYTHYLENE GLYCOL-BASED BIOMATERIAL

PEG has been widely used as a support biomaterial in cartilage tissue engineering. However, because of its low mechanical strength, it is commonly combined with several other natural or synthetic materials to achieve desired mechanical strength and compression modulus (Zhang et al. 2015). For example, human chondrocytes encased in PEG–albumin hydrogel and transplanted into the subcutaneous region in immunodeficient mice preserved chondrocyte genotypes expressing types I and II collagen and aggrecan (Scholz et al. 2010). PEG hydrogels prepared by photo-clickable reactions loaded with adolescent bovine chondrocytes accumulated increased quantities of sGAG and collagens (especially type II collagen) inside the hydrogels, confirming hydrogel breakdown (Neumann et al. 2016).When a high-strength (20 MPa) PEG hydrogel laden with chondrocyte cells was implanted subcutaneously into an osteochondral damage model in severe combined immunodeficiency (SCID) mice, demonstrated that the cells may grow with retaining their phenotypic characteristics in the hydrogel (Müller et al. 2006).

PLLA/ PLGA MATRICES

PLLA and PLGA polymeric blends are promising biomaterials for fabricating tissue engineering scaffolds possessing desired mechanical properties and architecture (Saoto et al. 2021). When polylactides, PLLA, and PLGA matrices were incorporated along with a chondrocyte/atelocollagen mixture and engrafted in nude mice subcutaneously, it was shown to maintain the 3D shape and the elevated level of types I and II collagen production in case of PLLA and PLGA scaffolds than polylactides (Tanaka et al. 2010). A compressive modulus of about 6 MPa in PLLA scaffolds with a porous microstructure combined with fibrin gel enhanced cell proliferation and mechanical properties when used in cartilage tissue engineering (Zhao et al. 2008).

POLYVINYL ALCOHOL-BASED BIOMATERIALS

PVA-based matrices have been recognized as promising biomaterials and suitable substrates for cartilage and associated joint tissue replacement through TE approach. Among the biomateriasls for cartilage TE application, PVA-based hybrid scaffolds which is increasingly matching with the biological and mechanical properties of native cartilage tissue and hence potential for CTE (Barbon et al. 2022). To enhance *in vitro* chondrocyte functions, a PVA sponge with macropores was created for the inclusion of cell-containing photocrosslinkable poly(ethylene glycol) diacrylate (PEGDA), PEGDA–methacrylated hyaluronic acid (PEGDA-MeHA; PHA), or PEGDA–methacrylated chondroitin sulphate (PEGDA-MeCS; PCS) within its pores. Load of chondrocytes embedded in PCS or PHA into macropores of sponge didn't alter the physiological phenotype of both the sponge and fillers. The mineralization by cells enhanced the mechanical characteristics of the PVA-PCS by 83.30% and PVA-PHA scaffolds by 73.76%. *In vivo* transplanataion of PVA-PCS and PVA-PHA remarkably enhanced the cartilage formation (Kim et al. 2017).

PCL-BASED BIOMATERIALS

PCL-derived biomaterials in various form such as porous, nanofibers, etc have been used in several biomedical applications such as sutures, wound dressings, and tissue engineering of cardiovascular, nerve, bone, blood vessel, and cartilage (Mondal et al. 2016) A 3D-printed layer-by-layer PCL deposition with chondrocyte cell-encapsulated alginate hydrogel scaffold was fabricated. Hydrogels having transforming growth factor-β (TGFβ) exhibited higher GAG deposition than the hydrogel without growth factor. The scaffold was implanted subcutaneously in female nude mice. The histological and immunohistochemical study of scaffold by Alcian blue and haematoxylin & eosin (H&E) staining showed an increase in regeneration of cartilage tissue and deposition of collagen in hydrogels having TGFβ (Kundu et al. 2015).

BIOMATERIALS FOR BONE DEFECT

In the case of defective bone tissue repair strategy, bone biomaterials should have osteoinductive and osteoconductive properties and be capable of integrating into the surrounding bone tissue which is referred to as osseointegration. In this strategy, numerous bioactive ceramic compounds are usually combined with synthetic and natural polymers as listed in the previous section to develop scaffolds. These polymer–ceramic composite biomaterials have made remarkable progress in the development of bone and related tissue engineering scaffolds. Besides, polymers and ceramics, some bioactive molecules, for example, cell signalling molecules like mechanical signals (elastic polymeric networks, e.g., hydrogels), bone morphogenetic protcin 2 (BMP-2), molecules with antimicrobial and anti-inflammation activities, are added to the bone scaffolds. The list of bioceramics used in bone tissue engineering scaffold is given in Table 3.3. The list of polymer-polymer blends and polymer-mineral composites which have been developed for BTE application are given in Tables 3.4 and 3.5.

TABLE 3.3
The List of Bioceramics Used in Bone Tissue Engineering Scaffolds

Type/Name of Bioceramics	Advantages	Disadvantages	References
Hydroxyapatite (HAp)	Excellent biocompatiblity, non-toxic and osteoconductive	Causes redness and soreness when injected into the joint	(Dorozhkin 2010)
Tricalcium phosphate e.g., beta-tricalcium phosphate (β-TCP)	Biocompatibe, lack of rejection, and helps in providing new tissue with calcium and phosphorus	α-TCP dissolves excessively and degrades quickly The rate of degradation and the pace of osteogenesis differ.	(Lee, Tripathy et al. 2017)
Akermanite (Ca, Si, Mg)	superior mechanical qualities, and a controlled rate of degradation	Poor fracture toughness	(Zadehnajar, Mirmusavi et al. 2021)
Bioactive glasses (BGs)	Osteogenic, osteo inductive property	Brittleness	(Fernandes, Gaddam et al. 2018)

TABLE 3.4
List of Polymer-Polymer Blends Used for BTE Application

Polymer-Polymer Blends	*In vitro/In vivo* Results of Using Polymer Blends in Bone Tissue Engineering	References
Collagen/ glycosaminoglycans	Increase the bone cells attachment and influence the osteoblast activity	(Angele, Abke et al. 2004), (Tierney, Jaasma et al. 2009)
Chitosan-gelatin	Improved the rat bone marrow derived MSCs adherence, spreading, and in vitro viability characteristics	(Lungu, Albu et al. 2011)
Collagen/dextran	Improved the colonisation with human osteoblast cells	(Mieszawska, Llamas et al. 2011)
Chitosan/alginate	Accelerated deposition of connective tissue, vascularization, and calcification of the matrix throughout the whole scaffold architecture.	(Albu, Trandafir et al. 2012)
PLGA/Tussah silk fibroin	Accelerated cell proliferation, adhesion and mineralization	(Shao, He et al. 2016)

TABLE 3.4 (Continued)
List of Polymer-Polymer Blends Used for BTE Application

Polymer-Polymer Blends	In vitro/In vivo Results of Using Polymer Blends in Bone Tissue Engineering	References
Alginate/cellulose nanocrystals/chitosan/gelatin composite scaffold	Cell attachment, differentiation, and proliferation were positively influenced	(Li, Chen et al. 2021)
Hyaluronic acid/PEG	Elevated CD31 and CD105 expression (actin expression) Enhanced cell-cell contact, invasion, and migration	(Hong, Song et al. 2013)
PCL-Chitosan	Rapid degradability, enhanced vascular remodelling, and without calcification or aneurysm formation of neotissues	(Fukunisshi, Best et al. 2016)
PLA/PCL/PEOT/PBT	Having the proper pore size, a stiffness or surface energy discrete gradient, and a much higher ALP activity	(Di Luca, Longoni et al. 2016)
Macroporous fibrin and 3D-printed wollastonite (containing 8% $MgSiO_3$)	Enticing bone marrow stem cells, cartilage promotion without the requirement for chondrogene cells, excellent osteoconductivity and bioresorbability, and being able to regenerate	(Shen, Dai et al. 2017)
Horseradish peroxidase (HRP)-cross-linked SF	Targeted activation of osteogenic and chondrogenic cell compartments, closely mimicked shape along with the development of an osteochondral-like tissue, and intricacy of the mechanical interactions between tissues	(Carnes, Gonyea et al. 2020)
CS-PEG	3% w/v and 7% w/v of PEGDA. Reports on ECM deposition and protracted cell viability of 94% are available. They reported ECM production Compressive modulus: 0.73–1.04 kPa (day 1, week 3)	(Smeriglio, Lai et al. 2015)
Photocrosslinking of PCL and bioactive polydopamine coating	polydopamine-coating enhanced bioactivity	(Zhang, George et al. 2014)
PLGA/PGA	Effects of proliferation and osteoblastic differentiation were visible	(Ge, Wang et al. 2009)

(*continued*)

TABLE 3.4 (Continued)
List of Polymer-Polymer Blends Used for BTE Application

Polymer-Polymer Blends	*In vitro/In vivo* Results of Using Polymer Blends in Bone Tissue Engineering	References
PEG/PU/BMSCs	High thermal stability, biodegradable, Biocompatible and excellent porosity of the matrix	(Geesala, Bar et al. 2016)
PLA/Tussah silk fibroin	Accelerated cell proliferation, adhesion and mineralization New bone formation	(Shao, He et al. 2016)

COMPOSITE AND NANOCOMPOSITE BIOMATERIALS

Composite materials comprised of bioactive ceramic materials and polymers possess desired properties necessary for developing scaffolds that can act as a suitable support matrix for bone tissue regeneration (Levett et al. 2014). Composite biomaterials are designed to bring the desirable properties of two or more biomaterials in a single platform, thereby improving its processability, fabrication, mechanical strength, biological performance, etc. The composite scaffolds when combined with bioactive signalling molecules and stem cells perform better in bioglass (BG) in comparison to general composite scaffolds, which are displayed in Table 3.6. Hydroxyapetite, β-TCP, and BG have been widely used in scaffold as bioactive ceramic materials because of their explicit biological interactions between scaffolds and body tissues.

The bioactive bioceramics are of great interest in BTE because of their composition match with the mineral phase of bone. Bioactive glasses can rapidly form bioactive hydroxycarbonated apatite layer that can easily bind to tissue in body fluid. Their properties can also be tailored appropriately so that they could release ions such as Si at levels that are able to activate gene transduction pathways, thereby enhancing osteogenesis and cell differentiation (Hench and Polak 2002; Jell and Stevens 2006; Tsigkou et al. 2007). Furthermore, inorganic component with nano-size is more bioactive in comparison to its micro-size. AP–collagen nanocomposite scaffolds are good examples which have shown promise than the corresponding scaffold with micro-size (Liao, Cui, and Zhu 2004). Sol-gel method is an another interesting route to make composite scaffold at the nanoscale. In an *in vitro* study, nano β-TCP-reinforced CS scaffold exhibited higher compressive strength and enhanced bioactivity in comparison to its counterpart micro-β-TCP-reinforced CS scaffold.

BIOMATERIAL PROCESSING

Many methods are adopted for processing the biomaterials aiming to enhance &/or modify their properties to make them appropriate for tissue engineering applications.

TABLE 3.5
List of Polymer-Mineral Composite Biomaterials Used for BTE Application

Polymer-Ceramic Composites	In vitro / In vivo Results of Using Composites in Bone Tissue Engineering	References
Chitosan/montmorillonite (MMT)/ hydroxyapatite (HAp)	Improved cell attachment and proliferation, and induced well-spread morphology	(Katti, Katti et al. 2008)
Chitosan/gelatin/Hap	Improved osteoblastic cell attachment and spreading	(Peter, Ganesh et al. 2010)
Collagen/silk fibroin/HAp	exhibited good biocompatibility with MG 63 cells	(Chen, Hu et al. 2014)
Pullulan/dextran/ nano-Hap particles	Encourage host mesenchymal stem cells to differentiate into bone cells and formation of bone	(Fricain, Schlaubitz et al. 2013)
Collagen/chitosan/HAp	Possess high histocompatibility and suitable as a bone substitute	(Becerra, Rodriguez et al. 2022)
Chitosan/gelatin/nSiO2	Facilitate better MG 63 cell proliferation inducing faster differentiation of osteoblasts	(Kavya, Jayakumar et al. 2013)
Silk/silica	Good hMSC proliferation rates as well as high cell viability; osteoinductive properties	(Mieszawska, Fourligas et al. 2010)
Collagen/porous calcium phosphate	Promoted the adhesion, dissemination, migration, proliferation, and differentiation of human bone marrow derived MSCs	(Zhou, Ye et al. 2014)
Fibrillar collagen/bioactive calcium phosphate silicate glass-ceramic	Increased osteogenic activity in human MG63 osteoblast cells	(Albu, Radev et al. 2013)
Chitosan-tricalcium phosphate-fucoidan scaffold	Osteogenic differentiation is enabled	(Puvaneswary, Talebian et al. 2015)
Chitosan–gelatin–siloxane	Increased ALP and bone-specific gene expression	(Nair, Gangadharan et al. 2015)
Graphene oxide/HAp/silk fibroin scaffold	Improved osteoblast differentiation and osteocalcin expression	(Wang, Chu et al. 2017)
Strontium HAp/chitosan nanohybrid scaffold	Cell proliferation and osteogenic differentiation are both boosted	(Lei, Xu et al. 2017)
Alginate/cellulose nanocrystals/ chitosan/gelatin composite scaffold	Cell attachment, differentiation, and proliferation were positively influenced	(Li, Chen et al. 2021)
HAp/gelatin/PVA	New bone growth enhanced	(Swain and Sarkar 2014)

(continued)

TABLE 3.5 (Continued)
List of Polymer-Mineral Composite biomaterials Used for BTE Application

Polymer-Ceramic Composites	In vitro / In vivo Results of Using Composites in Bone Tissue Engineering	References
Silk fibers/HAp	Induction of formation of new bone	(Jiang, Ran et al. 2018)
Gelatin/BG/Poly(3,4-ethylenedioxythiophene):poly(4-styrene sulfonate) and electrical stimulation	Stabilized scaffold structure and increased cellular activities MSCs achieved by adding PEDOT	(Shahini, Yazdimamaghani et al. 2014)
Collagen-glycosaminoglycan/ Bioactive glass	Promotes bone regeneration and vascularization of bone tissue graft	(Quinlan, Partap et al. 2015)
PLGA/gentamicin/Titanium dioxide	The antibacterial activity of the released gentamicin and scaffold supported osteoblast-like cells (MG-63)	(Rumian, Tiainen et al. 2016)
Gelatin/CMC cellulose/PVA/nHAp	Collagen type I, ALP, Runx2, and osteocalcin gene expression enhanced.	(Narayan, Agarwal et al. 2017)
HAp/gelatin/PVA	New bone growth enhanced	(Tontowi, Anindyajati et al. 2018)
Chitosan/nHAp -genipin	Encouraged proliferation and differentiation of osteoblasts	(Frohbergh, Katsman et al. 2012)
Collagen/PLLA/nHAp	Increased proliferation of osteoblasts	(Prabhakaran, Venugopal et al. 2009)
PLLA/PCL/HAp	Increased osteoblast proliferation and differentiation	(Qi, Ye et al. 2016)
Poly-hydroxybutyrate/ nHAp	Improved osteogenic phenotype, adhesion, and proliferation. Osteoid tissue development	(Chen, Song et al. 2017)
PLLA/Bioactive glass	More efficient cell division and osteogenic differentiation	(Shamsi, Karimi et al. 2017)
PCL/PLGA/TCP	Enhanced osteogenesis and Runx2 as its indicators	(Pati, Song et al. 2015)
PCL/HAp (85/15 wt%)	Promoted bone regeneration	(Youssef, Hollister et al. 2017)
PLGA-Tussah silk-GO	In addition to being an potential scaffold material for bone tissue regeneration, it also serves as a therapeutic patch for drug administration, treatment of cancer and biodegradability	(Shao, He et al. 2016)

Material	Description	Reference
DN hydrogel system (PGA/HAp)	Encourages cell development into porous structures, heals and makes it simple to cross-link damaged articular cartilage, biocompatibility, less toxic, and is reasonably inexpensive	(Zhu, Chen et al. 2018)
PLGA-TCP	Stimulated growth and guided development of endogenous MSCs for various formulations to fix various tissue abnormalities in the osteochondral area	(Ribeiro, Pina et al. 2019)
Fe3O4 nanoparticles/MBG/PCL	Had differentiation and proliferation characteristics	(Zhang, Zhao et al. 2014)
HAp and alpha-tricalcium phosphate/Collagen	New bone growth evolved	(Inzana, Olvera et al. 2014)
PLGA/Black phosphorus (BP)/SrCl$_2$	Scaffolds showed *in vivo* biocompatibility & bone regeneration capability in near-infrared irradiation in rats	(Wang, Shao et al. 2018)
n-HA/poly(D,L-lactide-co-glycolide) (PLAGA)	Allowed the formation of engineered bone tissue	(Lv, Deng et al. 2013)
Poly(D,L-Lactide) (PDLLA)/ BGs, CuO/ZnO	Cu- & Zn-doped BG in the PDLLA, composite prepared with enhanced bioactivity	(Bejarano, Detsch et al. 2017)
PLA/Bioactive organically modified glass (ormoglass)	Roughness, stiffness, morphology of the ormoglass coated fibers adjusted by varied experimental parameters	(Sachot, Mateos-Timoneda et al. 2015)
Collagen/HAp and alpha-tricalcium phosphate	New bone growth evolved	(Inzana, Olvera et al. 2014)
β-TCP/SrO and MgO scaffolds	Better bone growth than with β-TCP	(Tarafder, Davies et al. 2013)
HA/β-TCP	Promoted growth and differentiation of the osteoclasts	(Detsch, Schaefer et al. 2011)
Graphene oxide and nHAp	Elevated cell proliferation, expression of osteogenic and ALP gene	(Nie, Peng et al. 2017)
β-TCP/Iron-containing	Calcium phosphate (CaP) ceramics' bone conduction characteristics may be enhanced by iron	(Qu, Fu et al. 2019)

TABLE 3.6

Composite Biomaterials Derived from Polymer and Growth/Differentiation Factor/Electrical Stimulator

Material	Differentiation Factor	In vitro/In vivo Results	References
Silk fibroin	BMP-2	Triggered osteogenic response on human bone marrow stromal cells	(Karageorgiou, Meinel et al. 2004)
Collagen	Dexamethasone and collagen-D3	Promoted osteogenic activity in human osteoprogenitor cells	(Titorencu, Albu et al. 2012)
Collagen/hyaluronic acid/	BMP-4	Enhanced the MG63 osteoblast cells biocompatibility	(Lungu, Titorencu et al. 2011)
CMC/Zn-nHAp/ascorbic acid/	miR-15b	Osteoblast differentiation is enhanced	(Vimalraj, Partridge et al. 2014)
Biphasic calcium phosphate nanoparticles/collagen composite	Dexamethasone	Differentiation of osteoblasts is stimulated Runx2, ALP, IBSP, and BMP-2 expressions were upregulated.	(Chen, Kawazoe et al. 2018)
Collagen/chitosan/β-tricalcium phosphate composite loaded with PLGA	Raloxifene	Increased potential for cell growth and regeneration	(Zhang, Cheng et al. 2017)
Graphene oxide/chitosan/ hyaluronic acid	Simvastatin	Stimulated osteogenesis	(Unnithan, Sasikala et al. 2017)
Chitosan/CaPP	Pigeonite	Elevated cellular and molecular osteoblast differentiation. Increased bone mass density	(Dhivya, Keshav Narayan et al. 2018)
Chitosan/CMC/nHAp	Chrysin	Stimulated bone development and had a proliferative effect at the cellular and molecular levels	(Menon, Soundarya et al. 2018)

Material	Agent/Factor	Effect	Reference
PLLACL/collagen Collagen	Dexamethasone/**BMP-2** **Catecholamines and** Ca^{2+}	Depicted osteogenic differentiation Increased osteogenic expression of osteocalcin and osteopontin as well as cell adhesion, proliferation, differentiation enhanced	(Su, Su et al. 2012) (Dhand, Ong et al. 2016)
Fibrin	**BMP-2**	osteogenic differentiation potential was depicted	(Phillippi, Miller et al. 2008)
Mesoporous bioactive glass with PVA	**Dexamethasone**	Exhibited osteogenic differentiation as well as anti-inflammatory effects	(Wu, Luo et al. 2011)
HA and β-TCP	**Recombinant BMP-2**	Osteogenic differentiation and proliferative effects were observed	(Abarrategi, Moreno-Vicente et al. 2012)
Mesoporous bioactive glass/ alginate	**Dexamethasone**	Demonstrated osteogenic differentiation ability	(Luo, Wu et al. 2012)
PCL/Gelatin/HAp hydrogels	Fibrinogen Pluronic F-127	Showed elevated proliferation and differentiation	(Kang, Lee et al. 2016)
Poly(L/DL lactide) (PLDL)/ PCL	Osteogenon-drug	Osteogenon improved mineralization, cell adhesion and differentiation	(Rajzer, Menaszek et al. 2017)
HA/β-TCP	BMP-2	Possibility to apply for bone tissue regeneration	(Tateiwa, Nakagawa et al. 2021)
HA/Poly(D,L-lactic acid)- co-poly-(ethylene glycol)- co- poly(D,L-lactic acid) (PELA)	BMSCs/rhBMP-2	Potential for bone regeneration based on cell	(Kutikov, Skelly et al. 2015)
Transglutaminase cross-linked gelatin (TG-Gel)	BMP-2, mechanical signalling	On osteogenic differentiation, hydrogel hardness and **BMP-2** worked together synergistically	(Tan, Fang et al. 2014)

As described earlier, natural and synthetic polymers have their own advantages and disadvantages. Many of the limitations of these polymers can be overcome by biochemical and physical methods. Moreover, as discussed in the previous sections, no single polymer can satisfy all the properties necessary for any tissue engineering application and therefore, polymers are combined to form polymer–polymer blends, or combined with bioceramic material yielding polymer–ceramic composites biomaterials with improvised properties. Besides these strategies, currently, research interest is focused on developing biomimetic materials and nanomaterials through surface modification, thereby overcoming the limitation of single biomaterials which is the new trend in biomaterial field (Pasqui et al. 2014). These biomaterials have the ability to mediate cell–cell signalling and interaction during tissue regeneration process. Some of the important techniques for improving biomaterial properties are discussed as follows.

BIOCHEMICAL METHODS

In the process of biochemical modification, the poor mechanical properties of natural polymer, poor hydrophilicity and cell adhesion characteristics of synthetic materials are overcome by combining these polymers with a biological modifier, resulting in a biomaterial that exhibits higher tissue compatibility and facilitates cell growth and proliferation by providing necessary microenvironment (Aslan et al. 2006). Some of the important biological modifiers and their role in improving biomaterial properties are described as follows.

Different surface peptide bioactive molecules have been employed for improving chondrogenesis in porous biomaterials. Glutamic acid-Proline-Leucine-Gutamine-Leucine-Lysine-Methionine peptide which has specific attraction towards mesenchymal stem cells was conjugated with PCL and implanted at the cartilage defect site of a rat knee joint. The peptide sequence exhibited an enhanced MSCs recruitment, and thus promoted cartilage tissue regeneration at the defect site (Martens et al. 2003). Threonine-alanine-Threonine-Valine-Histidine-Leucine peptide loaded into polyethylene oxide/chitin/chitosan composite matrix and seeded with bovine knee chondrocytes promoted the chondrocytes proliferation, glycosaminoglycans secretion, and the production of collagen (Lan et al. 2020). The bovine knee chondrocytes seeded onto the surface of Cysteine-Aspartate-Proline-Glycine-Phenylalanine-Isoleuicne-Glycine-Serine-Arginine cross-linked with polyethylene oxide/Ch showed higher efficiency of cell adhesion and the maintenance of chondrocyte phenotype during culturing in a spinner flask bioreactor (Labet and Thielemans 2009). Alginate polymer can interact with cells through specific surface receptors, thereby facilitating cell migration and proliferation (Kim et al. 2011; Zhang et al. 2015). In an *in vivo* mice study, 3D alginate scaffold maintained functional phenotypes of porcine chondrocyte. The latter when encapsulated into alginate hydrogel made with gelatin microspheres exhibited higher proliferation and cartilage ECM formation. In another study, alginate hydrogels cross-linked with hyaluronate through carbodiimide chemistry using ethylenediamine as a cross-linking agent promoted chondrogenic differentiation of encapsulated ATDC5 isolated from mouse teratocarcinoma fibroblastic cells (Drury, Dennis, and Mooney 2004).

In an *in vitro* study, due to surface modification of a scaffold fabricated from CS/nano βTCP biomaterial upon crosslinking with genipin and tripolyphosphate, showed enhanced cell attachment, cell proliferation, cellular metabolic and ALP activities,. The genipin-cross-linked CS/nano β-TCP further enhanced cell adhesion, cell proliferation, and osteogenic differentiation capacity when the scaffold was surface coated with fibrin (having cell-binding ability) using ethyl-3-(3-dimethylaminopropyl) carbodimide as crosslinking agent (Siddiqui and Pramanik 2014). However, some studies have shown fibrin biomaterial as having non- or reduced chondrogenic characteristics (Deitzer 2006), whereas chondro-positive results were achieved when fibrin hydrogels were used by functionalizing with cartilage ECM. A fibrin hydrogel with exogenous TGF-β3 functionalized with cartilage ECM microparticles enhanced chondrogenesis, thereby synthesizing higher cartilage-like tissue in *in vivo* tests than the constructs loaded with gelatin microspheres used as a control (Almeida et al. 2016).

BG has specific biological and physiological characteristics. When BG 13–93 was used as a culture medium supplement, enhanced biochemical and mechanical characteristics of a regenerated cartilage indicated that it can be used as a medium substitute for neocartilage production (Jayabalan et al., 2011). The integration of BG into poly(hydroxybutyrate-co-hydroxyvalerate polymer enhanced hydrophilicity of the composites and cell adhesion and cell migration in the cartilage construct (Wu et al., 2013). HA incorporated in gelatin–methacrylamide hydrogels depicted natural functions of scaffolds in some cartilage properties including mechanical strength (Schuurman et al. 2013). The gelatin/HA-treated PLGA sponge scaffolds showed superior cells adhesion, proliferation, and ECM deposition than pure PLGA scaffolds (Chang et al. 2013).

A porous elastomeric poly-l-lactide-co-ε-caprolactone (PLCL) scaffold when cross-linked at the chitosan surface improved its wettability and the differentiation of bone marrow-derived MSCs into cartilage tissue without significant change in the physical elastomeric properties (Yang et al. 2012). In another study, Ch-modified PLCL scaffolds promoted cellular adhesion, proliferation, and also enhanced excretion of aggrecan and type-II collagen (Li et al. 2012). Ch–gelatin matrices crosslinked by water-soluble carbodiimide increased cartilage tissue regeneration (Whu et al. 2013).

Biochemical modification of nanomaterials can enhance the biocompatibility and bioactivity of the scaffolds. A functionalized nanofibrous scaffold promoted nucleus pulposus cell adhesion with less cytotoxicity and stimulated ECM synthesis (Dodge and Jimenez 2003). Electrospun PLLA nanofibrous membrane was subjected to oxygen plasma treatment for incorporating -COOH groups on its surface, followed by covalent grafting of covalent cationized gelatin molecules over the surface, using water-soluble carbodiimide as coupling agent (Chen et al., 2011). Embedding proteins, drugs, etc., in scaffold biomaterial not only mimics the structure of ECM but also mimics its function. In the process of cartilage repair, control of angiogenesis is important for the stability of immature construct. A biocompatible fibrin/hyaluronan scaffold loaded with nasal chondrocytes and functionalized with an antiangiogenic drug (bevacizumab) sequestrated vascular endothelial growth factor from the surrounding tissue was able to achieve controlled angiogenesis, thereby enhancing the rate of constructs survival and cartilage regeneration (Centola et al. 2013). The cartilage defect repair using scaffold is often associated with undesired terminal differentiation of bone marrow-derived MSCs, which can be inhibited by adding parathyroid hormone-related protein (Hammad et al. 2015). The administration of this protein with collagen–silk scaffold arrested this terminal differentiation that resulted in an enhanced chondrogenesis, thus improving cartilage repair and regeneration. A microfibrous poly (L-lactide) scaffold coupled with transforming growth factor-(TGF-) β1 showed higher GAGs deposition and total collagen with higher neo-ECM thickness by culturing bovine AFCs (Müller et al. 2006). In cartilage tissue engineering, cell adhesion-promoting polypeptides, owing to their lack of complementary or modulatory domains, are modified to increase their ability to promote cell adhesion (Cao et al., 2014).

Hydrogels are attractive biomaterials because of their structural similarity to the ECM of various tissues, and can be applied arthroscopically, which make it a potential candidate for minimally invasive treatment, and therefore have been widely studied (Jiang et al. 2006). Hydrogels are tunable, so their cartilage mimicking properties, degree and methods of cross-linking for a stable structure, and cell density in the hydrogel, etc., can be modified to make them suitable for cartilage tissue regeneration. The degree of cross-linking can control basic properties including swelling behaviour, stability, degradation rates, and porosity of the hydrogel (Khan and Ranjha 2014). Different cross-linking methods used are cross-linking covalently or non-covalently involving a chemical or physical reaction (Hu et al. 2019). Chemical cross-linking methods include photo-cross-linking, enzymatic cross-linking, ion- or pH-sensitive cross-linking, and click chemistry and often involve covalent bonding between polymer chains, whereas physical cross-linking is associated with a physical interaction between the chains or triggers chemical polymerizations. Copolymerization or free-radical polymerization cross-linking is another method that involves reacting hydrophilic monomers to multifunctional cross-linkers resulting in physical interactions and cross-link junctions. For example, the carbodiimide reaction uses N,N-(3-dimethylaminopropyl)-N-ethylcarbodiimide (EDC) reagent, thereby allowing cross-linking of water-soluble polymers with amide bonds. Click-cross-linked modified HA hydrogels showed chondrogenic differentiation and elevated GAG expression of stem cells derived from human periodontal ligament (Park et al. 2019). Similarly, enzymatic cross-linking of hydrogels offers rapid gelation under certain physiological conditions offering high specificity and low cytotoxicity (Nezhad-Mokhtari et al. 2019). The enzymatically cross-linked collagen-HA hydrogels supported chondrogenic differentiation of BMSCs and regeneration of hyaline cartilage (Zhang et al. 2020) both *in vitro* and *in vivo* in rats. In other studies, enzyme-cross-linked biomimetic hydrogels based on gelatin showed the formation of hyaline cartilage and GAG deposition in rabbit knee joint models (Tsai et al. 2020).

Interpenetrating network (IPN) is another approach for preparing hydrogel. In this approach, two or more polymers in the networks are partially interlaced on the molecular scale within the scaffold matrix (Parhi 2017). Multiple networks (IPN) are superior to single network because of their enhanced water content that reduces the mechanical strength and swelling ability (Ingavle et al. 2012; Dragan 2014). The IPN hydrogel approach (Nonoyama and Gong 2015) offers native cartilage-mimicking mechanical properties (Zhao et al. 2014), including stiffness, high wear resistance, and compression limit (Li, Zhang et al. 2020; Means et al. 2019). The double network (DN) approach has been applied by interpenetrating the damaged cartilage tissue, which increased equilibrium compressive modulus of the tissue and wear resistance, with maintenance of cartilage volume (Cooper et al. 2016). This type of hydrogels are also enzymatically cross-linked to repair cartilage through encapsulation of human articular chondrocytes, thereby obtaining highly cytocompatible hydrogels (Trachsel et al. 2019).

Natural biomaterials and coupled ECM proteins in hydrogels (e.g. gelatin, HA, and CS) are recognized to be good biomimetic materials for cartilage tissue engineering. A biomimetic cartilage ECM-like hydrogels with improved mechanical properties was resulted from CS, HA, and gelatin. Excellent mechanical, and GAG synthesis and cellular viability was obtained by hydrogel developed by combining cartilage-simulating collagen with HA and chondroitin sulfate (Jiang et al. 2018; Levett et al. 2014).

Physico-Chemical Method

Physico-chemical methods are usually used for the surface modification of metallic biomaterials. These methods are anodic oxidation, chemical etching, and thermal spraying. Anodic oxidation also known as anodization is the most simplest, cost effective and hence widely used to alter the metallic biomaterial surfaces. This method modifies the inclination and capacity to create a self-protective oxide layer on their surface, leading to the production of the intended oxide layer (Munir et al., 2020). complicated topographical based surfaces like oxide nanotubes and nano scale texture of porous surface coatings are formed. These nanostructures improve osteoblast cell adhesion and proliferation (Bayram et al., 2014). In chemical etching the metallic biomaterial surfaces acquire added functional groups when they come into contact with alkaline and acidic solutions biomaterials. The sol-gel method is a wet chemical technique that is typically applied to develop inorganic materials resulting from a colloidal suspension of inorganic or metal precursors like ceramics and metal oxides. In this method, a colloidal suspension aids as the pioneer for a combined system (or gel) of discrete particles, thereby enabling the combination of tiny molecules to produce a solid substance. The development of components of thin films, bulk solid, and different coatings in the process of sol-gel typically involves four major stages: (1) hydrolysis of inorganic precursor and condensation to develop particulate based sols; (2) sol particulate clustering to develop more firmer gel type structures; (3) removal of remaining liquid from the gel through drying; and (4) synthesis of structures and inorganic phases through sintering or heat treatment. Calcium phosphate coatings produced through sol-gel method have been found to increase new bone generation and osseointegration for biomedical applications, including orthopaedic and dental implants (Liu et al, 2003, Tache et al., 2004). Thermal spraying is an efficient coating method that is frequently used to modify the metallic biomaterial surfaces. (Ang et al., 2018). This method involves heating a coating material, using either chemical (combustion flame) or electrical (plasma or arc) means. In contrast to alternative coating methods like chemical vapour and physical vapour deposition, and electroplating, thermal spraying allows comparatively high deposition rates of thick coatings on large metallic surfaces, ranging from 50 µm to several millimetres (mm). The particles of the feedstock are heated and propelled through the nozzle towards the substrate during coating on metallic substrates. The thermal spraying method can be divided into three subclasses: (1) using a source of combustion like a flame, detonation gun or high-velocity based fuel spray; (2) coating of material by cold spraying process; and (3) film formation using electrical techniques, such as plasma or arc. The superiority of deposited layers on the metallic biomaterial surfaces may differ depending on the process used to coat particular biomaterials.

Physical alteration of the scaffold biomaterials is performed by using ultraviolet (UV) light irradiation, filtration, and compression, thereby enhancing the biomechanical property and porosity of biomaterials that can repair cartilage. It was shown in a study that a cartilage-derived matrix scaffold prevents cell-mediated contraction, and supports cell attachment when it was processed with UV light irradiation or dehydrothermal irradiation (Aslan et al. 2006). In another study, a glutaraldehyde cross-linked collagen scaffold enhanced the vascularization in a murine subcutaneous implantation model (Obermeier et al. 2011).

MECHANICAL METHODS

Mechanical techniques used for the modification of the surface of metallic biomaterials includes machining, grinding, polishing and blasting (Li et al., 2021). The surface is altered via mechanical processes that include shaping, removing, and subjecting the surface material to physical and attrition treatment. Through surface removal, these techniques aim to remove oxide layers and contaminants while producing specific topographies and roughness (Brunette et al., 2001). Grit blasting is a process that involves high-velocity bombardment of hard particles onto metallic surfaces. Hard particle impact causes metallic surfaces to flex plastically, removing materials like oxide coatings from the surface.

SURFACE NANO-MODIFICATION OF BIOMATERIALS

Surface modification can be used to create nanostructured surfaces on traditional biomaterials. The two classes of nano-functionalization procedures include in situ surface nano-functionalization and nano coating and film deposition, which are based on the methods used to modify surfaces. These methods are frequently combined to create surfaces with hybrid nanostructures, like nanostructured zones and coatings/films (Liu et al., 2010). Conventional methods for film deposition and coating encompass plasma spraying, sol–gel, chemical and physical vapor deposition cold spraying, self-assembly, and so forth; whereas, methods for in situ modification of surface comprise shot blasting, acid and alkali treatments, laser etching, micro-arc oxidation, ion implantation, anodic oxidation, and so forth (Liu et al., 2010).

IN VITRO CARTILAGE AND BONE TISSUE MODELS

Native cartilage and bone tissues with zonally stratified structures are important that can be achieved by combining multiple biomaterials with different characteristics and suitable fabrication techniques. For example, bioprinting offers controlled mixing of different bioinks following a layer-by-layer approach, thereby resulting in scaffold structures with a physical and chemical composition imitating cartilage defect area (Chuang et al. 2018; Fu et al. 2020). Similarly, biomimetic multiphasic structures with native osteochondral tissue properties have been fabricated (Longley et al. 2018). Mussel-inspired bilayer hydrogels looked promising in repairing osteochondral lesions in rabbit knee joints (Gan et al. 2019). Another example is the biphasic CAN-PAC hydrogel developed by thermally initiated free radical polymerization supporting regeneration of osteochondral defects in rats with low inflammatory response (Liao et al. 2017). Photo-cross-linked gelatin-hyaluronic acid (GEL-HAs) structures were fabricated by photocuring 3D printing technique for cartilage regeneration (Xia et al. 2018). *In vitro* and *in vivo*, encapsulated chondrocytes in scaffolds facilitated cartilage regeneration with a characteristic lacunae shape and cartilage-specific ECM. The bioprinting of biomimetic hydrogels revealed a strong interest in the use of functionalized natural components like GE, CS, and HA for cartilage (Xiongfa et al. 2018) constructing a sophisticated zonal microarchitecture of native hyaline cartilage and geometrically mimicking cartilage and osteochondral tissue interface constructs (Daly et al. 2017; Wu et al. 2021).

BIOMATERIAL DESIGN BY COMPUTATIONAL MODELLING

In general, a substantial number of iterations are required in multi-variant systems to obtain the desired scaffold biomaterial properties (Hautier, Jain, and Ong 2012), which can be achieved by computer-guided biomaterial design strategies (Zadpoor 2017). For example, a numerical model-based approach was used for designing of biomimetic soft network composites by selecting a biomaterial with desired mechanical strength for cartilage regeneration (Bas et al. 2018). It has been claimed that a mechanics-based model of tissue formation in biodegradable cell-seeded PEG-based cross-linked hydrogels has been developed (Sridhar et al. 2017). The alterations of osteoarthritis-induced articular cartilage deterioration and the remodelling of subchondral cortical as well as trabecular bones were studied using a finite element model.

EXERCISE

1. Define biomaterial and classify them with examples.
2. What are the ideal properties of biomaterials for their use in cartilage tissue engineering applications?
3. Name a few biomaterials used for cartilage regeneration along with their advantages, disadvantages, and diseases targeted.
4. Write the advantages and disadvantages of the use of hyaluronic acid in cartilage tissue engineering applications?
5. What are the polymers that contain the inherent RGD peptides? Describe any one of them from cartilage tissue regeneration perspective.
6. Name a synthetic polymer and write its importance in cartilage regeneration.
7. How collagen-based biomaterials help in cartilage disorders? How do they differ from chitosan-based biomaterials?
8. What are the effects of following composites in bone tissue engineering?

    i   Silk/HAp

    ii   PLGA/PGA

    iii Chitosan/CMC/nHAp

    iv Alginate/cellulose/chitosan/gelatin

9. Explain the importance of bioactive glass and transglutaminase cross-linked gelatin in bone tissue engineering.
10. Differentiate between natural and synthetic polymers.
11. Describe two important biological modifiers and their role in improving the biomaterial properties.
12. How does fibrin help in cartilage repair and regeneration?
13. Name a few scaffolding biomaterials that help in enhancing chondrogenesis and thereby importance in cartilage repair.
14. What is GAG? How does it help in the repair of bone and defects?
15. What is the role of hydrogels in bone and cartilage regeneration?
16. Give a few examples of *in vitro* cartilage and bone models.
17. Explain the importance of designing biomaterials by computational modelling?
18. What are the various strategy you can adopt for improving the properties of biomaterials? Explain one method in detail.
19. List out potential bioceramics and their characteristics.
20. Give two examples of natural biopolymers and their important characteristics for bone tissue engineering application

REFERENCES

Abarrategi, A., C. Moreno-Vicente, F. J. Martínez-Vázquez, A. Civantos, V. Ramos, J. V. Sanz-Casado, R. Martínez-Corriá, F. H. Perera, F. Mulero and P. Miranda. 2012. "Biological properties of solid free form designed ceramic scaffolds with BMP-2: In vitro and in vivo evaluation." *PloS One* 7 (3): e34117.

Acharya, C., S. K. Ghosh and S. Kundu. 2009. "Silk fibroin film from non-mulberry tropical tasar silkworms: A novel substrate for in vitro fibroblast culture." *Acta Biomaterialia* 5 (1): 429–437.

Agrawal, P., K. Pramanik and A. Biswas. 2018. "Chondrogenic differentiation of mesenchymal stem cells on silk fibroin: Chitosan–glucosamine scaffold in dynamic culture." *Regenerative Medicine* 13 (05): 545–558.

Agrawal, P., K. Pramanik, A. Biswas and R. K. Patra. 2018. "In vitro cartilage construct generation from silk fibroin-chitosan porous scaffold and umbilical cord blood derived human mesenchymal stem cells in dynamic culture condition." *Journal of Biomedical Materials Research Part A* 106 (2): 397–407.

Agrawal, P., K. Pramanik, V. Vishwanath, A. Biswas, A. Bissoyi and P. K. Patra. 2018. "Enhanced chondrogenesis of mesenchymal stem cells over silk fibroin/chitosan-chondroitin sulfate three dimensional scaffold in dynamic culture condition." *Journal of Biomedical Materials Research Part B: Applied Biomaterials* 106 (7): 2576–2587.

Aisenbrey, E. A. and S. J. Bryant. 2019. "The role of chondroitin sulfate in regulating hypertrophy during MSC chondrogenesis in a cartilage mimetic hydrogel under dynamic loading." *Biomaterials* 190–191: 51–62.

Albu, M., L. Radev, I. Titorenku and T. Vladkova. 2013. "Fibrillar collagen/bioactive calcium phosphate silicate glass-ceramic composites for bone tissue engineering." *Current Tissue Engineering* 2 (2): 119–132.

Albu, M., V. Trandafir, D. Suflet, G. Chitanu, P. Budrugeac and I. Titorencu. 2012. "Biocomposites based on collagen and phosphorylated dextran for bone regeneration." *Journal of Materials Research* 27 (7): 1086–1096.

Alinejad, Y., A. Adoungotchodo, E. Hui, F. Zehtabi and S. Lerouge. 2018. "An injectable chitosan/chondroitin sulfate hydrogel with tunable mechanical properties for cell therapy/tissue engineering." *International Journal of Biological Macromolecules* 113: 132–141.

Almeida, H., R. Eswaramoorthy, G. Cunniffe, C. Buckley, F. O'brien and D. Kelly. 2016. "Fibrin hydrogels functionalized with cartilage extracellular matrix and incorporating freshly isolated stromal cells as an injectable for cartilage regeneration." *Acta Biomaterialia* 36: 55–62.

Almqvist, K., L. Wang, J. Wang, D. Baeten, M. Cornelissen, R. Verdonk, E. Veys and G. Verbruggen. 2001. "Culture of chondrocytes in alginate surrounded by fibrin gel: Characteristics of the cells over a period of eight weeks." *Annals of the Rheumatic Diseases* 60 (8): 781–790.

Ang, A., R. Ahmed and C. C. Berndt. 2018. "Biomaterials: Thermal spray processes and applications." *Journal of Thermal Spray Technology* 27 (8): 1205–1211.

Angele, P., J. Abke, R. Kujat, H. Faltermeier, D. Schumann, M. Nerlich, B. Kinner, C. Englert, Z. Ruszczak and R. Mehrl. 2004. "Influence of different collagen species on physicochemical properties of crosslinked collagen matrices." *Biomaterials* 25 (14): 2831–2841.

Anisha, B. S., D. Sankar, A. Mohandas, K. P. Chennazhi, S. V. Nair and R. Jayakumar. et al. 2013 "Chitosan–hyaluronan/nano chondroitin sulfate ternary composite sponges for medical use." *Carbohydrate Polymers* 92(2): 1470–1476.

Ao, C., Y. Niu, X. Zhang, X. He, W. Zhang and C. Lu. 2017. "Fabrication and characterization of electrospun cellulose/nano-hydroxyapatite nanofibers for bone tissue engineering." *International Journal of Biological Macromolecules* 97: 568–573.

Armiento, A. R., M. J. Stoddart, M. Alini and D. Eglin. 2018. "Biomaterials for articular cartilage tissue engineering: Learning from biology." *Acta Biomaterialia* 65: 1–20.

Aslan, M., G. Şimşek and E. Dayi. 2006. "The effect of hyaluronic acid-supplemented bone graft in bone healing: Experimental study in rabbits." *Journal of Biomaterials Applications* 20 (3): 209–220.

Awad, H. A., M. Q. Wickham, H. A. Leddy, J. M. Gimble and F. Guilak. 2004. "Chondrogenic differentiation of adipose-derived adult stem cells in agarose, alginate, and gelatin scaffolds." *Biomaterials* 25 (16): 3211–3222.

Aydin, O., F. Korkusuz, P. Korkusuz, A. Tezcaner, E. Bilgic, V. Yaprakci and D. Keskin. 2015. "I n vitro and in vivo evaluation of doxycycline-chondroitin sulfate/PCL microspheres for intraarticular treatment of osteoarthritis." *Journal of Biomedical Materials Research Part B: Applied Biomaterials* 103 (6): 1238–1248.

Bai, X., S. Lü, Z. Cao, B. Ni, X. Wang, P. Ning, D. Ma, H. Wei and M. Liu. 2017. "Dual crosslinked chondroitin sulfate injectable hydrogel formed via continuous Diels-Alder (DA) click chemistry for bone repair." *Carbohydrate Polymers* 166: 123–130.

Baker, M. I., S. P. Walsh, Z. Schwartz and B. D. Boyan. 2012. "A review of polyvinyl alcohol and its uses in cartilage and orthopedic applications." *Journal of Biomedical Materials Research Part B: Applied Biomaterials* 100 (5): 1451–1457.

Bang, S., U. W. Jung and I. Noh. 2018. "Synthesis and biocompatibility characterizations of in situ chondroitin sulfate–gelatin hydrogel for tissue engineering." *Tissue Engineering and Regenerative Medicine* 15 (1): 25–35.

Barbon, S., E. Stocco, V. Macchi, M. Contran, F. Grandi, A. Borean, P. P. Parnigotto, A. Porzionato and R. De Caro. 2019. "Platelet-rich fibrin scaffolds for cartilage and tendon regenerative medicine: From bench to bedside." *International Journal of Molecular Sciences* 20 (7) 1–38.

Barbon, S. et al. 2022. "PVA-based hydrogels loaded with diclofenac for cartilage replacement." *Gels* 8(3): 143.

Bas, O., S. Lucarotti, D. D. Angella, N. J. Castro, C. Meinert, F. M. Wunner, E. Rank, G. Vozzi, T. J. Klein and I. Catelas. 2018. "Rational design and fabrication of multiphasic soft network composites for tissue engineering articular cartilage: A numerical model-based approach." *Chemical Engineering Journal* 340: 15–23.

Bayram, C., M. Demirbilek, E. Yalçın, M. Bozkurt, M. Doğan and E. B. Denkbaş. 2014. Osteoblast response on co-modified titanium surfaces via anodization and electrospinning. *Applied Surface Science* 288: 143–148.

Becerra, J., M. Rodriguez, D Leal, K. Noris-Suarez and G. Gonzalez. 2022. "Chitosan-collagen-hydroxyapatite membranes for tissue engineering." *Journal of Materials Science: Materials in Medicine* 33(2): 18.

Bejarano, J., R. Detsch, A. R. Boccaccini and H. Palza. 2017. "PDLLA scaffolds with Cu-and Zndoped bioactive glasses having multifunctional properties for bone regeneration." *Journal of Biomedical Materials Research Part A* 105 (3): 746–756.

Bello, A. B., D. Kim, D. Kim, H. Park and S.-H. Lee. 2020. "Engineering and functionalization of gelatin biomaterials: From cell culture to medical applications." *Tissue Engineering Part B: Reviews* 26 (2): 164–180.

Bendtsen, S. T., S. P. Quinnell and M. Wei. 2017. "Development of a novel alginate-polyvinyl alcohol-hydroxyapatite hydrogel for 3D bioprinting bone tissue engineered scaffolds." *Journal of Biomedical Materials Research Part A* 105 (5): 1457–1468.

Bharadwaz, A. and A. C. Jayasuriya. 2020. "Recent trends in the application of widely used natural and synthetic polymer nanocomposites in bone tissue regeneration." *Materials Science and Engineering C-Materials for Biological Applications* 110.

Bodick, N., T. Williamson, V. Strand, B. Senter, S. Kelley., R. Boyce and R. Lightfoot-Dunn. 2018. "Local effects following single and repeat intra-articular injections of triamcinolone acetonide extended-release: results from three nonclinical toxicity studies in dogs." *Rheumatology and Therapy* 5(2): 475–498.

Bonaventure, J., N. Kadhom, L. Cohen-Solal, K. Ng, J. Bourguignon, C. Lasselin and P. Freisinger. 1994. "Reexpression of cartilage-specific genes by dedifferentiated human articular chondrocytes cultured in alginate beads." *Experimental Cell Research* 212 (1): 97–104.

Bozkurt, M., M. D. Aşık, S. Gürsoy, M. Türk, S. Karahan, B. Gümüşkaya, M. Akkaya, M. E. Şimşek, N. Cay and M. Doğan. 2019. "Autologous stem cell-derived chondrocyte implantation with bio-targeted microspheres for the treatment of osteochondral defects." *Journal of Orthopaedic Surgery and Research* 14(1): 1–13.

Brunette, D. M., P. Tengvall, M. Textor and P. Thomsen. 2001. *Titanium in Medicine: Material Science, Surface Science, Engineering, Biological Responses and Medical Applications* (p. 232). Berlin: Springer.

Bulpitt, P. and D. Aeschlimann. 1999. "New strategy for chemical modification of hyaluronic acid: Preparation of functionalized derivatives and their use in the formation of novel biocompatible hydrogels." *Journal of Biomedical Materials Research* 47 (2): 152–169.

Cao, Z., C. Dou and S. Dong. 2014. "Scaffolding biomaterials for cartilage regeneration." *Journal of Nanomaterials* 2014: 1–8

Capuana, E., F. Lopresti, M. Ceraulo and V. La Carrubba. 2022. "Poly-l-Lactic Acid (PLLA)-based biomaterials for regenerative medicine: A review on processing and applications."*Polymers* (Basel) 14 (6): 1153.

Carnes, M. E., C. R. Gonyea, R. G. Mooney, J. W. Njihia, J. M. Coburn and G. D. Pins. 2020. "Horseradish peroxidase-catalyzed crosslinking of fibrin microthread scaffolds. " *Tissue Engineering Part C: Methods* 26 (6): 317–331.

Carossino, A. M., R. Recenti, R. Carossino, E. Piscitelli, A. Gozzini, V. Martineti, C. Mavilia, A. Franchi, D. Danielli and P. Aglietti. 2007. "Methodological models for in vitro amplification and maintenance of human articular chondrocytes from elderly patients." *Biogerontology* 8 (5): 483–498.

Catoira, M. C., L. Fusaro, D. Di Francesco, M. Ramella and F. Boccafoschi. 2019. "Overview of natural hydrogels for regenerative medicine applications." *Journal of Materials Science: Materials in Medicine* 30 (10): 1–10.

Cen, L., W. Liu, L. Cui, W. Zhang and Y. Cao. 2008. "Collagen tissue engineering: Development of novel biomaterials and applications." *Pediatric Research* 63 (5): 492–496.

Centola, M., F. Abbruzzese, C. Scotti, A. Barbero, G. Vadala, V. Denaro, I. Martin, M. Trombetta, A. Rainer and A. Marsano. 2013. "Scaffold-based delivery of a clinically relevant anti-angiogenic drug promotes the formation of in vivo stable cartilage." *Tissue Engineering Part A* 19 (17–18): 1960–1971.

Chan, Y. W., R. W. M. Ng, L. H. L. Liu, H. P. Chung, and W. I. Wei. 2011. "Reconstruction of circumferential pharyngeal defects after tumour resection: Reference or preference." *Journal of Plastic, Reconstructive & Aesthetic Surgery* 64(8): 1022–1028.

Chang, C. H., H. C. Liu, C. C. Lin, C. H. Chou and F. H. Lin. 2003. "Gelatin–chondroitin–hyaluronan tri-copolymer scaffold for cartilage tissue engineering." *Biomaterials* 24 (26): 4853–4858.

Chang, K. Y., L. H. Hung, I. M. Chu, C. S. Ko and Y. D. Lee. 2010. "The application of type II collagen and chondroitin sulfate grafted PCL porous scaffold in cartilage tissue engineering." *Journal of Biomedical Materials Research Part A: An Official Journal of the Society for Biomaterials, the Japanese Society for Biomaterials, and the Australian Society for Biomaterials and the Korean Society for Biomaterials* 92 (2): 712–723.

Chang, N. J., Y. R. Jhung, C. K. Yao and M. L. Yeh. 2013. "Hydrophilic gelatin and hyaluronic acid-treated PLGA scaffolds for cartilage tissue engineering." *Journal of Applied Biomaterials & Functional Materials* 11 (1): 45–52.

Chawla, D., T. Kaur, A. Joshi and N. Singh. 2020. "3D bioprinted alginate-gelatin based scaffolds for soft tissue engineering." *International Journal of Biological Macromolecules* 144: 560–567.

Chen, C.-H., C. Y. Kuo, Y. J. Wang and J. P. Chen. 2016. "Dual function of glucosamine in gelatin/hyaluronic acid cryogel to modulate scaffold mechanical properties and to maintain chondrogenic phenotype for cartilage tissue engineering." *International Journal of Molecular Sciences* 17(11): 1957.

Chen, F., S. Yu, B. Liu, Y. Ni, C. Yu, Y. Su, X. Zhu, X. Yu, Y. Zhou and D. Yan. 2016. "An injectable enzymatically crosslinked carboxymethylated pullulan/chondroitin sulfate hydrogel for cartilage tissue engineering." *Scientific Reports* 6 (1): 1–12.

Chen, H., D. He, Y. Zhu, W. Yu, M. Ramalingam and Z. Wu. 2019. "In situ osteochondral regeneration by controlled release of stromal cell-derived factor-1 chemokine from injectable biomaterials: a preclinical evaluation in animal model." *Journal of Biomaterials and Tissue Engineering* 9(7): 958–967.

Chen, J. P. and C. H. Su. 2011. "Surface modification of electrospun PLLA nanofibers by plasma treatment and cationized gelatin immobilization for cartilage tissue engineering." *Acta Biomaterialia* 7(1): 234–243.

Chen, L., J. Hu, J. Ran, X. Shen and H. Tong. 2014. "Preparation and evaluation of collagen-silk fibroin/hydroxyapatite nanocomposites for bone tissue engineering." *International Journal of Biological Macromolecules* 65: 1–7.

Chen, P., C. Xia, S. Mei, J. Wang, Z. Shan, X. Lin and S. Fan. 2016. "Intra-articular delivery of sinomenium encapsulated by chitosan microspheres and photo-crosslinked GelMA hydrogel ameliorates osteoarthritis by effectively regulating autophagy." *Biomaterials* 81: 1–13.

Chen, Y., N. Kawazoe and G. Chen. 2018. "Preparation of dexamethasone-loaded biphasic calcium phosphate nanoparticles/collagen porous composite scaffolds for bone tissue engineering." *Acta Biomaterialia* 67: 341–353.

Chen, Z., G. Griffanti, M. D. McKee and S. N. Nazhat. 2017. "Laminated electrospun nHA/PHB-composite scaffolds mimicking bone extracellular matrix for bone tissue engineering." *Materials Science and Engineering: C* 72: 341–351.

Chicatun, F., G. Griffanti, M. D. McKee and S. N. Nazhat. 2017. "Collagen/chitosan composite scaffolds for bone and cartilage tissue engineering." *Biomedical Composites* 163–198.

Choi, S., J. H. Kim, J. Ha, B. I. Jeong, Y. C. Jung, G. S. Lee, H. M. Woo and B. J. Kang. 2018. "Intra-articular injection of alginate-microencapsulated adipose tissue-derived mesenchymal stem cells for the treatment of osteoarthritis in rabbits." *Stem Cells International* 2018: 1–11.

Chuang, E. Y., C. W. Chiang, P. C. Wong and C. H. Chen. 2018. "Hydrogels for the application of articular cartilage tissue engineering: A review of hydrogels." *Advances in Materials Science and Engineering* 2018: 1–14.

Collin, E. C., O. Carroll, M. Kilcoyne, M. Peroglio, E. See, D. Hendig, M. Alini, S. Grad and A. Pandit. 2017. "Ageing affects chondroitin sulfates and their synthetic enzymes in the intervertebral disc." *Signal Transduction and Targeted Therapy* 2 (1): 1–8.

Collins, M. N. and C. Birkinshaw "Hyaluronic acid based scaffolds for tissue engineering--a review." (1879–1344 (Electronic)).

Cooper, B. G., R. C. Stewart, D. Burstein, B. D. Snyder and M. W. Grinstaff. 2016. "A tissue-penetrating double network restores the mechanical properties of degenerated articular cartilage." *Angewandte Chemie* 128 (13): 4298–4302.

Daly, A. C., F. E. Freeman, T. Gonzalez-Fernandez, S. E. Critchley, J. Nulty and D. J. Kelly. 2017. "3D bioprinting for cartilage and osteochondral tissue engineering." *Advanced Healthcare Materials* 6 (22): 1700298.

Dashtdar, H., M. R. Murali, A. A. Abbas, A. M. Suhaeb, L. Selvaratnam, L. X. Tay and T. Kamarul. 2015. "PVA-chitosan composite hydrogel versus alginate beads as a potential mesenchymal stem cell carrier for the treatment of focal cartilage defects." *Knee Surgery, Sports Traumatology, Arthroscopy* 23 (5): 1368–1377.

Deal, C. L. and R. W. Moskowitz. 1999. "Nutraceuticals as therapeutic agents in osteoarthritis: The role of glucosamine, chondroitin sulfate, and collagen hydrolysate." *Rheumatic Disease Clinics of North America* 25 (2): 379–395.

Deitzer, M. A. 2006. *Fibrin Gels: A Potential Biomaterial for the Chondrogenesis of Bone Marrow Mesenchymal Stem Cells*, University of Miami.

Deng, J., R. She, W. Huang, Z. Dong, G. Mo and B. Liu. 2013. "A silk fibroin/chitosan scaffold in combination with bone marrow-derived mesenchymal stem cells to repair cartilage defects in the rabbit knee." *Journal of Materials Science: Materials in Medicine* 24 (8): 2037–2046.

Derfoul, A., A. Miyoshi, D. Freeman and R. Tuan. 2007. "Glucosamine promotes chondrogenic phenotype in both chondrocytes and mesenchymal stem cells and inhibits MMP-13 expression and matrix degradation." *Osteoarthritis and Cartilage* 15 (6): 646–655.

Detsch, R., S. Schaefer, U. Deisinger, G. Ziegler, H. Seitz and B. Leukers. 2011. "In vitro-osteoclastic activity studies on surfaces of 3D printed calcium phosphate scaffolds." *Journal of Biomaterials Applications* 26 (3): 359–380.

Dhand, C., S. T. Ong, N. Dwivedi, S. M. Diaz, J. R. Venugopal, B. Navaneethan and R. Lakshminarayanan. 2016. "Bio-inspired in situ crosslinking and mineralization of electrospun collagen scaffolds for bone tissue engineering." *Biomaterials* 104: 323–338.

Dhivya, S., A. Keshav Narayan, R. Logith Kumar, S. Viji Chandran, M. Vairamani and N. Selvamurugan. 2018. "Proliferation and differentiation of mesenchymal stem cells on scaffolds containing chitosan, calcium polyphosphate and pigeonite for bone tissue engineering." *Cell Proliferation* 51(1): e12408.

Di Luca, A., A. Longoni, G. Criscenti, I. Lorenzo-Moldero, M. Klein-Gunnewiek, J. Vancso, C. van Blitterswijk, C. Mota and L. Moroni. 2016. "Surface energy and stiffness discrete gradients in additive manufactured scaffolds for osteochondral regeneration." *Biofabrication* 8 (1): 015014.

Djouad, F., L. M. Charbonnier, C. Bouffi, P. Louis-Plence, C. Bony, F. Apparailly, C. Cantos, C. Jorgensen and D. Noël. 2007. "Mesenchymal stem cells inhibit the differentiation of dendritic cells through an interleukin-6-dependent mechanism." *Stem Cells* 25 (8): 2025–2032.

Dodge, G. R. and S. Jimenez. 2003. "Glucosamine sulfate modulates the levels of aggrecan and matrix metalloproteinase-3 synthesized by cultured human osteoarthritis articular chondrocytes." *Osteoarthritis and Cartilage* 11 (6): 424–432.

Dominici, M., K. Le Blanc, I. Mueller, I. Slaper-Cortenbach, F. Marini, D. Krause, R. Deans, A. Keating, D. Prockop and E. Horwitz. 2006. "Minimal criteria for defining multipotent mesenchymal stromal cells. The international society for cellular therapy position statement." *Cytotherapy* 8 (4): 315–317.

Dorozhkin, S. V. 2010. "Bioceramics of calcium orthophosphates." *Biomaterials* 31 (7): 1465–1485.

Dragan, E. S. 2014. "Design and applications of interpenetrating polymer network hydrogels. A review." *Chemical Engineering Journal* 243: 572–590.

Drury, J. L., R. G. Dennis and D. J. Mooney. 2004. "The tensile properties of alginate hydrogels." *Biomaterials* 25 (16): 3187–3199.

Drury, J. L. and D. J. Mooney. 2003. "Hydrogels for tissue engineering: scaffold design variables and applications." *Biomaterials* 24 (24): 4337–4351.

Du, Y., H. Liu, Q. Yang, S. Wang, J. Wang, J. Ma, I. Noh, A. G. Mikos and S. Zhang. 2017. "Selective laser sintering scaffold with hierarchical architecture and gradient composition for osteochondral repair in rabbits." *Biomaterials* 137: 37–48.

Dutta, S. D., D. K. Patel and K. T. Lim. 2019. "Functional cellulose-based hydrogels as extracellular matrices for tissue engineering." *Journal of Biological Engineering* 13 1–19.

Echave, M. C., L. S. Burgo, J. L. Pedraz and G. Orive. 2017. "Gelatin as biomaterial for tissue engineering." *Current Pharmaceutical Design* 23 (24): 3567–3584.

Echave, M. C., R. Hernáez-Moya, L. Iturriaga, J. L. Pedraz, R. Lakshminarayanan, A. Dolatshahi-Pirouz and G. Orive. 2019. "Recent advances in gelatin-based therapeutics." *Expert Opinion on Biological Therapy* 19(8): 773–779.

Elango, J., J. Zhang, B. Bao, K. Palaniyandi, S. Wang, W. Wenhui and J. S. Robinson. 2016. "Rheological, biocompatibility and osteogenesis assessment of fish collagen scaffold for bone tissue engineering." *International Journal of Biological Macromolecules* 91: 51–59.

Enayati, M. S., T. Behzad, P. Sajkiewicz, M. Rafienia, R. Bagheri, L. Ghasemi-Mobarakeh, D. Kolbuk, Z. Pahlevanneshan and S. H. Bonakdar. 2018. "Development of electrospun poly (vinyl alcohol)-based bionanocomposite scaffolds for bone tissue engineering." *Journal of Biomedical Materials Research Part A* 106 (4): 1111–1120.

Erickson, G. R., J. M. Gimble, D. M. Franklin, H. E. Rice, H. Awad and F. Guilak. 2002. "Chondrogenic potential of adipose tissue-derived stromal cells in vitro and in vivo." *Biochemical and Biophysical Research Communications* 290 (2): 763–769.

Ezazi, N. Z., M. A. Shahbazi, Y. V. Shatalin, E. Nadal, E. Mäkilä, J. Salonen, M. Kemell, A. Correia, J. Hirvonen and H. A. Santos. 2018. "Conductive vancomycin-loaded mesoporous silica polypyrrole-based scaffolds for bone regeneration." *International Journal of Pharmaceutics* 536 (1): 241–250.

Fang, J., Y. Zhang, S. Yan, Z. Liu, S. He, L. Cui and J. Yin. 2014. "Poly (L-glutamic acid)/ chitosan polyelectrolyte complex porous microspheres as cell microcarriers for cartilage regeneration." *Acta Biomaterialia* 10(1): 276–288.

Fernandes, H. R., A. Gaddam, A. Rebelo, D. Brazete, G. E. Stan and J. M. Ferreira. 2018. "Bioactive glasses and glass-ceramics for healthcare applications in bone regeneration and tissue engineering." *Materials* 11(12): 2530.

Filová, E., Z. Tonar, V. Lukášová, M. Buzgo, A. Litvinec, M. Rampichová, J. Beznoska, M. Plencner, A. Staffa and J. Daňková. 2020. "Hydrogel containing anti-CD44-labeled microparticles, guide bone tissue formation in osteochondral defects in rabbits." *Nanomaterials* 10 (8): 1504.

Fomby, P., A. Cherlin, A. Hadjizadeh, C. Doillon, V. Sueblinvong, D. Weiss, J. Bates, T. Gilbert, W. Liles and C. Lutzko. 2010. "Stem cells and cell therapies in lung biology and diseases: Conference report." *Annals of the American Thoracic Society* 12 (3): 181–204.

Fourie, J., F. Taute, L. du Preez and D. de Beer. 2022. "Chitosan composite biomaterials for bone tissue engineering—a review, *Regenerative Engineering and Translational Medicine* 8: 1–21.

Fragonas, E., M. Valente, M. Pozzi-Mucelli, R. Toffanin, R. Rizzo, F. Silvestri and F. Vittur. 2000. "Articular cartilage repair in rabbits by using suspensions of allogenic chondrocytes in alginate." *Biomaterials* 21 (8): 795–801.

Müller, F. A., L. Müller, I. Hofmann, P. Greil, Magdalene, M. Wenzelb and R. Staudenmaier. 2006. "Cellulose-based scaffold materials for cartilage tissue engineering." Biomaterials 27(21): 3955–3963.

Freed, L., D. Grande, Z. Lingbin, J. Emmanual, J. Marquis and R. Langer. 1994. "Joint resurfacing using allograft chondrocytes and synthetic biodegradable polymer scaffolds." *Journal of Biomedical Materials Research* 28 (8): 891–899.

Freed, L., G. Vunjak-Novakovic and R. Langer. 1993. "Cultivation of cell-polymer cartilage implants in bioreactors." *Journal of Cellular Biochemistry* 51 (3): 257–264.

Fricain, J. C., S. Schlaubitz, C. Le Visage, I. Arnault, S. M. Derkaoui, R. Siadous, S. Catros, C. Lalande, R. Bareille and M. Renard. 2013. "A nano-hydroxyapatite–pullulan/dextran polysaccharide composite macroporous material for bone tissue engineering." *Biomaterials* 34 (12): 2947–2959.

Frohbergh, M. E., A. Katsman, G. P. Botta, P. Lazarovici, C. L. Schauer, U. G. Wegst and P. I. Lelkes. 2012. "Electrospun hydroxyapatite-containing chitosan nanofibers crosslinked with genipin for bone tissue engineering." *Biomaterials* 33(36): 9167–9178.

Fu, L., Z. Yang, C. Gao, H. Li, Z. Yuan, F. Wang, X. Sui, S. Liu and Q. Guo. 2020. "Advances and prospects in biomimetic multilayered scaffolds for articular cartilage regeneration." *Regenerative Biomaterials* 7 (6): 527–542.

Fukunishi, T., C. A. Best, T. Sugiura, T. Shoji, T. Yi, B. Udelsman, D. Ohst, C. S. Ong, H. Zhang and T. Shinoka. 2016. "Tissue-engineered small diameter arterial vascular grafts from cell-free nanofiber PCL/chitosan scaffolds in a sheep model." *PLoS One* 11 (7): e0158555.

Fussenegger, M., J. Meinhart, W. Hobling, W. Kullich, S. Funk and G. Bernatzky. 2003. "Stabilized autologous fibrin-chondrocyte constructs for cartilage repair in vivo." *Annals of Plastic Surgery* 51 (5): 493–498.

Gaharwar, A. K., S. A. Dammu, J. M. Canter, C.-J. Wu and G. Schmidt. 2011. "Highly extensible, tough, and elastomeric nanocomposite hydrogels from poly(ethylene glycol) and hydroxyapatite nanoparticles." *Biomacromolecules* 12 (5): 1641–1650.

Gan, D., Z. Wang, C. Xie, X. Wang, W. Xing, X. Ge, H. Yuan, K. Wang, H. Tan and X. Lu. 2019. "Mussel-inspired tough hydrogel with in situ nanohydroxyapatite mineralization for osteochondral defect repair." *Advanced Healthcare Materials* 8 (22): 1901103.

Gao, G., A. F. Schilling, K. Hubbell, T. Yonezawa, D. Truong, Y. Hong, G. Dai and X. Cui. 2015. "Improved properties of bone and cartilage tissue from 3D inkjet-bioprinted human mesenchymal stem cells by simultaneous deposition and photocrosslinking in PEG-GelMA." *Biotechnology Letters* 37 (11): 2349–2355.

Garakani, S. S., et al. 2020. "Fabrication of chitosan/agarose scaffolds containing extracellular matrix for tissue engineering applications." *International Journal of Biological Macromolecules* 143: 533–545.

Ge, Z., L. Wang, B. C. Heng, X.-F. Tian, K. Lu, V. Tai Weng Fan, J. F. Yeo, T. Cao and E. Tan. 2009. "Proliferation and differentiation of human osteoblasts within 3D printed poly-lactic-co-glycolic acid scaffolds." *Journal of Biomaterials Applications* 23 (6): 533–547.

Geesala, R., N. Bar, N. R. Dhoke, P. Basak and A. Das. 2016. "Porous polymer scaffold for on-site delivery of stem cells–protects from oxidative stress and potentiates wound tissue repair." *Biomaterials* 77: 1–13.

Gentile, P., V. Chiono, I. Carmagnola and P. V. Hatton. 2014. "An overview of poly (lactic-co-glycolic) acid (PLGA)-based biomaterials for bone tissue engineering." *International Journal of Molecular Sciences* 15 (3): 3640–3659.

Giuliani, C. 2019. "The flavonoid quercetin induces AP-1 activation in FRTL-5 thyroid cells." *Antioxidants* 8(5): 1–10.

Goa, K. L. and P. Benfield. 1994. "Hyaluronic acid." *Drugs* 47 (3): 536–566.

Goldenberg, I. S. 1959. "Catgut, silk, and silver--the story of surgical sutures." *Surgery* 46: 908–912.

Gong, Y., Y. Zhu, Y. Liu, Z. Ma, C. Gao and J. Shen. 2007. "Layer-by-layer assembly of chondroitin sulfate and collagen on aminolyzed poly (L-lactic acid) porous scaffolds to enhance their chondrogenesis." *Acta Biomaterialia* 3(5): 677–685.

Guarino, V., F. Causa, P. Taddei, M. Di Foggia, G. Ciapetti, D. Martini, C. Fagnano, N. Baldini and L. Ambrosio. 2008. "Polylactic acid fibre-reinforced polycaprolactone scaffolds for bone tissue engineering." *Biomaterials* 29 (27): 3662–3670.

Gui, X., Q. Li, J. Yu and Z. Jiang. 2017. "Injectable controlled release of SDF-1-loaded microspheres reduces cartilage degradation in a rabbit experimental osteoarthritis model." *Journal of Biomaterials and Tissue Engineering* 7(11): 1177–1183.

Gupta, R. C., R. Lall, A. Srivastava and A. Sinha. 2019. "Hyaluronic acid: molecular mechanisms and therapeutic trajectory." *Frontiers in Veterinary Science* 6: 1–24.

Halima, N. B. 2016. "Poly (vinyl alcohol): Review of its promising applications and insights into biodegradation." *RSC Advances* 6 (46): 39823–39832.

Hamad, K., M. Kaseem and F. Deri. 2012. "Preparation and characterization of binary and ternary blends with poly (lactic acid), polystyrene, and acrylonitrile-butadiene-styrene." *Journal of Biomaterials and Nanobiotechnology* 3: 405–412.

Hammad, Y. H., H. R. Magid and M. M. Sobhy. 2015. "Clinical and biochemical study of the comparative efficacy of topical versus oral glucosamine/chondroitin sulfate on osteoarthritis of the knee." *The Egyptian Rheumatologist* 37 (2): 85–91.

Han, L., J. L. Xu, X. Lu, D. L. Gan, Z. X. Wang, K. F. Wang, H. P. Zhang, H. P. Yuan and J. Weng. 2017. "Biohybrid methacrylated gelatin/polyacrylamide hydrogels for cartilage repair." *Journal of Materials Chemistry B* 5 (4): 731–741.

Han, L., N. Xu, S. Lv, J. Yin, D. Zheng and X. Li. 2021. "Enhanced in vitro and in vivo efficacy of alginate/silk protein/hyaluronic acid with polypeptide microsphere delivery for tissue regeneration of articular cartilage." *Journal of Biomedical Nanotechnology* 17 (5): 901–909.

Hanna, H., M. M., Lluis and F.M. Andre. 2018. "In vitro osteoblastic differentiation of mesenchymal stem cells generates cell layers with distinct properties." *Stem Cell Research & Therapy* 9, Article number: 203.

Hanson, R. R., L. R. Smalley, G. K. Huff, S. White and T. A. Hammad. 1997. "Oral treatment with a glucosamine-chondroitin sulfate compound for degenerative joint disease in horses: 25 cases." Equine Practice 19: 16–22.

Haq, M. A., Y. Su and D. Wang. 2017. "Mechanical properties of PNIPAM based hydrogels: A review." *Materials Science and Engineering: C* 70: 842–855.

Hassanajili, S., A. Karami-Pour, A. Oryan and T. Talaei-Khozani. 2019. "Preparation and characterization of PLA/PCL/HA composite scaffolds using indirect 3D printing for bone tissue engineering." *Materials Science and Engineering: C* 104: 109960.

Hautier, G., A. Jain and S. P. Ong. 2012. "From the computer to the laboratory: materials discovery and design using first-principles calculations." *Journal of Materials Science* 47 (21): 7317–7340.

Hench, L. L. and J. M. Polak. 2002. "Third-generation biomedical materials." *Science* 295 (5557): 1014–1017.

Hendrickson, D. A., A. J. Nixon, D. A. Grande, R. J. Todhunter, R. M. Minor, H. Erb and G. Lust. 1994. "Chondrocyte-fibrin matrix transplants for resurfacing extensive articular cartilage defects." *Journal of Orthopaedic Research* 12 (4): 485–497.

Heydari, Z., D. Mohebbi-Kalhori and M. S. Afarani. 2017. "Engineered electrospun polycaprolactone (PCL)/octacalcium phosphate (OCP) scaffold for bone tissue engineering." *Materials Science and Engineering: C* 81: 127–132.

Hoemann, C. D., J. Sun, A. Legare, M. D. McKee and M. D. Buschmann. 2005. "Tissue engineering of cartilage using an injectable and adhesive chitosan-based cell-delivery vehicle." *Osteoarthritis and Cartilage* 13(4): 318–329.

Hong, S., S.-J. Song, J. Y. Lee, H. Jang, J. Choi, K. Sun and Y. Park. 2013. "Cellular behavior in micropatterned hydrogels by bioprinting system depended on the cell types and cellular interaction." *Journal of Bioscience and Bioengineering* 116 (2): 224–230.

Hou, K.-T., T. Y. Liu, M. Y. Chiang, C. Y. Chen, S. J. Chang and S. Y. Chen. 2020. "Cartilage tissue-mimetic pellets with multifunctional magnetic hyaluronic acid-graft-amphiphilic gelatin microcapsules for chondrogenic stimulation." *Polymers* 12(4): 785.

Hu, W., Z. Wang, Y. Xiao, S. Zhang and J. Wang. 2019. "Advances in crosslinking strategies of biomedical hydrogels." *Biomaterials Science* 7 (3): 843–855.

Hu, X., D. Li, F. Zhou and C. Gao. 2011. "Biological hydrogel synthesized from hyaluronic acid, gelatin and chondroitin sulfate by click chemistry." *Acta Biomaterialia* 7 (4): 1618–1626.

Hubbe, M. A., P. Tayeb, M. Joyce, P. Tyagi, M. Kehoe, K. Dimic-Misic and L. Pal. 2017. "Rheology of nanocellulose-rich aqueous suspensions: A review." *Bioresources* 12 (4): 9556–9661.

Hunziker, E. B. 2002. "Articular cartilage repair: Basic science and clinical progress. A review of the current status and prospects." *Osteoarthritis and Cartilage* 10 (6): 432–463.

Hutmacher, D. W. 2000. "Scaffolds in tissue engineering bone and cartilage." *Biomaterials* 21 (24): 2529–2543.

Hwang, N. S., S. Varghese, H. J. Lee, P. Theprungsirikul, A. Canver, B. Sharma and J. Elisseeff. 2007. "Response of zonal chondrocytes to extracellular matrix-hydrogels." *FEBS Letters* 581 (22): 4172–4178.

Hwang, N. S., S. Varghese and J. Elisseeff. 2007. "Cartilage tissue engineering: directed differentiation of embryonic stem cells in three-dimensional hydrogel culture." *Stem Cell Assays* 407: 351–373.

Ingavle, G. C., N. H. Dormer, S. H. Gehrke and M. S. Detamore. 2012. "Using chondroitin sulfate to improve the viability and biosynthesis of chondrocytes encapsulated in interpenetrating network (IPN) hydrogels of agarose and poly (ethylene glycol) diacrylate." *Journal of Materials Science: Materials in Medicine* 23 (1): 157–170.

Inzana, J. A., D. Olvera, S. M. Fuller, J. P. Kelly, O. A. Graeve, E. M. Schwarz, S. L. Kates and H. A. Awad. 2014. "3D printing of composite calcium phosphate and collagen scaffolds for bone regeneration." *Biomaterials* 35 (13): 4026–4034.

Islam, M. S., M. S. Rahman, T. Ahmad, S. Biswas, P. Haque, and M. M. Rahman. 2020. Chitosan and chitosan-based biomaterials for wound management. *Handbook of Chitin and Chitosan. Volume 3: Chitin and Chitosan based Polymer Materials for Various Applications*: 721–759.

Islam, M. S., M. Shahruzzaman, S. Biswas, M. N. Sakib, and T. U. Rashid. 2020. "Chitosan based bioactive materials in tissue engineering applications-A review." *Bioactive Materials*, 5 (1): 164–183.

Isobe, N., T. Komamiya, S. Kimura, U. J. Kim and M. Wada. 2018. "Cellulose hydrogel with tunable shape and mechanical properties: From rigid cylinder to soft scaffold." 117: 625–631.

Jayabalan, P., A. R. Tan, M. N. Rahaman, B. S. Bal, C. T. Hung and J. L. Cook. 2011. "Bioactive glass 13-93 as a subchondral substrate for tissue-engineered osteochondral constructs: A pilot study". *Clinical Orthopaedics and Related Research* 469 (10): 2754–2763 doi:10.1007/s11999-011-1818-x

Jell, G. and M. Stevens. 2006. "Gene activation by bioactive glasses." *Journal of Materials Science: Materials in Medicine* 17 (11): 997–1002.

Jia, S., J. Wang, T. Zhang, W. Pan, Z. Li, X. He, C. Yang, Q. Wu, W. Sun and Z. Xiong. 2018. "Multilayered scaffold with a compact interfacial layer enhances osteochondral defect repair." *ACS Applied Materials & Interfaces* 10 (24): 20296–20305.

Jiang, P., J. Ran, P. Yan, L. Zheng, X. Shen and H. Tong. 2018. "Rational design of a high-strength bone scaffold platform based on in situ hybridization of bacterial cellulose/nano-hydroxyapatite framework and silk fibroin reinforcing phase." *Journal of Biomaterials Science Polymer Edition* 29(2): 107–124.

Jiang, T., W. I. Abdel-Fattah and C. T. Laurencin. 2006. "In vitro evaluation of chitosan/poly (lactic acid-glycolic acid) sintered microsphere scaffolds for bone tissue engineering." *Biomaterials* 27 (28): 4894–4903.

Jiang, X., J. Liu, Q. Liu, Z. Lu, L. Zheng, J. Zhao and X. Zhang. 2018. "Therapy for cartilage defects: Functional ectopic cartilage constructed by cartilage-simulating collagen, chondroitin sulfate and hyaluronic acid (CCH) hybrid hydrogel with allogeneic chondrocytes." *Biomaterials Science* 6 (6): 1616–1626.

Johnson, K., D. A. Hulse, R. C. Hart, D. Kochevar and Q. Chu. 2001. "Effects of an orally administered mixture of chondroitin sulfate, glucosamine hydrochloride and manganese ascorbate on synovial fluid chondroitin sulfate 3B3 and 7D4 epitope in a canine cruciate ligament transection model of osteoarthritis." *Osteoarthritis and Cartilage* 9(1): 14–21.

Ju, J., X. Peng, K. Huang, L. Li, X. Liu, C. Chitrakar and T. Kuang. 2019. "High-performance porous PLLA-based scaffolds for bone tissue engineering: Preparation, characterization, and in vitro and in vivo evaluation." *Polymer* 180: 121707.

Kamel, S., N. Ali, K. Jahangir, S. Shah and A. El-Gendy. 2008. "Pharmaceutical significance of cellulose: A review." *Express Polymer Letters* 2 (11): 758–778.

Kang, H.-W., S. J. Lee, I. K. Ko, C. Kengla, J. J. Yoo and A. Atala. 2016. "A 3D bioprinting system to produce human-scale tissue constructs with structural integrity." *Nature Biotechnology* 34 (3): 312–319.

Kanikireddy, V., K. Varaprasad, T. Jayaramudu, C. Karthikeyan and R. Sadiku. 2020. "Carboxymethyl cellulose-based materials for infection control and wound healing: A review." *International Journal of Biological Macromolecules* 164: 963–975.

Karageorgiou, V., L. Meinel, S. Hofmann, A. Malhotra, V. Volloch and D. Kaplan. 2004. "Bone morphogenetic protein-2 decorated silk fibroin films induce osteogenic differentiation of human bone marrow stromal cells." *Journal of Biomedical Materials Research Part A: An Official Journal of the Society for Biomaterials, the Japanese Society for Biomaterials, and the Australian Society for Biomaterials and the Korean Society for Biomaterials* 71 (3): 528–537.

Katti, K. S., D. R. Katti and R. Dash. 2008. "Synthesis and characterization of a novel chitosan/montmorillonite/hydroxyapatite nanocomposite for bone tissue engineering." *Biomedical Materials* 3 (3): 034122.

Kavya, K., R. Jayakumar, S. Nair and K. P. Chennazhi. 2013. "Fabrication and characterization of chitosan/gelatin/nSiO2 composite scaffold for bone tissue engineering." *International Journal of Biological Macromolecules* 59: 255–263.

Keller, L., A. Regiel-Futyra, M. Gimeno, S. Eap, G. Mendoza, V. Andreu, Q. Wagner, A. Kyziol, V. Sebastian, G. Stochel, M. Arruebo and N. Benkirane-Jessel. 2017. "Chitosan-based nanocomposites for the repair of bone defects." *Nanomedicine* 13 (7): 2231–2240.

Khaled, E., M. Saleh, S. Hindocha, M. Griffin and W. S. Khan. 2011. "Suppl 2: tissue engineering for bone production-stem cells, gene therapy and scaffolds." *The Open Orthopaedics Journal* 5: 289.

Khan, S. and N. M. Ranjha. 2014. "Effect of degree of cross-linking on swelling and on drug release of low viscous chitosan/poly (vinyl alcohol) hydrogels." *Polymer Bulletin* 71 (8): 2133–2158.

Khatab, S., M. J. Leijs, G. van Buul, J. Haeck, N. Kops, M. Nieboer, P. K. Bos, J. A. N. Verhaar, M. Bernsen and G. J. V. M. van Osch. 2020. "MSC encapsulation in alginate microcapsules prolongs survival after intra-articular injection, a longitudinal in vivo cell and bead integrity tracking study." *Cell Biology and Toxicology* 36 (6): 553–570.

Kim, C., O. H. Jeon, D. H. Kim, J. J. Chae, L. Shores, N. Bernstein and J. H. Elisseeff. 2016. "Local delivery of a carbohydrate analog for reducing arthritic inflammation and rebuilding cartilage." *Biomaterials* 83: 93–101.

Kim, H. D., Y. Lee, Y. Kim, Y. Hwang and N. S. Hwang. 2017. "Biomimetically reinforced polyvinyl alcohol-based hybrid scaffolds for cartilage tissue engineering." *Polymers* 9 (12): 655.

Kim, I. L., R. L. Mauck and J. A. Burdick. 2011. "Hydrogel design for cartilage tissue engineering: A case study with hyaluronic acid." *Biomaterials* 32 (34): 8771–8782.

Knudson, W., B. Casey, Y. Nishida, W. Eger, K. E. Kuettner and C. B. Knudson. 2000. "Hyaluronan oligosaccharides perturb cartilage matrix homeostasis and induce chondrocytic chondrolysis." *Arthritis Rheum* 43 (5): 1165–1174.

Kon, E., Delcogliano, M., Filardo, G., Busacca, M., Di Martino, A., & Marcacci, M. (2011). Novel nano-composite multilayered biomaterial for osteochondral regeneration: A pilot clinical trial. *The American Journal of Sports Medicine*, 39 (6): 1180–1190.

Kuiper, N. and A. Sharma. 2015. "A detailed quantitative outcome measure of glycosaminoglycans in human articular cartilage for cell therapy and tissue engineering strategies." *Osteoarthritis and Cartilage* 23 (12): 2233–2241.

Kundu, B., R. Rajkhowa, S. C. Kundu and X. Wang. 2013. "Silk fibroin biomaterials for tissue regenerations." *Advanced Drug Delivery Reviews* 65 (4): 457–470.

Kundu, J., J. H. Shim, J. Jang, S. W. Kim and D. W. Cho. 2015. "An additive manufacturing-based PCL–alginate–chondrocyte bioprinted scaffold for cartilage tissue engineering." *Journal of Tissue Engineering and Regenerative Medicine* 9 (11): 1286–1297.

Kuroda, R., K. Ishida, T. Matsumoto, T. Akisue, H. Fujioka, K. Mizuno, H. Ohgushi, S. Wakitani and M. Kurosaka. 2007. "Treatment of a full-thickness articular cartilage defect in the femoral condyle of an athlete with autologous bone-marrow stromal cells." *Osteoarthritis and Cartilage* 15 (2): 226–231.

Kutikov, A. B., J. D. Skelly, D. C. Ayers and J. Song. 2015. "Templated repair of long bone defects in rats with bioactive spiral-wrapped electrospun amphiphilic polymer/hydroxy-apatite scaffolds." *ACS Applied Materials & Interfaces* 7 (8): 4890–4901.

Kuznetsov, S. A., A. Hailu-Lazmi, N. Cherman, L. F. Castro, P. G. Robey and R. Gorodetsky. 2019. "In vivo formation of stable hyaline cartilage by naive human bone marrow stromal cells with modified fibrin microbeads." *Stem Cells Translational Medicine* 8 (6): 586–592.

Labet, M. and W. Thielemans. 2009. "Synthesis of polycaprolactone: A review." *Chemical Society Reviews* 38 (12): 3484–3504.

Lam, A., S. Reuveny, J. Li, J. Hui, W. Birch and S. Oh. 2020. "Human early mesenchymal stromal cells delivered on biodegradable polycaprolactone based microcarriers result in improved cartilage formation." *Cytotherapy* 22 (5): S97.

Lan, W., M. Xu, X. Zhang, L. Zhao, D. Huang, X. Wei and W. Chen. 2020. "Biomimetic poly-vinyl alcohol/type II collagen hydrogels for cartilage tissue engineering." *Journal of Biomaterials Science, Polymer Edition* 31 (9): 1179–1198.

Lanao, R. P. F., A. M. Jonker, J. G. Wolke, J. A. Jansen, J. C. van Hest and S. C. Leeuwenburgh. 2013. "Physicochemical properties and applications of poly (lactic-co-glycolic acid) for use in bone regeneration." *Tissue Engineering Part B: Reviews* 19 (4): 380–390.

Larsen, M., V. V. Artym, J. A. Green and K. M. Yamada. 2006. "The matrix reorganized: Extracellular matrix remodeling and integrin signaling." *Current Opinion in Cell Biology* 18 (5): 463–471.

Lee, C., A. Grodzinsky, H. P. Hsu and M. Spector. 2003. "Effects of a cultured autologous chondrocyte-seeded type II collagen scaffold on the healing of a chondral defect in a canine model." *Journal of Orthopaedic Research* 21 (2): 272–281.

Lee, C. H., A. Singla and Y. Lee. 2001. "Biomedical applications of collagen." *Interantional Journal of Pharmaceutics* 221 (1–2): 1–22.

Lee, C.-T.,C. P. Huang and Y. D. Lee. 2006. "Preparation of amphiphilic poly (L-lactide)-graft-chondroitin sulfate copolymer self-aggregates and its aggregation behavior." *Biomacromolecules* 7(4): 1179–1186.

Lee, D. H., N. Tripathy, J. H. Shin, J. E. Song, J. G. Cha, K. D. Min, C. H. Park and G. Khang. 2017. "Enhanced osteogenesis of β-tricalcium phosphate reinforced silk fibroin scaffold for bone tissue biofabrication." *International Journal of Biological Macromolecules* 95: 14–23.

Leferink, A. M., W. Hendrikson, J. Rouwkema, M. Karperien, C. Van Blitterswijk and L. Moroni. 2016. "Increased cell seeding efficiency in bioplotted three-dimensional PEOT/PBT scaffolds." *Journal of Tissue Engineering and Regenerative Medicine* 10 (8): 679–689.

Lei, Y., Z. Xu, Q. Ke, W. Yin, Y. Chen, C. Zhang and Y. Guo. 2017. "Strontium hydroxyapatite/chitosan nanohybrid scaffolds with enhanced osteoinductivity for bone tissue engineering." *Materials Science and Engineering: C* 72: 134–142.

Leslie, S. K., D. J. Cohen, S. L. Hyzy, C. R. Dosier, A. Nicolini, J. Sedlaczek and B. D. Boyan. 2018. "Microencapsulated rabbit adipose stem cells initiate tissue regeneration in a rabbit ear defect model." *Journal of Tissue Engineering and Regenerative Medicine* 12(7): 1742–1753.

Levengood, S. K. L. and M. Zhang. 2014. "Chitosan-based scaffolds for bone tissue engineering." *Journal of Materials Chemistry B* 2 (21): 3161–3184.

Levett, P. A., F. P. Melchels, K. Schrobback, D. W. Hutmacher, J. Malda and T. J. Klein. 2014. "A biomimetic extracellular matrix for cartilage tissue engineering centered on photocurable gelatin, hyaluronic acid and chondroitin sulfate." *Acta Biomaterialia* 10 (1): 214–223.

Li, M., J. You, J. You, Q. Qin, M. Liu, Y. Yang, K. Jia, Y. Zhang and Y. Zhou. 2023. "A comprehensive review on silk fibroin as a persuasive biomaterial for bone tissue engineering." *International Journal of Molecular Science*, 24(3): 2660.

Li, B., Y. Gao, L. Guo, Y. Fan, N. Kawazoe, H. Fan, X. Zhang and G. Chen. 2018. "Synthesis of photo-reactive poly (vinyl alcohol) and construction of scaffold-free cartilage like pellets in vitro." *Regenerative Biomaterials* 5 (3): 159–166.

Li, C., L. Wang, Z. Yang, G. Kim, H. Chen and Z. Ge. 2012. "A viscoelastic chitosan-modified three-dimensional porous poly (L-lactide-co-ε-caprolactone) scaffold for cartilage tissue engineering." *Journal of Biomaterials Science, Polymer Edition* 23 (1–4): 405–424.

Li, F. Y., V. X. Truong, H. Thissen, J. E. Frith and J. S. Forsythe. 2017. "Microfluidic encapsulation of human mesenchymal stem cells for articular cartilage tissue regeneration." *Acs Applied Materials & Interfaces* 9 (10): 8589–8601.

Li, J., P. Zhou, S. Attarilar and H. Shi. 2021. "Innovative surface modification procedures to achieve micro/nano-graded Ti-based biomedical alloys and implants." *Coatings*, 11 (6): 1–31.

Li, L., F. Yu, L. Zheng, R. Wang, W. Yan, Z. Wang, J. Xu, J. Wu, D. Shi and L. Zhu. 2019. "Natural hydrogels for cartilage regeneration: Modification, preparation and application." *Journal of Orthopaedic Translation* 17: 26–41.

Li, L., K. Zhang, T. Wang, P. Wang, B. Xue, Y. Cao, L. Zhu and Q. Jiang. 2020. "Biofabrication of a biomimetic supramolecular-polymer double network hydrogel for cartilage regeneration." *Materials & Design* 189: 108492.

Li, T., B. Liu, Y. Jiang, Y. Lou, K. Chen and D. Zhang. 2020. "L-polylactic acid porous microspheres enhance the mechanical properties and in vivo stability of degummed silk/silk fibroin/gelatin scaffold." *Biomedical Materials* 16 (1): 015025.

Li, Z., H. R. Ramay, K. D. Hauch, D. Xiao and M. Zhang. 2005. "Chitosan–alginate hybrid scaffolds for bone tissue engineering." *Biomaterials* 26 (18): 3919–3928.

Li, Z., X. Chen, C. Bao, C. Liu, D. Li, Q. Lin. 2021. "Fabrication and evaluation of alginate/bacterial cellulose nanocrystals–chitosan–gelatin composite scaffolds." *Molecules* 26(16): 5003.

Liao, J., T. Tian, S. Shi, X. Xie, Q. Ma, G. Li and Y. Lin. 2017. "The fabrication of biomimetic biphasic CAN-PAC hydrogel with a seamless interfacial layer applied in osteochondral defect repair." *Bone Research* 5 (1): 1–15.

Liao, S., F. Cui and Y. Zhu. 2004. "Osteoblasts adherence and migration through three-dimensional porous mineralized collagen based composite: nHAC/PLA." *Journal of Bioactive and Compatible Polymers* 19 (2): 117–130.

Lin, S. J., Y. C. Chan, Z. C. Su, W. L. Yeh, P. L. Lai and I. M. Chu. 2021. "Growth factor-loaded microspheres in mPEG-polypeptide hydrogel system for articular cartilage repair." *Journal of Biomedical Materials Research Part A* 109(12): 2516–2526.

Lippiello, L., J. Woodward, R. Karpman and T. A. Hammad. 2000. "In vivo chondroprotection and metabolic synergy of glucosamine and chondroitin sulfate." *Clinical Orthopaedics and Related Research* 381: 229–240.

Liu, J., C. Qi, K. Tao, J. Zhang, J. Zhang, L. Xu, X. Jiang, Y. Zhang, L. Huang, Q. Li, H. Xie, J. Gao, X. Shuai, G. Wang, Z. Wang and L. Wang. 2016. "Sericin/Dextran inject-able hydrogel as an optically trackable drug delivery system for malignant melanoma treatment." *ACS Applied Materials & Interfaces* 8 (10): 6411–6422.

Liu, J. X., D. Z. Yang, F. Shi and Y. J. 2003. "Sol–gel deposited TiO2 film on NiTi surgical alloy for biocompatibility improvement." *Thin Solid Films* 429 (1–2): 225–230.

Liu, P., L. Gu, L. Ren, J. Chen, T. Li, X. Wang, J. Yang, C. Chen and L. Sun. 2019. "Intra-articular injection of etoricoxib-loaded PLGA-PEG-PLGA triblock copolymeric nanoparticles attenuates osteoarthritis progression." *American Journal of Translational Research* 11 (11): 6775.

Liu, R., Y. Chen, L. Liu, Y. Gong, M. Wang, S. Li, C. Chen and B. Yu. 2018. "Long-term delivery of rhIGF-1 from biodegradable poly (lactic acid)/hydroxyapatite@ Eudragit double-layer microspheres for prevention of bone loss and articular degeneration in C57BL/6 mice." *Journal of Materials Chemistry B* 6 (19): 3085–3095.

Longley, R., A. M. Ferreira and P. Gentile. 2018. "Recent approaches to the manufacturing of biomimetic multi-phasic scaffolds for osteochondral regeneration." *International Journal of Molecular Sciences* 19 (6): 1755.

Lubiatowski, P., J. Kruczynski, A. Gradys, T. Trzeciak and J. Jaroszewski. 2006. "Articular cartilage repair by means of biodegradable scaffolds." *Transplantation Proceedings* 38 (1): 320–322.

Lungu, A., M. Albu, N. Florea, I. Stancu, E. Vasile and H. Iovu. 2011. "The influence of glycosaminoglycan type on the collagen-glycosaminoglycan porous scaffolds." *Digest Journal of Nanomaterials and Biostructures* 6 (4): 1867–1875.

Lungu, A., I. Titorencu, M. Albu, N. Florea, E. Vasile, H. Iovu, V. Jinga and M. Simionescu. 2011. "The effect of BMP-4 loaded in 3D collagen-hyaluronic acid scaffolds on biocom-patibility assessed with MG 63 osteoblast-like cells." *Digest Journal of Nanomaterials Biostructures* 6: 1897–1908.

Luo, Y., C. Wu, A. Lode and M. Gelinsky. 2012. "Hierarchical mesoporous bioactive glass/ alginate composite scaffolds fabricated by three-dimensional plotting for bone tissue engineering." *Biofabrication* 5 (1): 015005.

Lv, Q., M. Deng, B. D. Ulery, L. S. Nair and C. T. Laurencin. 2013. "Nano-ceramic composite scaffolds for bioreactor-based bone engineering." *Clinical Orthopaedics and Related Research* 471 (8): 2422–2433.

Ma, D. K., Y. S. Wang and W. J. Dai. 2018. "Silk fibroin-based biomaterials for musculoskel-etal tissue engineering." *Materials Science & Engineering C-Materials for Biological Applications* 89: 456–469.

Mallick, S. P., K. Pal, A. Rastogi and P. Srivastava. 2016. "Evaluation of poly (L-lactide) and chitosan composite scaffolds for cartilage tissue regeneration." *Designed Monomers and Polymers* 19(3): 271–282.

Mankin, H. J., H. Dorfman, L. Lippiello and A. Zarins. 1971. "Biochemical and metabolic abnormalities in articular cartilage from osteo-arthritic human hips: II. Correlation of morphology with biochemical and metabolic data." *Journal of Bone and Joint Surgery. American Volume* 53(3): 523–537.

Marcacci, M., M. Berruto, D. Brocchetta, A. Delcogliano, D. Ghinelli, A. Gobbi, E. Kon, L. Pederzini, D. Rosa and G. L. Sacchetti. 2005. "Articular cartilage engineering with Hyalograft® C: 3-year clinical results." *Clinical Orthopaedics and Related Research* 435: 96–105.

Marques, C. F., G. S. Diogo, S. Pina, J. M. Oliveira, T. H. Silva and R. L. Reis. 2019. "Collagen-based bioinks for hard tissue engineering applications: A comprehensive review." *Journal of Materials Science-Materials in Medicine* 30 (3) 1–12.

Martens, P. J., S. J. Bryant and K. S. Anseth. 2003. "Tailoring the degradation of hydrogels formed from multivinyl poly (ethylene glycol) and poly (vinyl alcohol) macromers for cartilage tissue engineering." *Biomacromolecules* 4 (2): 283–292.

Mazaki, T., Y. Shiozaki, K. Yamane, A. Yoshida, M. Nakamura, Y. Yoshida, D. Zhou, T. Kitajima, M. Tanaka and Y. Ito. 2014. "A novel, visible light-induced, rapidly cross-linkable gelatin scaffold for osteochondral tissue engineering." *Scientific Reports* 4 (1): 1–10.

Means, A. K., C. S. Shrode, L. V. Whitney, D. A. Ehrhardt and M. A. Grunlan. 2019. "Double network hydrogels that mimic the modulus, strength, and lubricity of cartilage." *Biomacromolecules* 20 (5): 2034–2042.

Mehrali, M., A. Thakur, C. P. Pennisi, S. Talebian, A. Arpanaei, M. Nikkhah and A. Dolatshahi-Pirouz. 2017. "Nanoreinforced hydrogels for tissue engineering: biomaterials that are compatible with load-bearing and electroactive tissues." *Advanced Materials* 29 (8): 1603612.

Menon, A. H., S. P. Soundarya, V. Sanjay, S. V. Chandran, K. Balagangadharan and N. Selvamurugan. 2018. "Sustained release of chrysin from chitosan-based scaffolds promotes mesenchymal stem cell proliferation and osteoblast differentiation." *Carbohydrate Polymers* 195: 356–367.

Mierisch, C. M., H. A. Wilson, M. A. Turner, T. A. Milbrandt, L. Berthoux, M.-L. Hammarskjöld, D. Rekosh, G. Balian and D. R. Diduch. 2003. "Chondrocyte transplantation into articular cartilage defects with use of calcium alginate: The fate of the cells." *JBJS* 85 (9): 1757–1767.

Mieszawska, A. J., N. Fourligas, I. Georgakoudi, N. M. Ouhib, D. J. Belton, C. C. Perry and D. L. Kaplan. 2010. "Osteoinductive silk–silica composite biomaterials for bone regeneration." *Biomaterials* 31 (34): 8902–8910.

Mieszawska, A. J., J. G. Llamas, C. A. Vaiana, M. P. Kadakia, R. R. Naik and D. L. Kaplan. 2011. "Clay enriched silk biomaterials for bone formation." *Acta Biomaterialia* 7 (8): 3036–3041.

Mondal, D., M. Griffith and S. S. Venkatraman. 2016. "Polycaprolactone-based biomaterials for tissue engineering and drug delivery: Current scenario and challenges." *International Journal of Polymeric Materials and Polymeric Biomaterials* 65 (5): 255–265.

Miron, R. J., M. Fujioka-Kobayashi, M. Hernandez, U. Kandalam, Y. Zhang, S. Ghanaati and J. Choukroun. 2017. "Injectable platelet rich fibrin (i-PRF): opportunities in regenerative dentistry?" *Clinical Oral Investigations* 21 (8): 2619–2627.

Moran, J. M., D. Pazzano and L. J. Bonassar. 2003. "Characterization of polylactic acid–polyglycolic acid composites for cartilage tissue engineering." *Tissue Engineering* 9 (1): 63–70.

Morille, M., K. Toupet, C. N. Montero-Menei, C. Jorgensen and D. Noël. 2016. "PLGA-based microcarriers induce mesenchymal stem cell chondrogenesis and stimulate cartilage repair in osteoarthritis." *Biomaterials* 88: 60–69.

Mozumder, M. S., A. Mairpady and A. H. I. Mourad. 2017. "Polymeric nanobiocomposites for biomedical applications." *Journal of Biomedical Materials Research Part B: Applied Biomaterials* 105(5): 1241–1259.

Mueller-Rath, R., Gavénis, K., Andereya, S., Mumme, T., Albrand, M., Stoffel, M., ... & Schneider, U. (2010). "Condensed cellular seeded collagen gel as an improved biomaterial for tissue engineering of articular cartilage." *Bio-Medical Materials and Engineering*, 20 (6): 317–328.

Müller, F. A., L. Müller, I. Hofmann, P. Greil, M. M. Wenzel and R. Staudenmaier. 2006. "Cellulose-based scaffold materials for cartilage tissue engineering." *Biomaterials* 27 (21): 3955–3963.

Munir, K., A. Biesiekierski, C. Wen and Y. Li. 2020. Surface modifications of metallic biomaterials. In *Metallic Biomaterials Processing and Medical Device Manufacturing* (pp. 387–424). Woodhead Publishing.

Muzzarelli, R. A., J. Boudrant, D. Meyer, N. Manno, M. DeMarchis and M. G. Paoletti. 2012. "Current views on fungal chitin/chitosan, human chitinases, food preservation, glucans, pectins and inulin: A tribute to Henri Braconnot, precursor of the carbohydrate polymers science, on the chitin bicentennial." *Carbohydrate Polymers* 87(2): 995–1012.

Naeimi, M., M. Fathi, M. Rafienia and S. Bonakdar. 2014. "Silk fibroin-chondroitin sulfate-alginate porous scaffolds: Structural properties and in vitro studies." *Journal of Applied Polymer Science* 131(21: 1–9).

Naghizadeh, Z., A. Karkhaneh, H. Nokhbatolfoghahaei, S. Farzad-Mohajeri, M. Rezai-Rad, M. M. Dehghan and A. Khojasteh. 2021. "Cartilage regeneration with dual-drug-releasing injectable hydrogel/microparticle system: In vitro and in vivo study." *Journal of Cellular Physiology* 236(3): 2194–2204.

Nair, B. P., D. Gangadharan, N. Mohan, B. Sumathi and P. D. Nair. 2015. "Hybrid scaffold bearing polymer-siloxane Schiff base linkage for bone tissue engineering." *Materials Science and Engineering: C* 52: 333–342.

Namkaew, J., N. Sawaddee and S. Yodmuang. 2019. "Polyvinyl alcohol-carboxymethyl cellulose scaffolds for cartilage tissue formation." *2019 12th Biomedical Engineering International Conference (BMEiCON)*, IEEE.

Narayan, R., T. Agarwal, D. Mishra, S. Maji, S. Mohanty, A. Mukhopadhyay and T. K. Maiti. 2017. "Ectopic vascularized bone formation by human mesenchymal stem cell microtissues in a biocomposite scaffold." *Colloids and Surfaces B: Biointerfaces* 160: 661–670.

Necas, J., L. Bartosikova, P. Brauner and J. Kolar. 2008. "Hyaluronic acid (hyaluronan): A review." *Veterinarni Medicina* 53 (8): 397–411.

Neumann, A. J., T. Quinn and S. J. Bryant. 2016. "Nondestructive evaluation of a new hydrolytically degradable and photo-clickable PEG hydrogel for cartilage tissue engineering." *Acta Biomaterialia* 39: 1–11.

Nezhad-Mokhtari, P., M. Ghorbani, L. Roshangar and J. S. Rad. 2019. "Chemical gelling of hydrogels-based biological macromolecules for tissue engineering: Photo-and enzymatic-crosslinking methods." *International Journal of Biological Macromolecules* 139: 760–772.

Ngadimin, K. D., A. Stokes, P. Gentile and A. M. Ferreira. 2021. "Biomimetic hydrogels designed for cartilage tissue engineering." *Biomaterials Science* 9 (12): 4246–4259.

Nguyen, L. H., A. K. Kudva, N. S. Saxena and K. Roy. 2011. "Engineering articular cartilage with spatially-varying matrix composition and mechanical properties from a single stem cell population using a multi-layered hydrogel." *Biomaterials* 32 (29): 6946–6952.

Ni, P., S. Fu, M. Fan, G. Guo, S. Shi, J. Peng, F. Luo and Z. Qian. 2011. "Preparation of poly (ethylene glycol)/polylactide hybrid fibrous scaffolds for bone tissue engineering." *International Journal of Nanomedicine* 6: 3065.

Nie, W., C. Peng, X. Zhou, L. Chen, W. Wang, Y. Zhang and C. He. 2017. "Three-dimensional porous scaffold by self-assembly of reduced graphene oxide and nano-hydroxyapatite composites for bone tissue engineering." *Carbon* 116: 325–337.

Nonoyama, T. and J. P. Gong. 2015. "Double-network hydrogel and its potential biomedical application: A review." *Proceedings of the Institution of Mechanical Engineers, Part H: Journal of Engineering in Medicine* 229 (12): 853–863.

O'Sullivan, A. C. 1997. "Cellulose: The structure slowly unravels." *Cellulose* 4 (3): 173–207.

Obermeier, B., F. Wurm, C. Mangold and H. Frey. 2011. "Multifunctional poly (ethylene glycol) s." *Angewandte Chemie International Edition* 50 (35): 7988–7997.

Ochi, M., Y. Uchio, K. Kawasaki, S. Wakitani and J. Iwasa. 2002. "Transplantation of cartilage-like tissue made by tissue engineering in the treatment of cartilage defects of the knee." *The Journal of Bone and Joint Surgery. British Volume* 84 (4): 571–578.

Oliveira, A. S., O. Seidi, N. Ribeiro, R. Colaço and A. P. Serro. 2019. "Tribomechanical comparison between PVA hydrogels obtained using different processing conditions and human cartilage." *Materials* 12 (20): 3413.

Ossendorf, C., C. Kaps, P. C. Kreuz, G. R. Burmester, M. Sittinger and C. Erggelet. 2007. "Treatment of posttraumatic and focal osteoarthritic cartilage defects of the knee with autologous polymer-based three-dimensional chondrocyte grafts: 2-year clinical results." *Arthritis Research & Therapy* 9 (2): 1–11.

Pahoff, S., C. Meinert, O. Bas, L. Nguyen, T. J. Klein and D. W. Hutmacher. 2019. "Effect of gelatin source and photoinitiator type on chondrocyte redifferentiation in gelatin methacryloyl-based tissue-engineered cartilage constructs." *Journal of Materials Chemistry B* 7 (10): 1761–1772.

Paige, K. T., L. G. Cima, M. J. Yaremchuk, B. L. Schloo, J. P. Vacanti and C. A. Vacanti. 1996. "De novo cartilage generation using calcium alginate-chondrocyte constructs." *Plastic and Reconstructive Surgery* 97 (1): 168–178.

Parenteau-Bareil, R., R. Gauvin and F. Berthod. 2010. "Collagen-based biomaterials for tissue engineering applications." *Materials* 3 (3): 1863–1887.

Parhi, R. 2017. "Cross-linked hydrogel for pharmaceutical applications: A review." *Advanced Pharmaceutical Bulletin* 7 (4): 515–530.

Park, S. H., J. Y. Seo, J. Y. Park, Y. B. Ji, K. Kim, H. S. Choi, S. Choi, J. H. Kim, B. H. Min and M. S. Kim. 2019. "An injectable, click-crosslinked, cytomodulin-modified hyaluronic acid hydrogel for cartilage tissue engineering." *NPG Asia Materials* 11 (1): 1–16.

Pasqui, D., P. Torricelli, M. De Cagna, M. Fini and R. Barbucci. 2014. "Carboxymethyl cellulose—hydroxyapatite hybrid hydrogel as a composite material for bone tissue engineering applications." *Journal of Biomedical Materials Research Part A* 102 (5): 1568–1579.

Pati, F., T.-H. Song, G. Rijal, J. Jang, S. W. Kim and D. W. Cho. 2015. "Ornamenting 3D printed scaffolds with cell-laid extracellular matrix for bone tissue regeneration." *Biomaterials* 37: 230–241.

Patil, T., D. Patel, S. Dutta, K. Ganguly, T. Santra and K. Lim. 2020. "Bioactive electrospun nanocomposite scaffolds of poly (lactic acid)/cellulose nanocrystals for bone tissue engineering." *International Journal of Biological Macromolecules* 162: 1429–1441.

Pavelká, K., J. Gatterová, M. Olejarová, S. Machacek, G. Giacovelli and L. C. Rovati. 2002. "Glucosamine sulfate use and delay of progression of knee osteoarthritis: a 3-year, randomized, placebo-controlled, double-blind study." *Archives of Internal Medicine* 162 (18): 2113–2123.

Peretti, G. M., M. A. Randolph, M. T. Villa, M. S. Buragas and M. J. Yaremchuk. 2000. "Cell-based tissue-engineered allogeneic implant for cartilage repair." *Tissue Engineering* 6 (5): 567–576.

Peter, M., N. Ganesh, N. Selvamurugan, S. Nair, T. Furuike, H. Tamura and R. Jayakumar. 2010. "Preparation and characterization of chitosan–gelatin/nanohydroxyapatite composite scaffolds for tissue engineering applications." *Carbohydrate Polymers* 80 (3): 687–694.

Peterson, L., M. Brittberg, I. Kiviranta, E. L. Akerlund and A. Lindahl. 2002. "Autologous chondrocyte transplantation – Biomechanics and long-term durability." *American Journal of Sports Medicine* 30 (1): 2–12.

Phillippi, J. A., E. Miller, L. Weiss, J. Huard, A. Waggoner and P. Campbell. 2008. "Microenvironments engineered by inkjet bioprinting spatially direct adult stem cells toward muscle-and bone-like subpopulations." *Stem Cells* 26 (1): 127–134.

Poole, A. R., T. Kojima, T. Yasuda, F. Mwale, M. Kobayashi and S. Laverty. 2001. "Composition and structure of articular cartilage: A template for tissue repair." *Clinical Orthopaedics and Related Research* 391: S26–S33.

Prabhakaran, M. P., J. Venugopal and S. Ramakrishna. 2009. "Electrospun nanostructured scaffolds for bone tissue engineering." *Acta Biomaterialia* 5(8): 2884–2893.

Puthucheary, Z. A., J. Rawal, M. McPhail, B. Connolly, G. Ratnayake, P. Chan, N. S. Hopkinson, R. Phadke, T. Dew and P. S. Sidhu. 2013. "Acute skeletal muscle wasting in critical illness." *Jama* 310 (15): 1591–1600.

Puvaneswary, S., S. Talebian, H. B. Raghavendran, M. R. Murali, M. Mehrali, A. M. Afifi and T. Kamarul. 2015. "Fabrication and in vitro biological activity of βTCP-Chitosan-Fucoidan composite for bone tissue engineering." *Carbohydrate Polymers* 134: 799–807.

Qi, C., J. Liu, Y. Jin, L. Xu, G. Wang, Z. Wang and L. Wang. 2018. "Photo-crosslinkable, injectable sericin hydrogel as 3D biomimetic extracellular matrix for minimally invasive repairing cartilage." *Biomaterials* 163: 89–104.

Qi, H., Z. Ye, H. Ren, N. Chen, Q. Zeng, X. Wu and T. Lu. 2016. "Bioactivity assessment of PLLA/PCL/HAP electrospun nanofibrous scaffolds for bone tissue engineering." *Life Sciences* 148: 139–144.

Qi, X., X. Hu, W. Wei, H. Yu, J. Li, J. Zhang and W. Dong. 2015. "Investigation of Salecan/poly(vinyl alcohol) hydrogels prepared by freeze/thaw method." *Carbohydrate Polymers* 118: 60–69.

Qu, H., H. Fu, Z. Han and Y. Sun. 2019. "Biomaterials for bone tissue engineering scaffolds: A review." *RSC Advances* 9 (45): 26252–26262.

Quinlan, E., S. Partap, M. M. Azevedo, G. Jell, M. M. Stevens and F. J. O'Brien. 2015. "Hypoxia-mimicking bioactive glass/collagen glycosaminoglycan composite scaffolds to enhance angiogenesis and bone repair." *Biomaterials* 52: 358–366.

Rajzer, I., E. Menaszek and O. Castano. 2017. "Electrospun polymer scaffolds modified with drugs for tissue engineering." *Materials Science and Engineering: C* 77: 493–499.

Ratanavaraporn, J., K. Soontornvipart, S. Shuangshoti, S. Shuangshoti and S. Damrongsakkul. 2017. "Localized delivery of curcumin from injectable gelatin/Thai silk fibroin microspheres for anti-inflammatory treatment of osteoarthritis in a rat model." *Inflammopharmacology* 25 (2): 211–221.

Ribeiro, V. P., A. da Silva Morais, F. R. Maia, R. F. Canadas, J. B. Costa, A. L. Oliveira and R. L. Reis. 2018. "Combinatory approach for developing silk fibroin scaffolds for cartilage regeneration." *Acta Biomaterialia* 72: 167–181.

Ribeiro, V. P., S. Pina, J. o. B. Costa, I. F. Cengiz, L. García-Fernández, M. d. M. Fernández-Gutiérrez, O. C. Paiva, A. L. Oliveira, J. San-Román and J. M. Oliveira. 2019. "Enzymatically cross-linked silk fibroin-based hierarchical scaffolds for osteochondral regeneration." *ACS Applied Materials & Interfaces* 11 (4): 3781–3799.

Rowley, J. A., G. Madlambayan and D. J. Mooney. 1999. "Alginate hydrogels as synthetic extracellular matrix materials." *Biomaterials* 20 (1): 45–53.

Rudnik-Jansen, I., K. Schrijver, N. Woike, A. Tellegen, S. Versteeg, P. Emans and L. Creemers. 2019. "Intra-articular injection of triamcinolone acetonide releasing biomaterial microspheres inhibits pain and inflammation in an acute arthritis model." *Drug Delivery* 26(1): 226–236.

Rumian, Ł., H. Tiainen, U. Cibor, M. Krok-Borkowicz, M. Brzychczy-Włoch, H. J. Haugen and E. Pamuła. 2016. "Ceramic scaffolds enriched with gentamicin loaded poly (lactide-co-glycolide) microparticles for prevention and treatment of bone tissue infections." *Materials Science and Engineering: C* 69: 856–864.

Sachot, N., M. A. Mateos-Timoneda, J. A. Planell, A. H. Velders, M. Lewandowska, E. Engel and O. Castano. 2015. "Towards 4th generation biomaterials: A covalent hybrid polymer–ormoglass architecture." *Nanoscale* 7 (37): 15349–15361.

Sala, R. L., M. Y. Kwon, M. Kim, S. E. Gullbrand, E. A. Henning, R. L. Mauck, E. R. Camargo and J. A. Burdick "(*) Thermosensitive poly(N-vinylcaprolactam) injectable hydrogels for cartilage tissue engineering." (1937–335X (Electronic)).

Salati, M. A., J. Khazai, A. M. Tahmuri, A. Samadi, A. Taghizadeh, M. Taghizadeh, P. Zarrintaj, J. D. Ramsey, S. Habibzadeh and F. Seidi. 2020. "Agarose-based biomaterials: Opportunities and challenges in cartilage tissue engineering." *Polymers* 12 (5): 1150.

Salgado, C., L. Guenee, R. Černý, E. Allemann and O. Jordan. 2020. "Nano wet milled celecoxib extended release microparticles for local management of chronic inflammation." *International Journal of Pharmaceutics* 589: 119783.

Samantaray, P. K., A. Little, D. M. Haddleton, T. McNally, B. Tan, Z. Sun and C. Wan. 2020. "Poly (glycolic acid)(PGA): A versatile building block expanding high performance and sustainable bioplastic applications." *Green Chemistry* 22(13): 4055–4081.

Sawatjui, N., T. Damrongrungruang, W. Leeanansaksiri, P. Jearanaikoon, S. Hongeng and T. Limpaiboon. 2015. "Silk fibroin/gelatin-chondroitin sulfate-hyaluronic acid effectively enhances in vitro chondrogenesis of bone marrow mesenchymal stem cells." *Materials Science & Engineering C-Materials for Biological Applications* 52: 90–96.

Sawitzke, A. D., H. Shi, M. F. Finco, D. D. Dunlop, C. O. Bingham III, C. L. Harris and D. O. Clegg. 2008. "The effect of glucosamine and/or chondroitin sulfate on the progression of knee osteoarthritis: a report from the glucosamine/chondroitin arthritis intervention trial." *Arthritis & Rheumatism: Official Journal of the American College of Rheumatology* 58(10): 3183–3191.

Scholz, B., C. Kinzelmann, K. Benz, J. Mollenhauer, H. Wurst and B. Schlosshauer. 2010. "Suppression of adverse angiogenesis in an albumin-based hydrogel for articular cartilage and intervertebral disc regeneration." *European Cell Material* 20 (24): 2010.2018.

Scott, M. 1983. "32,000 years of sutures." *NATNews* 20 (5): 15–17.

Selmi, T. A. S., P. Verdonk, P. Chambat, F. Dubrana, J.-F. Potel, L. Barnouin and P. Neyret. 2008. "Autologous chondrocyte implantation in a novel alginate-agarose hydrogel: Outcome at two years." *The Journal of Bone and Joint Surgery. British Volume* 90 (5): 597–604.

Shahini, A., M. Yazdimamaghani, K. J. Walker, M. A. Eastman, H. Hatami-Marbini, B. J. Smith, J. L. Ricci, S. V. Madihally, D. Vashaee and L. Tayebi. 2014. "3D conductive nanocomposite scaffold for bone tissue engineering." *International Journal of Nanomedicine* 9: 167.

Shamsi, M., M. Karimi, M. Ghollasi, N. Nezafati, M. Shahrousvand, M. Kamali and A. Salimi. 2017. "In vitro proliferation and differentiation of human bone marrow mesenchymal stem cells into osteoblasts on nanocomposite scaffolds based on bioactive glass (64SiO(2)-31CaO-5P(2)O(5))-poly-l-lactic acid nanofibers fabricated by electrospinning method." *Materials Science & Engineering. C, Materials for Biological Applications* 78: 114–123.

Shao, W., J. He, Q. Han, F. Sang, Q. Wang, L. Chen and B. Ding. 2016. "A biomimetic multilayer nanofiber fabric fabricated by electrospinning and textile technology from polylactic acid and Tussah silk fibroin as a scaffold for bone tissue engineering." *Materials Science and Engineering: C* 67: 599–610.

Shao, W., J. He, F. Sang, Q. Wang, L. Chen, S. Cui and B. Ding. 2016. "Enhanced bone formation in electrospun poly (l-lactic-co-glycolic acid)–tussah silk fibroin ultrafine nanofiber scaffolds incorporated with graphene oxide." *Materials Science and Engineering: C* 62: 823–834.

Schuurman, W., P. A. Levett, M. W. Pot, P. R. van Weeren, W. J. Dhert, D. W. Hutmacher, ... and J. Malda. 2013. "Gelatin-methacrylamide hydrogels as potential biomaterials for fabrication of tissue-engineered cartilage constructs." *Macromolecular Bioscience*, 13(5), 551–561.

Shen, T., Y. Dai, X. Li, S. Xu, Z. Gou and C. Gao. 2017. "Regeneration of the osteochondral defect by a wollastonite and macroporous fibrin biphasic scaffold." *ACS Biomaterials Science & Engineering* 4 (6): 1942–1953.

Siddiqui, N. and K. Pramanik. 2014. "Effects of micro and nano β-TCP fillers in freeze-gelled chitosan scaffolds for bone tissue engineering." *Journal of Applied Polymer Science* 131 (21) 1–10.

Sims, C. D., P. Butler, Y. Cao, R. Casanova, M. A. Randolph, A. Black, C. A. Vacanti and M. J. Yaremchuk. 1998. "Tissue engineered neocartilage using plasma derived polymer substrates and chondrocytes." *Plastic and Reconstructive Surgery* 101 (6): 1580–1585.

Singh, Y. P., N. Bhardwaj and B. B. Mandal. 2016. "Potential of agarose/silk fibroin blended hydrogel for in vitro cartilage tissue engineering." *ACS Applied Materials & Interfaces* 8 (33): 21236–21249.

Sittinger, M., D. Reitzel, M. Dauner, H. Hierlemann, C. Hammer, E. Kastenbauer and J. Bujia. 1996. "Resorbable polyesters in cartilage engineering: affinity and biocompatibility of polymer fiber structures to chondrocytes." *Journal of Biomedical Materials Research* 33(2): 57–63.

Sivandzade, F. and S. Mashayekhan. 2018. "Design and fabrication of injectable microcarriers composed of acellular cartilage matrix and chitosan." *Journal of Biomaterials Science, Polymer Edition* 29 (6): 683–700.

Skaalure, S. C., S. O. Dimson, A. M. Pennington and S. J. Bryant. 2014. "Semi-interpenetrating networks of hyaluronic acid in degradable PEG hydrogels for cartilage tissue engineering." *Acta Biomaterialia* 10(8): 3409–3420.

Skaalure, S. C., S. Chu and S. J. Bryant. 2015. "An enzyme-sensitive PEG hydrogel based on aggrecan catabolism for cartilage tissue engineering." *Advanced Healthcare Materials* 4 (3): 420–431.

Smeriglio, P., J. H. Lai, F. Yang and N. Bhutani. 2015. "3D hydrogel scaffolds for articular chondrocyte culture and cartilage generation." *JoVE (Journal of Visualized Experiments)* 104: e53085.

Soundarya, S. P., A. H. Menon, S. V. Chandran and N. Selvamurugan. 2018. "Bone tissue engineering: Scaffold preparation using chitosan and other biomaterials with different design and fabrication techniques." *International Journal of Biological Macromolecules* 119: 1228–1239.

Sowjanya, J., J. Singh, T. Mohita, S. Sarvanan, A. Moorthi, N. Srinivasan and N. Selvamurugan. 2013. "Biocomposite scaffolds containing chitosan/alginate/nano-silica for bone tissue engineering." *Colloids and Surfaces B: Biointerfaces* 109: 294–300.

Spain, T. L., C. M. Agrawal and K. A. Athanasiou. 1998. "New technique to extend the useful life of a biodegradable cartilage implant." *Tissue Engineering* 4 (4): 343–352.

Spicer, C. D. 2020. "Hydrogel scaffolds for tissue engineering: The importance of polymer choice." *Polymer Chemistry* 11 (2): 184–219.

Sridhar, B. V., J. L. Brock, J. S. Silver, J. L. Leight, M. A. Randolph and K. S. Anseth. 2015. "Development of a cellularly degradable PEG hydrogel to promote articular cartilage extracellular matrix deposition." *Advanced Healthcare Materials* 4 (5): 702–713.

Sridhar, S. L., M. C. Schneider, S. Chu, G. De Roucy, S. J. Bryant and F. J. Vernerey. 2017. "Heterogeneity is key to hydrogel-based cartilage tissue regeneration." *Soft Matter* 13 (28): 4841–4855.

Stevens, K. R., J. S. Miller, B. L. Blakely, C. S. Chen and S. N. Bhatia. 2015. "Degradable hydrogels derived from PEG-diacrylamide for hepatic tissue engineering." *Journal of Biomedical Materials Research Part A* 103 (10): 3331–3338.

Su, X., L. Wei, Z. Xu, L. Qin, J. Yang, Y. Zou, Y. Zhao Chen and N. Hu. 2023. "Evaluation and application of silk fibroin based biomaterials to promote cartilage regeneration in osteoarthritis therapy." *Biomedicines* 11(8): 2244.

Su, Y., et al. 2012. "Controlled release of bone morphogenetic protein 2 and dexamethasone loaded in core–shell PLLACL–collagen fibers for use in bone tissue engineering." *Acta Biomaterialia* 8(2): 763–771.

Sultankulov, B., D. Berillo, K. Sultankulova, T. Tokay and A. Saparov. 2019. "Progress in the development of chitosan-based biomaterials for tissue engineering and regenerative medicine." *Biomolecules* 9(9): 470.

Sun, J. and H. Tan. 2013. "Alginate-based biomaterials for regenerative medicine applications." *Materials* 6 (4): 1285–1309.

Sun, Q., L. Zhang, T. Xu, J. Ying, B. Xia, H. Jing and P. Tong. 2018. "Combined use of adipose derived stem cells and TGF-β3 microspheres promotes articular cartilage regeneration in vivo." *Biotechnic & Histochemistry* 93(3): 168–176.

Swain, S. K. and D. Sarkar. 2014. "Fabrication, bioactivity, in vitro cytotoxicity and cell viability of cryo-treated nanohydroxyapatite–gelatin–polyvinyl alcohol macroporous scaffold." *Journal of Asian Ceramic Societies* 2(3): 241–247.

Taché, A., L. Gan, D. Deporter, R. M. Pilliar. 2004. Effect of surface chemistry on the rate of osseointegration of sintered porous-surfaced Ti-6Al-4V implants. *International Journal of Oral & Maxillofacial Implants* 19: 19–29.

Tan, S., J. Y. Fang, Z. Yang, M. E. Nimni and B. Han. 2014. "The synergetic effect of hydrogel stiffness and growth factor on osteogenic differentiation." *Biomaterials* 35 (20): 5294–5306.

Tanaka, Y., H. Yamaoka, S. Nishizawa, S. Nagata, T. Ogasawara, Y. Asawa, Y. Fujihara, T. Takato and K. Hoshi. 2010. "The optimization of porous polymeric scaffolds for chondrocyte/atelocollagen based tissue-engineered cartilage." *Biomaterials* 31 (16): 4506–4516.

Tang, X.-J., L. Gui and X.-Y. Lü. 2008. "Hard tissue compatibility of natural hydroxyapatite/chitosan composite." *Biomedical Materials* 3 (4): 044115.

Tarafder, S., V. K. Balla, N. M. Davies, A. Bandyopadhyay and S. Bose. 2013. "Microwave-sintered 3D printed tricalcium phosphate scaffolds for bone tissue engineering." *Journal of Tissue Engineering and Regenerative Medicine* 7 (8): 631–641.

Tarafder, S., N. M. Davies, A. Bandyopadhyay and S. Bose. 2013. "3D printed tricalcium phosphate bone tissue engineering scaffolds: Effect of SrO and MgO doping on in vivo osteogenesis in a rat distal femoral defect model." *Biomaterials Science* 1 (12): 1250–1259.

Tateiwa, D., S. Nakagawa, H. Tsukazaki, R. Okada, J. Kodama, J. Kushioka and T. Kaito. 2021. "A novel BMP-2–loaded hydroxyapatite/beta-tricalcium phosphate microsphere/hydrogel composite for bone regeneration." *Scientific Reports* 11(1): 16924.

Tayeb, A. H., E. Amini, S. Ghasemi and M. Tajvidi. 2018. "Cellulose nanomaterials—binding properties and applications: A review." *Molecules* 23 (10): 2684.

Theodosakis, J., B. Adderly and B. Fox. 1997. *The Arthritis Cure*, New York: St, Martins Press.

Thorpe, C., R. Stark, A. Goodship and H. Birch. 2010. "Mechanical properties of the equine superficial digital flexor tendon relate to specific collagen cross-link levels." *Equine Veterinary Journal* 42: 538–543.

Tierney, C. M., M. J. Jaasma and F. J. O'Brien. 2009. "Osteoblast activity on collagen-GAG scaffolds is affected by collagen and GAG concentrations." *Journal of Biomedical Materials Research Part A: An Official Journal of the Society for Biomaterials, the Japanese Society for Biomaterials, and the Australian Society for Biomaterials and the Korean Society for Biomaterials* 91 (1): 92–101.

Titorencu, I., M. G. Albu, F. Anton, A. Georgescu and V. V. Jinga. 2012. "Collagen—Dexamethasone and collagen-D3 scaffolds for bone tissue engineering." *Molecular Crystals and Liquid Crystals* 555 (1): 208–217.

Tognana, E., R. F. Padera, F. Chen, G. Vunjak-Novakovic and L. E. Freed. 2005. "Development and remodeling of engineered cartilage-explant composites in vitro and in vivo." *Osteoarthritis and Cartilage* 13 (10): 896–905.

Tontowi, A. E., A. Anindyajati, R. Tangkudung and P. Dewo. 2018. Biocomposite of Hydroxyapatite/Gelatin/PVA for bone graft application. 2018 1st international conference on bioinformatics, Biotechnology, and Biomedical Engineering-Bioinformatics and Biomedical Engineering, IEEE.

Torgbo, S. and P. Sukyai. 2018. "Bacterial cellulose-based scaffold materials for bone tissue engineering." *Applied Materials Today* 11: 34–49.

Trachsel, L., C. Johnbosco, T. Lang, E. M. Benetti and M. Zenobi-Wong. 2019. "Double-network hydrogels including enzymatically crosslinked poly-(2-alkyl-2-oxazoline)s for 3D bioprinting of cartilage-engineering constructs." *Biomacromolecules* 20 (12): 4502–4511.

Tsai, C.-C., S.-H. Kuo, T.-Y. Lu, N.-C. Cheng, M.-Y. Shie and J. Yu. 2020. "Enzyme-cross-linked gelatin hydrogel enriched with an articular cartilage extracellular matrix and human adipose-derived stem cells for hyaline cartilage regeneration of rabbits." *ACS Biomaterials Science & Engineering* 6 (9): 5110–5119.

Tsigkou, O., L. Hench, A. Boccaccini, J. Polak and M. Stevens. 2007. "Enhanced differentiation and mineralization of human fetal osteoblasts on PDLLA containing bioglass® composite films in the absence of osteogenic supplements." *Journal of Biomedical Materials Research Part A* 80 (4): 837–851.

Tsukuda, Y., T. Onodera, M. Ito, Y. Izumisawa, Y. Kasahara, T. Igarashi and N. Iwasaki. 2015. "Therapeutic effects of intra-articular ultra-purified low endotoxin alginate administration on an experimental canine osteoarthritis model." *Journal of Biomedical Materials Research Part A* 103(11): 3441–3448.

Türk, S., I. Altınsoy, G. Ç. Efe, M. İpek, M. Özacar and C. Bindal. 2018. "3D porous collagen/functionalized multiwalled carbon nanotube/chitosan/hydroxyapatite composite scaffolds for bone tissue engineering." *Materials Science and Engineering: C* 92: 757–768.

Unnithan, A. R., A. R. K. Sasikala, C. H. Park and C. S. Kim. 2017. "A unique scaffold for bone tissue engineering: An osteogenic combination of graphene oxide–hyaluronic acid–chitosan with simvastatin." *Journal of Industrial and Engineering Chemistry* 46: 182–191.

Vangsness Jr, C. T., W. Spiker and J. Erickson. 2009. "A review of evidence-based medicine for glucosamine and chondroitin sulfate use in knee osteoarthritis." *Arthroscopy: The Journal of Arthroscopic & Related Surgery* 25(1): 86–94.

Van Susante, J. L., P. Buma, L. Schuman, G. N. Homminga, W. B. van den Berg and R. P. Veth. 1999. "Resurfacing potential of heterologous chondrocytes suspended in fibrin glue in large full-thickness defects of femoral articular cartilage: an experimental study in the goat." *Biomaterials* 20 (13): 1167–1175.

Varghese, S., N. S. Hwang, A. C. Canver, P. Theprungsirikul, D. W. Lin and J. Elisseeff. 2008. "Chondroitin sulfate based niches for chondrogenic differentiation of mesenchymal stem cells." *Matrix Biology* 27(1): 12–21.

Vayas, R., R. Reyes, M. Rodríguez-Évora, C. Del Rosario, A. Delgado and C. Évora. 2017. "Evaluation of the effectiveness of a bMSC and BMP-2 polymeric trilayer system in cartilage repair." *Biomedical Materials* 12(4): 045001.

Vimalraj, S., N. C. Partridge and N. Selvamurugan. 2014. "A positive role of microRNA-15b on regulation of osteoblast differentiation." *Journal of Cellular Physiology* 229(9): 1236–1244.

Vinatier, C., O. Gauthier, A. Fatimi, C. Merceron, M. Masson, A. Moreau, F. Moreau, B. Fellah, P. Weiss and J. Guicheux. 2009. "An injectable cellulose-based hydrogel for the transfer of autologous nasal chondrocytes in articular cartilage defects." *Biotechnology and Bioengineering* 102 (4): 1259–1267.

Vinatier, C., O. Gauthier, M. Masson, O. Malard, A. Moreau, B. H. Fellah, M. Bilban, R. Spaethe, G. Daculsi and J. Guicheux. 2009. "Nasal chondrocytes and fibrin sealant for cartilage tissue engineering." *Journal of Biomedical Materials Research Part A* 89a (1): 176–185.

Wakitani, S., T. Goto, S. J. Pineda, R. G. Young, J. M. Mansour, A. I. Caplan and V. M. Goldberg. 1994. "Mesenchymal cell-based repair of large, full-thickness defects of articular cartilage." *The Journal of Bone and Joint Surgery. American Volume* 76 (4): 579–592.

Wakitani, S., T. Goto, R. G. Young, J. M. Mansour, V. M. Goldberg and A. I. Caplan. 1998. "Repair of large full-thickness articular cartilage defects with allograft articular chondrocytes embedded in a collagen gel." *Tissue Engineering* 4 (4): 429–444.

Wang, D. A., S. Varghese, B. Sharma, I. Strehin, S. Fermanian, J. Gorham, D. H. Fairbrother, B. Cascio and J. H. Elisseeff. 2007. "Multifunctional chondroitin sulphate for cartilage tissue–biomaterial integration." *Nature Materials* 6 (5): 385–392.

Wang, G. L., X. D. Hu, W. Lin, C. C. Dong and H. Wu. 2011. "Electrospun PLGA-silk fibroin-collagen nanofibrous scaffolds for nerve tissue engineering." *Vitro Cellular & Developmental Biology-Animal* 47 (3): 234–240.

Wang, J., Q. Yang, N. Cheng, X. Tao, Z. Zhang, X. Sun and Q. Zhang. 2016. "Collagen/silk fibroin composite scaffold incorporated with PLGA microsphere for cartilage repair." *Materials Science and Engineering: C* 61: 705–711.

Wang, L. S., C. Du, W. S. Toh, A. C. A. Wan, S. J. Gao and M. Kurisawa. 2014. "Modulation of chondrocyte functions and stiffness-dependent cartilage repair using an injectable enzymatically crosslinked hydrogel with tunable mechanical properties." *Biomaterials* 35 (7): 2207–2217.

Wang, Q., Y. Chu, J. He, W. Shao, Y. Zhou, K. Qi and S. Cui. 2017. "A graded graphene oxide-hydroxyapatite/silk fibroin biomimetic scaffold for bone tissue engineering." *Materials Science and Engineering: C* 80: 232–242.

Wang, X., J. Shao, M. Abd El Raouf, H. Xie, H. Huang, H. Wang, P. K. Chu, X.-F. Yu, Y. Yang and A. M. AbdEl-Aal. 2018. "Near-infrared light-triggered drug delivery system based on black phosphorus for in vivo bone regeneration." *Biomaterials* 179: 164–174.

Wang, Y., U. J. Kim, D. J. Blasioli, H. J. Kim and D. L. Kaplan. 2005. "In vitro cartilage tissue engineering with 3D porous aqueous-derived silk scaffolds and mesenchymal stem cells." *Biomaterials* 26(34): 7082–7094.

Wang, Y., X. Yuan, K. Yu, H. Meng, Y. Zheng, J. Peng, S. Lu, X. Liu, Y. Xie and K. Qiao. 2018. "Fabrication of nanofibrous microcarriers mimicking extracellular matrix for functional microtissue formation and cartilage regeneration." *Biomaterials* 171: 118–132.

Wang, Y., L. Zhang, M. Hu, H. Liu, W. Wen, H. Xiao and Y. Niu. 2008. "Synthesis and characterization of collagen-chitosan-hydroxyapatite artificial bone matrix." *Journal of Biomedical Materials Research Part A: An Official Journal of the Society for Biomaterials, the Japanese Society for Biomaterials, and the Australian Society for Biomaterials and the Korean Society for Biomaterials* 86 (1): 244–252.

Wei, F., S. Liu, M. Chen, G. Tian, K. Zha, Z. Yang and Q. Guo. 2021. "Host response to biomaterials for cartilage tissue engineering: key to remodeling." *Frontiers in Bioengineering and Biotechnology* 9: 664592.

Wendels, S. and L. Avérous. 2021. "Biobased polyurethanes for biomedical applications." *Bioactive Materials* 6(4): 1083–1106.

Whu, S. W., K.-C. Hung, K.-H. Hsieh, C.-H. Chen, C.-L. Tsai and S.-h. Hsu. 2013. "In vitro and in vivo evaluation of chitosan–gelatin scaffolds for cartilage tissue engineering." *Materials Science and Engineering*: C 33 (5): 2855–2863.

Wilke, M. M., D. V. Nydam and A. J. Nixon. 2007. "Enhanced early chondrogenesis in articular defects following arthroscopic mesenchymal stem cell implantation in an equine model." *Journal of Orthopaedic Research* 25 (7): 913–925.

Wong, C. C., C. H. Chen, W. P. Chan, L. H. Chiu, W. P. Ho, F. J. Hsieh, Y. T. Chen and T. L. Yang. 2017. "Single-Stage cartilage repair using platelet-rich fibrin scaffolds with autologous cartilaginous grafts." *American Journal of Sports Medicine* 45 (13): 3128–3142.

Wu, C., Y. Luo, G. Cuniberti, Y. Xiao and M. Gelinsky. 2011. "Three-dimensional printing of hierarchical and tough mesoporous bioactive glass scaffolds with a controllable pore architecture, excellent mechanical strength and mineralization ability." *Acta Biomaterialia* 7 (6): 2644–2650.

Wu, C. C., S. Y. Sheu, L. H. Hsu, K. C. Yang, C. C. Tseng and T. F. Kuo. 2017. "Intra-articular injection of platelet-rich fibrin releasates in combination with bone marrow-derived mesenchymal stem cells in the treatment of articular cartilage defects: An in vivo study in rabbits." *Journal of Biomedical Materials Research Part B: Applied Biomaterials* 105 (6): 1536–1543.

Wu, Y., P. Kennedy, N. Bonazza, Y. Yu, A. Dhawan and I. Ozbolat. 2021. "Three-dimensional bioprinting of articular cartilage: A systematic review." *Cartilage* 12 (1): 76–92.

Xia, H., D. Zhao, H. Zhu, Y. Hua, K. Xiao, Y. Xu, Y. Liu, W. Chen, Y. Liu and W. Zhang. 2018. "Lyophilized scaffolds fabricated from 3D-printed photocurable natural hydrogel for cartilage regeneration." *ACS Applied Materials & Interfaces* 10 (37): 31704–31715.

Xiongfa, J., Z. Hao, Z. Liming and X. Jun. 2018. "Recent advances in 3D bioprinting for the regeneration of functional cartilage." *Regenerative Medicine* 13 (1): 73–87.

Xiao, H., W. Huang, K. Xiong, S. Ruan, C. Yuan, G. Mo, R. Tian, S. Zhou, R. She, P. Ye, et al. 2019. "Osteochondral repair using scaffolds with gradient pore sizes constructed with silk fibroin, chitosan, and nano-hydroxyapatite." *International Journal of Nanomedicine* 14: 2011–2027.

Xu, Y., J. Peng, G. Richards, S. Lu and D. Eglin. 2019. "Optimization of electrospray fabrication of stem cell–embedded alginate–gelatin microspheres and their assembly in 3D-printed poly (ε-caprolactone) scaffold for cartilage tissue engineering." *Journal of Orthopaedic Translation* 18: 128–141.

Yang, B., C. Wang, Y. Zhang, L. Ye, Y. Qian, Y. Shu, J. Wang, J. Li and F. Yao. 2015. "A thermoresponsive poly(N-vinylcaprolactam-co-sulfobetaine methacrylate) zwitterionic hydrogel exhibiting switchable anti-biofouling and cytocompatibility11Electronic supplementary information (ESI) available: Preparation parameters of P(VCL-co-SBMA) hydrogels (Table S1); GPC traces of the copolymers (Fig. S11); Fluorescence microscopic images of HUVECs cell detachment from the surfaces of the TCPS, the PVCL hydrogel, the P(VCL-co-SBMA) hydrogels, and the PSBMA hydrogel at 25 °C for 0, 30, 60, and 120 min (Fig. S21). See DOI: 10.1039/c5py00123d." *Polymer Chemistry* 6 (18): 3431–3442.

Yang, L., Y. Liu, X. Shou, D. Ni, T. Kong and Y. Zhao. 2020. "Bio-inspired lubricant drug delivery particles for the treatment of osteoarthritis." *Nanoscale* 12 (32): 17093–17102.

Yang, S., L. Jang, S. Kim, J. Yang, K. Yang, S. W. Cho and J. Y. Lee. 2016. "Polypyrrole/ alginate hybrid hydrogels: electrically conductive and soft biomaterials for human mesenchymal stem cell culture and potential neural tissue engineering applications." *Macromolecular Bioscience* 16 (11): 1653–1661.

Yang, Z., Y. Wu, C. Li, T. Zhang, Y. Zou, J. H. Hui, Z. Ge and E. H. Lee. 2012. "Improved mesenchymal stem cells attachment and in vitro cartilage tissue formation on chitosan-modified poly (L-lactide-co-epsilon-caprolactone) scaffold." *Tissue Engineering Part A* 18 (3–4): 242–251.

Yao, Q., B. Wei, Y. Guo, C. Jin, X. Du, C. Yan, J. Yan, W. Hu, Y. Xu and Z. Zhou. 2015. "Design, construction and mechanical testing of digital 3D anatomical data-based PCL–HA bone tissue engineering scaffold." *Journal of Materials Science: Materials in Medicine* 26 (1): 1–9.

Yin, H., Y. Wang, X. Sun, G. Cui, Z. Sun, P. Chen, Y. Xu, X. Yuan, H. Meng and W. Xu. 2018. "Functional tissue-engineered microtissue derived from cartilage extracellular matrix for articular cartilage regeneration." *Acta Biomaterialia* 77: 127–141.

Yin, H., Y. Wang, Z. Sun, X. Sun, Y. Xu, P. Li, H. Meng, X. Yu, B. Xiao and T. Fan. 2016. "Induction of mesenchymal stem cell chondrogenic differentiation and functional cartilage microtissue formation for in vivo cartilage regeneration by cartilage extracellular matrix-derived particles." *Acta Biomaterialia* 33: 96–109.

Yin, N., M. D. Stilwell, T. M. Santos, H. Wang and D. B. Weibel. 2015. "Agarose particle-templated porous bacterial cellulose and its application in cartilage growth in vitro." *Acta Biomaterialia* 12: 129–138.

Yokoyama, A., T. C. Somervaille, K. S. Smith, O. Rozenblatt-Rosen, M. Meyerson and M. L. Cleary. 2005. "The menin tumor suppressor protein is an essential oncogenic cofactor for MLL-associated leukemogenesis." *Cell* 123(2): 207–218.

Youssef, A., S. J. Hollister and P. D. Dalton. 2017. "Additive manufacturing of polymer melts for implantable medical devices and scaffolds." *Biofabrication* 9 (1): 012002.

Yu, F., X. Cao, L. Zeng, Q. Zhang and X. Chen. 2013. "An interpenetrating HA/G/CS biomimic hydrogel via Diels–Alder click chemistry for cartilage tissue engineering." *Carbohydrate Polymers* 97 (1): 188–195.

Yu, X., H. Zhang, Y. Miao, S. Xiong and Y. Hu. 2022. "Recent strategies of collagen-based biomaterials for cartilage repair: From structure cognition to function endowment." *Journal of Leather Science and Engineering* 4 (1): 1–23.

Zadehnajar, P., M. H. Mirmusavi, S. Soleymani Eil Bakhtiari, H. R. Bakhsheshi-Rad, S. Karbasi, S. RamaKrishna and F. Berto. 2021. "Recent advances on akermanite calcium-silicate ceramic for biomedical applications." *International Journal of Applied Ceramic Technology* 18(6): 1901–1920.

Zadpoor, A. A. 2017. Mechanics of additively manufactured biomaterials, *Elsevier*. 70: 1–6.

Zarrintaj, P., S. Manouchehri, Z. Ahmadi, M. R. Saeb, A. M. Urbanska, D. L. Kaplan and M. Mozafari. 2018. "Agarose-based biomaterials for tissue engineering." *Carbohydrate Polymers* 187: 66–84.

Zeng, Y., X. Li, X. Liu, Y. Yang, Z. Zhou, J. Fan and H. Jiang. 2021. "PLLA porous microsphere-reinforced silk-based scaffolds for auricular cartilage regeneration." *ACS Omega* 6 (4): 3372–3383.

Zhang, C., M. R. Salick, T. M. Cordie, T. Ellingham, Y. Dan and L.-S. Turng. 2015. "Incorporation of poly (ethylene glycol) grafted cellulose nanocrystals in poly (lactic acid) electrospun nanocomposite fibers as potential scaffolds for bone tissue engineering." *Materials Science and Engineering: C* 49: 463–471.

Zhang, D., O. J. George, K. M. Petersen, A. C. Jimenez-Vergara, M. S. Hahn and M. A. Grunlan. 2014. "A bioactive "self-fitting" shape memory polymer scaffold with potential to treat cranio-maxillo facial bone defects." *Acta Biomaterialia* 10 (11): 4597–4605.

Zhang, J., S. Zhao, M. Zhu, Y. Zhu, Y. Zhang, Z. Liu and C. Zhang. 2014. "3D-printed magnetic Fe 3 O 4/MBG/PCL composite scaffolds with multifunctionality of bone regeneration, local anticancer drug delivery and hyperthermia." *Journal of Materials Chemistry B* 2 (43): 7583–7595.

Zhang, L., K. Li, W. Xiao, L. Zheng, Y. Xiao, H. Fan and X. Zhang. 2011. "Preparation of collagen–chondroitin sulfate–hyaluronic acid hybrid hydrogel scaffolds and cell compatibility in vitro." *Carbohydrate Polymers* 84(1): 118–125.

Zhang, M.-L., J. Cheng, Y. C. Xiao, R. F. Yin and X. Feng. 2017. "Raloxifene microsphere-embedded collagen/chitosan/β-tricalcium phosphate scaffold for effective bone tissue engineering." *International Journal of Pharmaceutics* 518(1–2): 80–85.

Zhang, X., Y. Shi, Z. Zhang, Z. Yang and G. Huang. 2018. "Intra-articular delivery of tetramethylpyrazine microspheres with enhanced articular cavity retention for treating osteoarthritis." *Asian Journal of Pharmaceutical Sciences* 13(3): 229–238.

Zhang, Y., Y. Cao, H. Zhao, L. Zhang, T. Ni, Y. Liu, Z. An, M. Liu and R. Pei. 2020. "An injectable BMSC-laden enzyme-catalyzed crosslinking collagen-hyaluronic acid hydrogel for cartilage repair and regeneration." *Journal of Materials Chemistry B* 8 (19): 4237–4244.

Zhang, Y. P., H. X. Yang, H. L. Shao and X. C. Hu. 2010. "Antheraea pernyi silk fiber: A potential resource for artificially biospinning spider dragline silk." *Journal of Biomedicine and Biotechnology*: 1–8.

Zhang, Z., M. J. Gupte, X. Jin and P. X. Ma. 2015. "Injectable peptide decorated functional nanofibrous hollow microspheres to direct stem cell differentiation and tissue regeneration." *Advanced Functional Materials* 25(3): 350–360.

Zhao, H., L. Ma, Y. Gong and C. Gao. 2008. "A polylactide/fibrin gel composite scaffold for cartilage tissue engineering: Fabrication and an in vitro evaluation." *Journal of Materials Science: Materials in Medicine* 20(1): 135–143.

Zhao, Y., T. Nakajima, J. J. Yang, T. Kurokawa, J. Liu, J. Lu, S. Mizumoto, K. Sugahara, N. Kitamura and K. Yasuda. 2014. "Proteoglycans and glycosaminoglycans improve toughness of biocompatible double network hydrogels." *Advanced Materials* 26 (3): 436–442.

Zhao, Y., X. Zhao, R. Zhang, Y. Huang, Y. Li, M. Shan, X. Zhong, Y. Xing, M. Wang and Y. Zhang. 2020. "Cartilage extracellular matrix scaffold with kartogenin-encapsulated PLGA microspheres for cartilage regeneration." *Frontiers in Bioengineering and Biotechnology* 8: 600103.

Zheng, Y., J. Yang, J. Liang, X. Xu, W. Cui, L. Deng and H. Zhang. 2019. "Bioinspired hyaluronic acid/phosphorylcholine polymer with enhanced lubrication and anti-inflammation." *Biomacromolecules* 20 (11): 4135–4142.

Zhou, C., X. Ye, Y. Fan, F. Qing, H. Chen and X. Zhang. 2014. "Synthesis and characterization of CaP/Col composite scaffolds for load-bearing bone tissue engineering." *Composites Part B: Engineering* 62: 242–248.

Zhou, F., X. Zhang, D. Cai, J. Li, Q. Mu, W. Zhang, S. Zhu, Y. Jiang, W. Shen, S. Zhang and H. W. Ouyang. 2017. "Silk fibroin-chondroitin sulfate scaffold with immuno-inhibition property for articular cartilage repair." *Acta Biomaterialia* 63: 64–75.

Zhou, F., Y. Hong, X. Zhang, L. Yang, J. Li, D. Jiang and S. Zhang. 2018. "Tough hydrogel with enhanced tissue integration and in situ forming capability for osteochondral defect repair." *Applied Materials Today* 13: 32–44.

Zhou, Y. S., K. L. Liang, S. Y. Zhao, C. Zhang, J. Li, H. J. Yang, X. Liu, X. Z. Yin, D. Z. Chen, W. L. Xu and P. Xiao. 2018. "Photopolymerized maleilated chitosan/methacrylated silk fibroin micro/nanocomposite hydrogels as potential scaffolds for cartilage tissue engineering." *International Journal of Biological Macromolecules* 108: 383–390.

Zhu, W., H. T. Cui, B. Boualam, F. Masood, E. Flynn, R. D. Rao, Z. Y. Zhang and L. G. Zhang. 2018. "3D bioprinting mesenchymal stem cell-laden construct with core-shell nanospheres for cartilage tissue engineering." *Nanotechnology* 29 (18) 1–30.

Zhu, X., T. Chen, B. Feng, J. Weng, K. Duan, J. Wang and X. Lu. 2018. Biomimetic Bacterial Cellulose-Enhanced Double-Network Hydrogel with Excellent Mechanical Properties Applied for the Osteochondral Defect Repair *ACS Biomaterials Science and Engineering*. 4(10) 3534–3544.

Zhu, Z., Y.-M. Wang, J. Yang and X.-S. Luo. 2017. "Hyaluronic acid: A versatile biomaterial in tissue engineering." *Plastic and Aesthetic Research* 4: 219.

Zignego, D. L., A. A. Jutila, M. K. Gelbke, D. M. Gannon and R. K. June. 2014. "The mechanical microenvironment of high concentration agarose for applying deformation to primary chondrocytes." *Journal of Biomechanics* 47 (9): 2143–2148.

4 Advances in Fabrication of Tissue Scaffolds

INTRODUCTION

In bone and cartilage tissue engineering, scaffolds, the artificial extra-cellular matrices, play a vital role to repair and regenerate the damaged bone and cartilage tissues. Scaffold builds the backbone for the cellular and tissue structure, delivers essential biofactors for cell growth, and guides cell differentiation and constructive remoulding process of the damaged bone and cartilage tissue, resulting in successful repair of these lost tissues. It offers the necessary structural support, shape stability of the defect site, microenvironment for cell attachment, proliferation, and differentiation and maintains differentiated tissue function in *both in vitro* and *in vivo* conditions. The challenge of the scaffolding systems is to retain the cells in an appropriate 3D architecture for a desired period of time and to transmit molecular signals to the cells suitably both in spatial and temporal fashion, and therefore to facilitate cell growth and formation of desired tissue structures as well as to manufacture the scaffolds in a reproducible and cost-effective manner on a commercial scale. So, scaffold should have a set of desired properties such as pore size, porosity, mechanical strength, nanofibrous architecture, and 3D hierarchical structures, etc. In this context, scaffold fabrication plays a vital role in achieving appropriate 3D scaffold with desired structures and fibrous architecture. This has prompted for the development of a number of fabrication techniques and significant progress in these techniques has been achieved keeping in view the bone and cartilage tissue . This chapter provides the basic concept and function of scaffold towards tissue regeneration and discusses the progress in the scaffold fabrication techniques, starting from the conventional salt leaching to the advanced techniques such as 3D printing. The chapter also highlights the fabrication of 3D nanofibrous scaffold by the advanced electrospinning technology and more recent fabrication strategies of combining 3D printing and electrospinning.

SCAFFOLD: CONCEPT AND FUNCTIONS

Scaffolds are porous solid structures that are designed to promote cellular growth, proliferation, and extra-cellular matrix (ECM) synthesis. They can be applied to substitute a portion of a living system or function in close contact with the living tissue.

DOI: 10.1201/9781003245353-4

These porous biomaterial structures are seeded with the cells and are capable of and supporting three-dimensional tissue formation under *in vitro* and *in vivo* conditions. In general, they find various uses in bone and cartilage, and related substitutes, drug delivery systems, implantable electronic devices, hybrid artificial organs, tendon, and ligament replacements (Hutmacher 2001). The primary functions of the engineered scaffolds are the following: (i) allow cellular movement and cell attachment and guide cell differentiation; (ii) sustain cells and provide biochemical factors, biomechanical and electrical stimuli to alter the behaviour of the cell phase; (iii) facilitate the transport of cell nutrients, gases and metabolic by-products; and (iv) provide sufficient mechanical support while promoting chondrogenesis, osteogenesis, osteoconduction, and even osteoinduction for the ECM formation (Chen et al. 2021).

FABRICATION OF SCAFFOLDS

Depending on the type of tissue engineering application, scaffolds should have specific vital features such as biocompatibility, thereby avoiding undesirable reaction to host tissue upon implantation; outstanding surface interaction to permit cell adhesion, migration, growth, and differentiation; desired pore size and pore interconnectivity with controlled biodegradability, thereby facilitating cell penetration, vascularization, and neotissue formation; and adequate mechanical properties to provide necessary cues in order to regulate the function and structure of the regenerated tissue and their maintenance during the tissue remodelling process, upkeep the development of ECM by stimulating the cell function, and the ability to transact the necessary bimolecular signals to the cells (Zhao et al. 2018). The scaffold should have features and a structure comparable to that of the organ or tissue it replaces.

Keeping the above factors in view, many methods have been established to fabricate scaffolds with two-dimensional (2D) or 3D porous architectures with controlled porosity, *viz.*, solvent casting, gas foaming, freeze drying, salt or particulate leaching, freeze gelation, and self-assembly. These techniques are considered as conventional scaffold fabrication techniques. However, these fabricated scaffolds have limitations, such as they are not able to effectively mimic the structure or architecture of the natural ECM, thereby lacking in generating functional tissues. To overcome these drawbacks, many advanced techniques have been developed, including the additive manufacturing (3D printing), electrospinning, and combined systems for fabricating scaffolds with the desired architecture that can replicate the ECM, thereby enabling them to facilitate functional ECM formation, cellular interactions, structural stability, and transport of nutrients, gases, and generated waste (Subia et al. 2010). Among these, additive manufacturing techniques hold the most potential applications for fabricating bone and related tissue scaffolds. The various scaffold fabrication methods are described in the following section.

SOLVENT CASTING

Solvent casting is a simple and inexpensive technique for fabricating 3D porous polymeric scaffold. This process involves the solvent evaporation to forming scaffolds which is performed in two ways: (i) an appropriate mould is immersed into the polymeric solution and allowed for adequate time to draw off the solution, which results in the formation of a layer of polymeric membranes, and (ii) the polymer solution is added into a mould, and the solvent is evaporated, which creates a film of polymeric crust sticking to the mould (Lu et al. 2004). This method suffers from the toxic residual solvent that leads to denaturation of protein and will be harmful to the cells and the tissue during the *in vitro* and *in vivo* experiments. Complete removal of this toxic solvent may be achieved by vacuum drying of the scaffold, which is very time consuming. To avoid this difficulty, the method is combined with particulate leaching technique for fabricating scaffolds (Mikos, Bao et al. 1993; Mikos, Sarakinos et al. 1993).

SOLVENT CASTING/PARTICULATE LEACHING

Salt leaching is the most simplest and common scaffold fabrication technique and it was developed by Mikos et al. in 1994 (Plikk et al. 2009). In this process, polymer is dissolved in a suitable solvent and the soluble salt particles, the so-called porogens, with appropriate size are added to the polymer solution to create pores in the scaffold. Various inorganic salts like sodium chloride (common salt, NaCl), potassium chloride (KCl), ammonium carbonate, and sugars (e.g. glucose), which are highly soluble in water and insoluble in organic solvents, can be used as porogens. Among these, sodium chloride has been widely used because of its low cost and easy availability. The resulting polymer solution is cast into a suitable mould (Zhang et al. 2017; Duan et al. 2019) followed by the evaporation of the solvent, resulting in a highly porous sponge-like structure. The porous structures are immersed in water to leach out the porogen and then freeze-dried. The requirement of a small quantity of polymer to get the final scaffold product and, without involving any complex, machinery are the main advantages of this technique, which make it especially suitable for manufacturing scaffold at its development stage. However, poor pore interconnectivity due to non-uniform pore size distribution and porosity control, low mechanical strength, and the requirement of highly toxic solvents are the significant drawbacks of this technique. However, the properties of the scaffold can be modified by adjusting the amount, size, and shape of the salt particles (porogens) added (Plikk et al. 2009).

Similar to the simple salt leaching technique, in this fabrication method also, the polymer is dissolved in a volatile solvent. Then water-soluble porogens like NaCl, KCl, sugar, and wax particles are mixed with the polymer solution and cast into a mould with the desired form. A porous scaffold structure is obtained after solvent lyophilization or evaporation, as the porogen particles dissolving in water are leached out. In this method, the type and concentration of the polymers, amount, size and shape of the porogens, are the crucial factors that influence the pore size and porosity. This process is shown in Figure 4.1. The advantage and disadvantages of this fabrication method are as follows.

Advantages:

- Simple setup and inexpensive
- Sufficient control of porosity and pore size by polymer/porogen ratio
- Particle size regulation of the extra porogen
- Significantly connected pores

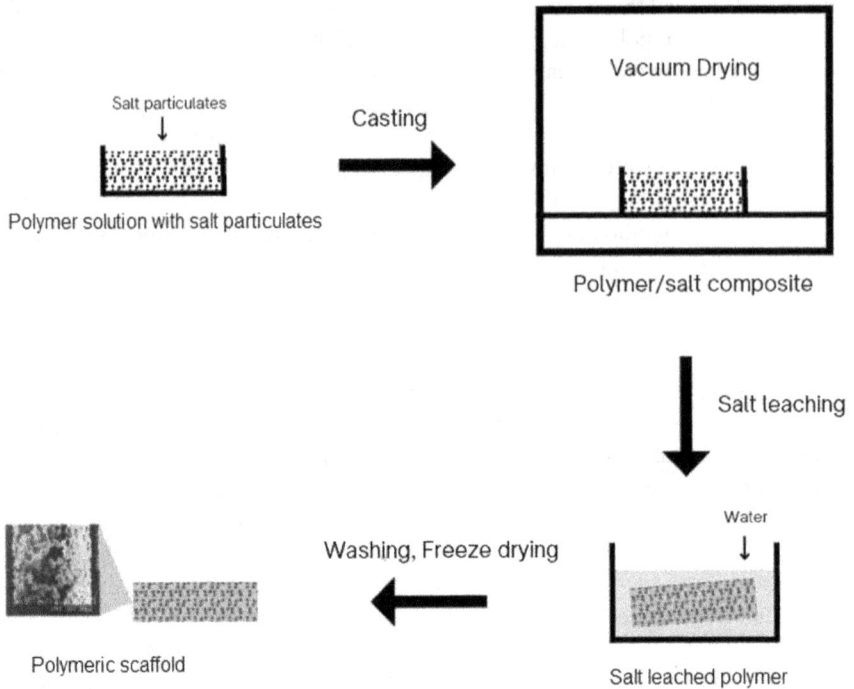

FIGURE 4.1   Solvent casting/particle leaching.

Disadvantages

- Thermal deprivation of polymer solution
- Toxicity risk due to residual solvent
- Irregular crystal shape of the porogen
- Accurate control of porosity and pore size is difficult.

Polyethylene oxide (PEO) and polycaprolactone (PCL) porous scaffolds were manufactured by Reignier and Huneault for cartilage tissue engineering application. They performed particulate leaching by improving concentrations of salt and altering polymers. The achieved porosity of scaffolds was extended from 75% to 88 % by adjusting the volume fraction of salt particles and the ratio of PCL/PEO blend (Zhao et al. 2018). Maji et al. (2016) developed a 3D porous scaffold for bone tissue regrowth from bioactive glass nanoparticles prepared by the sol-gel method (Maji et al. 2016). The porosity of the scaffold is >80% which gives optimal environment for the bone tissue growth. Similarly, for bone regeneration hydroxyapatite based porous scaffold was prepared by slip-casting process and the porosity of the scaffold was measured as 85% (Cyster et al. 2005).

GAS FOAMING

Gas foaming is a unique method for preparing porous scaffolds without any solvent or high temperature, which is detrimental to the cells, surrounding tissues, and various bioactive molecules present in the scaffold. The basic principle of this method involves the nucleation–growth mechanism of gas bubbles, thereby creating a porous structure. The various steps involved in this method include the following: (i) the porogens are dispersed in the polymeric matrix. Although the porogens may be of different types such as chemical blowing agent, for example, sodium bicarbonate (Na_HCO_3), which decomposes either the substance or the agent into inert gas by chemical reaction or by physical blowing agent like inert nitrogen or CO_2 gas, the latter being widely used; (ii) polymer blocks are exposed to high pressure (800 psi) CO_2 while allowing gas bubbles to pass through the polymer system, thereby forming a 3D porous structure, in which the amount of porogen (gas) dissolved in the polymer influences the porosity and pores of the scaffolds; (iii) finally, the hardening of the polymer matrix occurs (Subia et al. 2010; Costantini and Barbetta 2018). Figure 4.2 shows the gas foaming method for scaffold fabrication.

Specialized equipment to handle high-pressure porogen gas is the main drawback of this method. Furthermore, the process is limited to a few polymers. This method produces spongy structures with a porosity of up to 85% and a pore size range of 30–700 μm (Sultana and Wang 2008). The inclusion of particle leaching method in

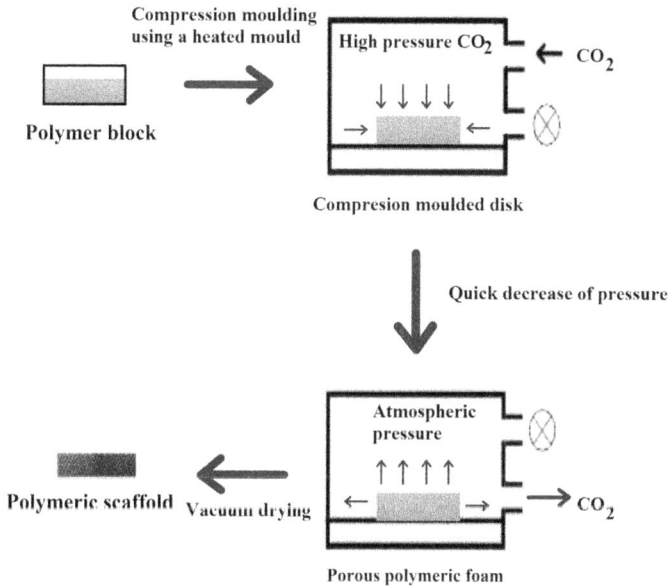

FIGURE 4.2 Gas foaming method for scaffold fabrication.

the gas foaming process facilitates the formation of open pores on the surface of a scaffold and the porosity of the scaffolds can be controlled using porogens like sugar, salts, and wax, with appropriate size. This method is suitable for semicrystalline and amorphous polymers (Manavitehrani et al. 2019).

In a study, PLGA scaffold was developed by gas foaming method, where in, the porogen was removed by foaming after the polymer had reached saturation with CO_2 under high pressure, leaving behind a visibly interconnected pore structure (Huang et al. 2005). In another experiment, a gelatin/PVP polymer porous structure was developed using gas foaming technique for the bone tissue engineering (BTE) application (Mishra et al. 2019). Gas foaming technique was also used to develop a biodegradable poly (propylene carbonate) porous scaffold with pore sizes between 100 and 500 μm (Manavitehrani et al. 2019).

PHASE SEPARATION

Phase separation technique works on the principle of separating phases including the one with low polymer concentration, called polymer lean phase, and the other one with high polymer concentration, called polymer-rich or polymer-dense phase. The polymer lean phase generally leads to the formation of pores in the scaffold matrix, whereas the polymer-rich phase forms a solidified material. Various strategies have been adopted to induce phase separation. Phase separation can be achieved by different ways, including the (i) thermally induced phase separation (TIPS)—this process involves the change in temperature that leads to deviations in the Gibbs free energy and solubility of a solution, thereby de-mixing it and creating a multiphase system; (ii) non-solvent-induced phase separation—which involves a ternary system comprising a solvent, a non-solvent, and a polymer, in which phase separation occurs by adding a non-solvent into the polymer solution, for example, an extremely porous polybenzimidazole-based isolator was developed by employing a simple non-solvent induced phase separation procedure (NIPS) with water, ethanol, chloroform, and ethyl acetate as the coagulation bath solvents (Wang, He et al. 2019); and (iii) chemically induced phase separation—which takes place in systems involving a monomer that undergoes condensation polymerization and a non-reactive polymer.

THERMALLY INDUCED PHASE SEPARATION

TIPS is one of the most suitable techniques to fabricate scaffold with tunable properties including highly porous 3D structure with controllable architecture without the involvement of any complex or expensive equipment and therefore easily implementable in a cost-effective manner (Pavia et al. 2016). Initially, this technique was developed for the purpose of fabricating microporous membrane (Schugens et al. 1996). This process induces the polymeric system to be separated into two distinct phases which are initiated by temperature variations. Basically, phase separation occurs by dropping the temperature of the polymer solution, which results in a polymer-rich and a polymer-lean phase. The polymer-rich phase is transformed into the porous structure following the removal of the solvent by an evaporation process or a vacuum-assisted sublimation, which influences the final porosity of the obtained scaffold (Kasoju et al. 2016). Polymeric porous scaffolds with porosity higher than 95% (Lou et al. 2016) and pore diameters in the range of ~1 to 100 µm (Schugens et al. 1996) can be obtained.

TIPS can also incorporate small bioactive molecules into the scaffolds structures and avoid harsh chemical or thermal environments. Compared to the salt leaching technique, scaffolds fabricated by this method often offer good mechanical properties. The ideal morphology, pore size, and degree of interconnected pores of the scaffolds, which are important in tissue regeneration, can be achieved by carefully choosing processing parameters like the molecular weight and concentration of the polymer used, quenching temperature and rate of cooling, solvent and non-solvent ratio, and additives (Akbarzadeh and Yousefi 2014; Lombardo et al. 2019). Besides, other vital features such as biodegradability and mechanical properties (La Carrubba et al. 2008; Molladavoodi et al. 2013; Zeinali et al. 2020) can be controlled together with the advantage of no residual solvent, thereby ensuring the biocompatibility of the fabricated scaffold (Akbarzadeh and Yousefi 2014). However, the major limitation of this technique is the precise control over the pore size of the fabricated scaffolds, although the process is simple and cost-effective (Kim et al. 2016).

Liquid–liquid phase separation occurs when the temperature of the solution is decreased to the upper critical solution temperature. When a non-solvent is added, the polymer solution experiences phase separation producing the polymer-dense and polymer-lean phases. The subsequent removal of excess solvent results in the formation of open pore structure. In solid–liquid phase separation at the freezing temperatures, the polymer solution and solvent crystallize, and the polymer is separated from the crystallized solvent that involves the nucleation and growth mechanism. Interconnected pores are produced following the sublimation of solvent. Frozen polymer solution forms a porous structure by freeze-drying or freeze gelation for solvent removal, which is described below.

Many advanced fabrication techniques have been established by combining TIPS with other scaffold fabrication techniques, such as electrospinning (Farzamfar et al. 2019), particulate leaching (Szustakiewicz et al. 2019; Yao et al. 2020), and 3D printing (Yousefi et al. 2018; Zhu et al. 2020).

Freeze-Drying

Freeze-drying also known as lyophilization is a technique that is typically used to fabricate 3D scaffold with a porous architecture. The process of freeze-drying occurs in three stages: (i) dissolution of polymer in a suitable solvent; (ii) freezing of the polymer solution in a deep freezer, with liquid nitrogen under controlled freezing conditions; and (iii) primary and secondary drying. During the cooling of polymer solution to the freezing point, the solutes are separated in the ice phase, yielding a porous structure surrounding the ice crystals (Roseti et al. 2017). In primary drying, a low temperature and high vacuum atmosphere initiate the sublimation process of frozen solution and the phase-separated mixture is retained after the sublimation of the solvent. Pores are generated within the polymer solution

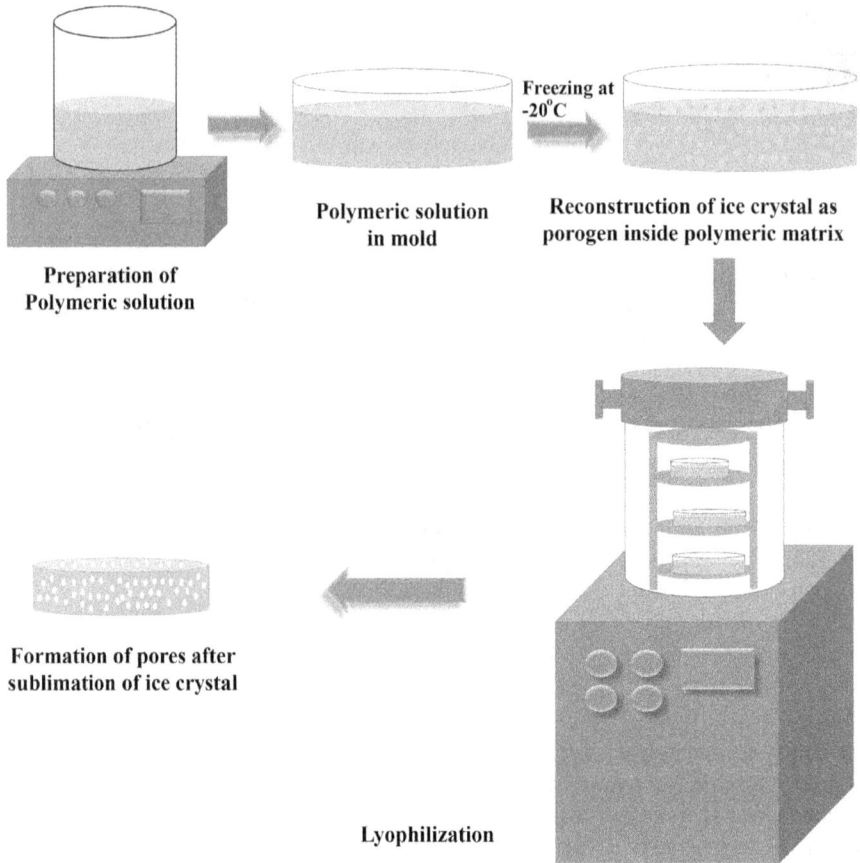

FIGURE 4.3 A schematic diagram of the freeze-drying process for fabrication of porous scaffold.

upon freezing and removing ice crystals of the solvent. These solvent crystals function as the porogen, and the size of pores can be regulated by adjusting the polymer solution concentration, freezing temperature, freezing rate (Nail et al. 2002), presence of impurities, and orientation inside the lyophilizer. Secondary drying involves the desorption of unbound solvent molecules, which results in a completely dried porous matrix. The major advantage of this method is its ability of avoiding high temperature that can reduce the activity of the integrated biological factors. The other advantage is that the desired pore size can be achieved by controlling and modifying the method of freezing (Aranaz et al. 2014). A schematic diagram of the freeze-drying technique for the fabrication of porous scaffold is shown in Figure 4.3.

This method has the advantages like minimum damage to scaffold property, helps to maintain biological activity of scaffolds, usable in water-based polymer systems, and controlled pore morphology with 3D structures, all of which together makes this method in combination with other scaffold fabrication techniques, for example, particulate leaching, more efficient. Furthermore, to create nanofibrous scaffolds, it can be combined with an additive manufacturing process. In spite of having these advantages and being widely used for manufacturing scaffold, this method has many disadvantages, including the small and non-uniform pore size (15–35 μm), low mechanical strength, high processing time, high cost of equipment, high energy consumption, and use of toxic solvent and difficulty in the removal of the residual solvent (Tomihata and Ikada 1997).

Freeze-drying method was used for the fabrication of scaffold in numerous applications (Nasiri and Mashayekhan 2017). Chitosan–alginate composite using fucoidan was developed by freeze-drying method for BTE application (Venkatesan, Bhatnagar, and Kim 2014). Silk fibroin and chitosan blend scaffolds with different polymer ratio were freeze dried to develop porous scaffolds suitable for bone tissue engineering applications (Vishwanath, Pramanik et al. 2016).

FREEZE GELATION

Freeze gelation based on the principle of TIPS is a unique and easy method for fabricating a 3D scaffold. In this process, the polymer solution is frozen and the frozen solution is dipped in a gelation environment at a temperature below the freezing point of the polymer solution. The resulting porous matrix is formed without the freeze-drying as it becomes a gel before the drying stage. Figure 4.4 shows a typical freeze gelation method. The ice crystals are formed in the polymer solution at 272 K. Gelation does not occur until the temperature goes below the freezing point. The gel undergoes mild heating to melt the ice crystals and then dried, resulting a highly porous structure with pores that match the size and shape of the ice crystals formed during the freezing (Lozinsky and Okay 2014). This method overcomes the limitations of residual solvent and high energy and time consumption that are associated with

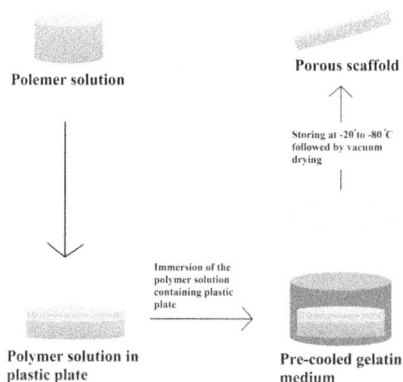

FIGURE 4.4   Freeze gelation method of fabrication of scaffold.

TABLE 4.1

Difference between Freeze-Drying and Freeze Gelation

Freeze-Drying	Freeze Gelation
It works on the principle of sublimation of frozen solvent.	An appropriate gelation medium is required for the polymer sample preparation.
The frozen scaffolds are placed in low temperature (–110 °C) vacuum conditions— so called lyophilization.	The frozen polymer solution is immersed in a prechilled gelation medium.
The frozen solvent is removed which helps in the formation of pores.	The freeze-gelled polymer solution is vacuum dried for solvent evaporation resulting in porous structure.
Requires long process time	Requires less process time
High energy cost	Low energy cost
High residual solvent	Low residual solvent
Comparatively uniform pore distribution	Uneven pore distribution and brittle scaffolds

the freeze-drying method, it is cost-effective, and produces zero shrinkage crack-free scaffolds. It is a quick and easy process that doesn't require a separate leaching step or high temperatures (Siddiqui Ma 2014). However, uneven pore distribution and brittle scaffolds are the drawbacks of this method. Freeze gelation has been used to fabricate many scaffolds from various types of polymers and their composites such as CH, silk, CH/alginate/carboxy methyl cellulose, CH-TCP, and CH/PGA in broad areas of tissue engineering applications. A comparison between the freeze-drying and freeze gelation process is shown in Table 4.1.

Self-Assembly

Self-assembly is an effective and novel approach to fabricate nanofibrous biomimetic composite scaffolds that have potential BTE applications. This process occurs spontaneously as a consequence of various non-covalent interactions, *viz.*, electrostatic, van der Waals, ionic, hydrogen, hydrophobic interactions, and coordination bonds, by which a disordered system constituting pre-existing components transforms into an ordered structure under a certain condition of nature, but without any external influence (Erkal 2012). For example, phospholipids, which are one of the vital cell membrane components, have the ability to self-assemble into many highly organized structures, namely, vesicles, tubules, and micelles in the aqueous solution, because of possessing natural amphiphilic structures (Ma 2008). For example, in a study, a pH-influenced self-assembly method for a peptide amphiphile has been shown to create nanofibres for BTE application (Webber and Pashuck 2021). Basement membrane RADA16-I/RGD peptides, collagen/chitosan-phosphoric acid biocomposites, and peptide amphiphiles have been investigated for developing biocomposites for bone tissue regeneration (Seminole 2008). Another example of self-assembly technique is the conversion of polyphenylene dendrimers into micrometre-long nanofibres (Liu et al. 2002; Liu et al. 2003).

ELECTROSPINNING (ES)

Electrospinning is known to exist for a long time and the primary objective was to make it useful for fabricating non-woven fabric products in the early 1930s (Morton 1902; Formhals 1934). The concept of this method was on the basis of usual spinning machine used in textile industry. In later stages, the technique has been rejuvenated to make it suitable for tissue engineering research with the aim of producing fine polymer fibres with uniform diameter at nano scale. In recent years, electrospinning technique has gained much attraction to fabricate the nanofibrous tissue scaffold with structural similarity with the collagen fibres of the bone tissue, thereby promoting cell adhesion because of their high surface to volume ratio, therefore accommodating higher cell population, and providing high porosity with the desired pore size and enhancing the mechanical properties of the scaffold (Wahid et al. 2018; Ranganathan et al. 2019). The ES method was discovered by Marley and Cooleis in 1902. This is a widely used technique for fabricating nanofibres from polymer solution using electrostatic field (Teo and Ramakrishna 2006).

Principle

This technique involves the charging of polymer solution applying high voltage, causing interaction between the surface tension of the solution and electrostatic forces forming droplets on the spinneret to eject and to continuously stretch the created viscoelastic polymer jet. The electrostatic repulsions between the surface charges and the solvent evaporation resulting in the deposition of polymer fibres over the collector, which is kept at the opposite polarity, cause the electrified jet to constantly elongate, thereby generating a non-oven solid fibre (Reneker et al. 2000; Yarin, Koombhongse, and Reneker 2001; Huang et al. 2003; Mitchell 2015).

Electrospinning Process

A schematic diagram of a typical electrospinning set-up is presented in Figure 4.5. A basic ES system is made up of four major components: a spinneret (normally a needle with a sharp tip) connected to a syringe pump, a high-voltage power supply system, and a grounded (conductive) plate collector, which can be either static (plate) or moving (wheel) (rotating drum or mandrel). When the force created by the electric field exceeds the surface tension of the polymer solution, the syringe pump forces the polymer solution via a capillary, thereby generating a pendant droplets known as the Taylor cone at the tip of the needle and subsequently electrified polymer jets are ejected. These charged jets are elongated along a straight line and bend due to electrical instability, thereby becoming thin. The solvent evaporates during the travel of the polymer jets towards the collector, and then the jets get solidified into non-woven nanofibers that are randomly deposited on the grounded collector (Li, Xie et al. 2016).

Depending on the collector design, oriented fibres can also be produced (Theron, Zussman, and Yarin 2001; Deitzel et al. 2002; Matthews et al. 2002). The created non-woven mat is an efficient platform for tissue regeneration because it possesses a very high specific surface area and a multiscale pore size distribution that ranges from nano- to micrometres (Doshi and Reneker 1995). The ES technique has been widely used for fabricating nanofibrous polymers and biocomposite scaffolds to

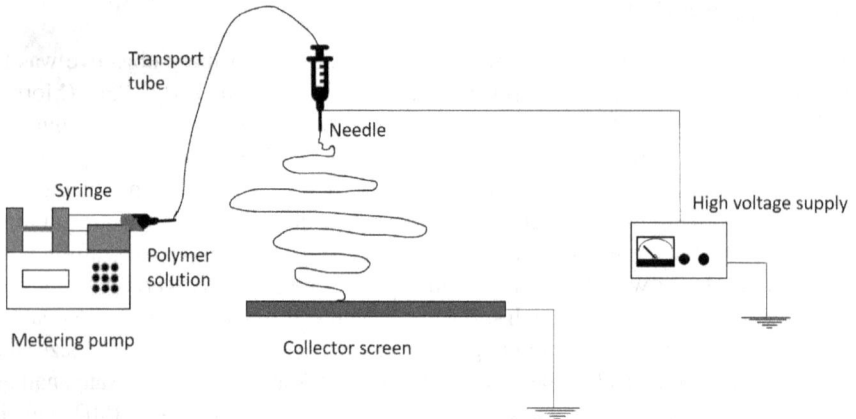

FIGURE 4.5 Schematic diagram of a electrospinning set-up for fabrication of a nanofibrous scaffold.

regenerate bone and cartilage tissue (Yoshimoto et al. 2003; Li et al. 2006; Yu et al. 2017; Maghdouri-White et al. 2018).

Electrospinning Parameters

The process of electrospinning is governed by many parameters that influence the nanofibre formation. These parameters are of three types: (i) solution parameters which include surface tension, conductivity, concentration, solvent volatility, and viscosity; (ii) process parameters such as tip or nozzle diameter, feed rate, electrostatic potential or applied voltage, tip-to-collector distance (working distance), and (iii) environmental parameters like temperature, pressure, humidity, air velocity, etc. The type of solvent system and polymer also influence the spinnability of polymer. The solvents used are ethanol, methanol, hexafluoroisopropanol (HFIP) and the solvent is selected based on its solubility, boiling point, and dielectric constant (Beachley and Wen 2009).

Viscosity and Concentration of the Polymer Solution

When a polymer of higher molecular weight is dissolved in a solvent, the viscosity of the solution is higher than that with a lower molecular weight. The polymer must have adequate molecular weight, and the polymer solution of sufficient viscosity is necessary for electrospinning to occur. A low-viscosity polymer solution creates beads in the fibre, whereas polymer solution with high viscosity forms morphologically homogeneous nanofibres with higher fibre diameter and lesser or without bead formation. Polymer solution with a higher concentration increases the fibre diameter.

Solution Conductivity

In ES technique the polymer solution is stretched due to repulsion of the surface charges. So, the polymer solution with high conductivity enables the generated ES jet to carry more charges and produce fibre with decreased diameter. The polymer solution with higher conductivity can be achieved by the addition of ions, for example, salt.

Surface Tension

Electrospinning starts when the electrically charged polymer solution overcomes its surface tension, which depends on the polymer type and voltage applied. The polymer solution with higher surface tension increases the interaction between the solvent and polymer molecules, leading to the spreading of the solvent over the entangled polymer under the influence of charges. This decreases the affinity of the solvent molecules to come closer by the influence of surface tension. Surface tension of the polymer solution does not have any influence on the fibre morphology, but polymer solution with high surface tension makes the jets unstable.

Solvent Volatility

The solvent should have sufficient volatility to allow the formation of dry fibres. If the solvent is less volatile, the fibres will be moist, resulting in a polymer film rather than separated fibres due to solvent deposition along with the fibre (Beachley and Wen 2009).

Process Parameters

Voltage

The application of high voltage inducing the required charges on the polymer solution along with the applied electric field is an essential component that initiates the fibre formation in ES. The applied electric field also influences the nanofibre diameter produced in this technique. Typically, for initiation of jet formation, more than 6kV either high negative or positive voltage is required to cause the polymer solution drop at the tip of the needle to form the Taylor cone (He and Wane 2004).

Feed Rate

The feed rate determines the amount of polymer solution available for electrospinning. With a given voltage, an appropriate feed rate is needed for maintaining a stable Taylor cone. However, a very high feed rate may increase the fibre diameter or bead size (He and Wane 2004).

Distance between Tip and Collector

This is one of the important parameters that has a great influence on the electrospun fibre formation. The more gap or distance between the nozzle tip and the collector results in the formation of thinner fibres. The ES jet must be given enough time to travel from its source to the collector for the removal of the solvents by evaporation in order to generate distinct fibres. The lesser distance between the needle tip and the collector may lead to incomplete solvent removal because of insufficient time for the polymeric jets to pass through before it reaches the collecting plate resulting in the formation of wet fibres or fibre film (Ding et al. 2006)

Environmental Parameters

Temperature and Humidity

Temperature influences the solvent's volatility inside the ES chamber, resulting in fine fibre. Humidity is important to form dry and distinct fibres. Water condensation may take place on the fibre surface when ES is performed under high humid condition. This may influence the morphology of the generated fibre especially when volatile solvent is used to dissolve the polymer to be used for ES.

Air Velocity inside the Chamber

The air velocity inside the electrospinning chamber has a vital role to play in the collection of the fibre on the collector. An adequate air flow rate needs to be maintained to allow the complete deposition of the generated fibre on the collector. It also controls the voltage between the electrodes at desired level.

Pressure

Maintaining pressure at the desired level is important as it directly influences the polymer feed rate (Webber and Pashuck 2021) to the ES process and it also determines how fast the polymer solution is forced to exit the needle tip.

Advantages and Disadvantages of Electrospinning Technique

The ES methods have numerous advantages compared to the other scaffold fabrication techniques such as complete solvent removal, fibre diameter matching the ECM diameter, and higher cellular adhesion. In spite of having all these advantages, there are still significant challenges in this technique to fabricate complex 3D scaffold with desired internal pore structures, which make its application limited in the biomedical field (Ma 2008; Lu, Li and Chen 2013). The major disadvantages are: (i) energy-intensive process; (ii) high risk of using high voltage; (iii) lack of providing 3D scaffolds with interconnecting pore network, thus requiring appropriate designing of the collector; (iv) frequent choking of the needle tip, poor cell infiltration in the interior of the scaffolds because of smaller pore size; (v) limited to single fibre formation at a time; (vi) lack of mechanical property for load-bearing applications; (vii) limitation in using diverse polymers (Shi et al. 2015); (viii) toxicity effect due to chemical residue in fibres (Khorshidi et al. 2016; Kishan and Cosgriff-Hernandez 2017); and (ix) low fibre manufacturing rate, typically less than 0.3 g/h. Each needle usually can generate a single jet each time. Further, the scaffold with increased thickness can be achieved by simply increasing the ES time; however, it may take many hours to get an enhanced thickness of scaffold by ≈0.14 mm, which is the consequence of loss of electrostatic force when the collector is insulated with the nanofibres collected on it (Kishan et al. 2017).

ADVANCED ELECTROSPINNING TECHNIQUES

To overcome the various drawbacks of the needle-based ES technique as described above (Singh 2017), in recent years some needleless or nozzle-free and multi-needle ES techniques have been developed, which are described here (Shi et al. 2015).

Multi-Jet or Multi-Nozzle Electrospinning

The productivity of needle-based electrospinning process can be enhanced by increasing the number of needles in place of single one (Theron et al. 2005; Varesano et al. 2010). This is known as multi-needle or multi-jet ES. This type of ES set-up is complex, requiring a large working space to avoid the interferences between the adjacent polymer jets and also a regular cleaning system for each needle nozzle to avoid the choking or blockage of nozzles during fibre production. To overcome these drawbacks, porous tubes with large drilled holes have been considered as alternative fibre generators to achieve improved productivity of electrospun fibres (Teo et al. 2005). The pores conveyed polymer solutions to the tube surface, in which the polymer solution dropping under the influence of high electric field are drawn into polymer jets. This ES technology occupies lesser space than the multi-jet ES and it also involves a simple operation. However, there is still a challenge related to the interferences among the polymer jets (Theron et al. 2005).

Needleless Electrospinning

In recent decades, needless ES techniques have come up as a promising alternative technology for large-scale nanofibre production with a compact space. These methods are described in the following section.

Upward Needleless ES Technique

A typical two-layer fluid ES technique is shown in Figure 4.6. This technique consists of two layers: the upper layer containing the polymer solution to be spun and the lower layer is a ferromagnetic suspension. In this electrospinning process, a normal magnetic field is applied that produces stable vertical spikes, disrupting the interlayer

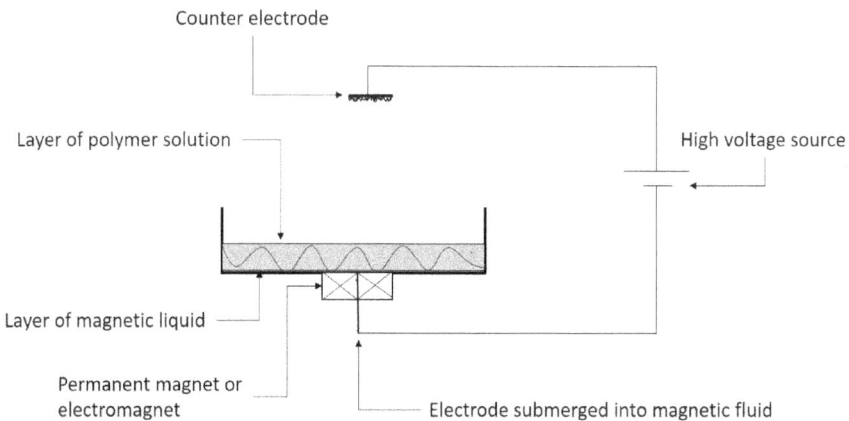

A two-layer fluid electrospinning setup

FIGURE 4.6   A two-layer fluid electrospinning set-up.

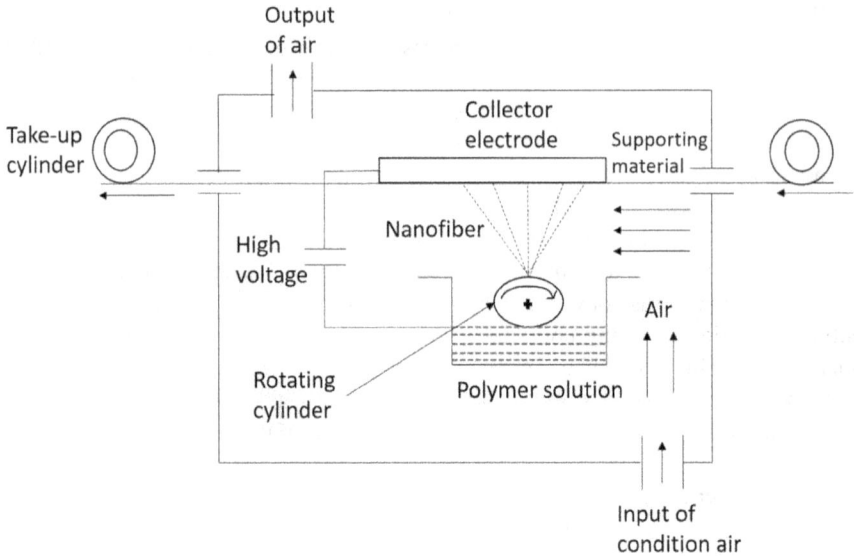

FIGURE 4.7   Free liquid surface electrospinning.

interface. When a high voltage is simultaneously applied to the fluid, numerous polymer jets are ejected in the upward direction and then deposited in the collector (Niu et al. 2011). The major limitations associated with this ES technique are its complicated set-up, generation of nanofibres with large and wide variation in diameter, and inability to provide scaffolds with 3D complex design.

Free Liquid Surface Electrospinning

Jirsak et al. developed the needless ES method in 2005 and this is the most promising one that can produce nanofibres directly from the open liquid surface at an industrial scale (Jirsak et al. 2005). The technique uses a rotating roller which acts as the generator of nanofibre, submerged in the polymer solution to be electrospun and rotates in a gentle motion, leading to the loading of the polymer solution onto the upper roller surface. Numerous polymer jets are ejected from the roller surface upwards under the influence of a high voltage, and the resulting nanofibres are collected in the grounded collector (Lukas et al. 2008). Figure 4.7 shows a schematic illustration of this technique. One of the free liquid surface electrospinning techniques was developed by Elmarco Co. and the system is marketed under the brand name "Nanospider TM".

Other Modified Electrospinning Devices

Various other ES processes have been established with the aim of fabricating nanofibrous scaffolds for bone and other tissue engineering applications. These include solution electrospinning (Ji et al. 2006; Muerza-Cascante et al. 2015), melt electrospinning (Asran, Henning, and Michler 2010), multi-axial electrospinning (Chen and Lv 2015; Khalf and Madihally 2017), and modified collector electrospinning

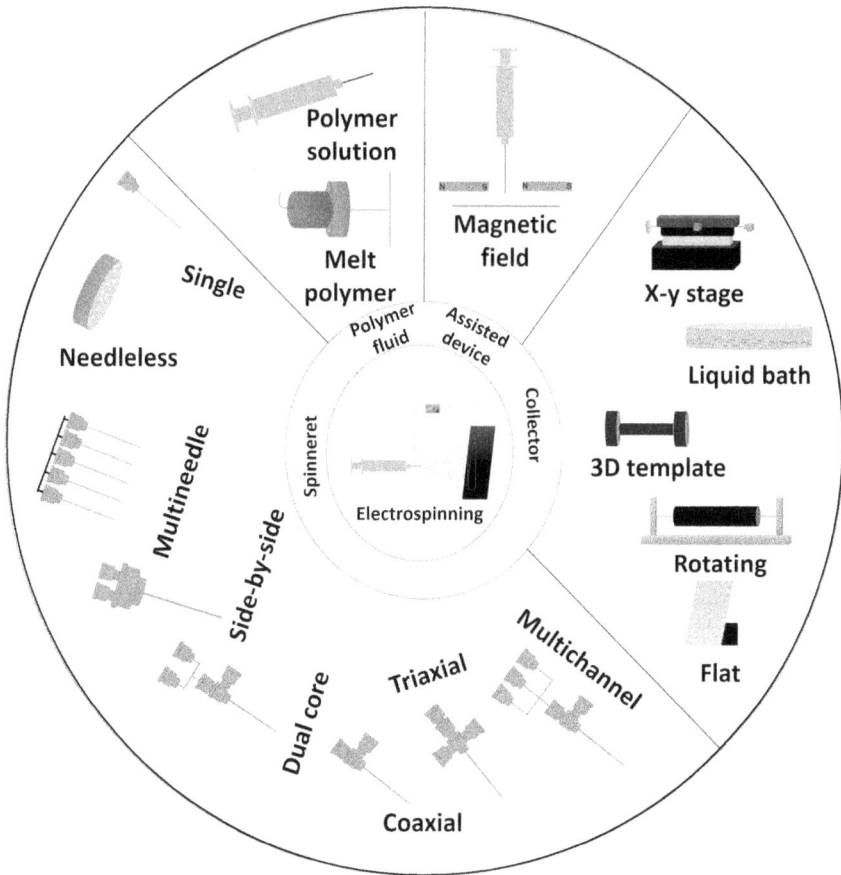

FIGURE 4.8 Pictorial representation of a simple electrospinning technique and its various customized configurations.

(Teo et al. 2005; Udomluck et al. 2019). The incredibly flexible scaffold construction method, the so-called electrospinning, uses spinning in conjunction with an electric field to draw polymer solutions either into microfibres or into nanofibres and has been widely investigated in tissue engineering research. However, the challenge prevailing in this technique has led to a modification in ES set-up that employs an opposite connection or a dual-electrode with positive and negative voltage. The addition of an assisted magnetic or electric field and modification in the spinneret or collector have been proposed in the literature (Rim et al. 2013) for further improvement in the ES process. Figure 4.8 presents a simple ES and its various customized configurations. Some of the modified ES processes are also described in the following section.

Melt Electrospinning

Melt electrospinning is an emerging ES technique used for fabricating scaffolds with 3D structure under solvent-free environment, thereby avoiding volatility and toxicity issues associated with solution ES system (Asran et al. 2010; Muerza-Cascante et al. 2015). This method produces nanofibre from the molten polymer in a diameter ranging typically 270–500 nm, and is subsequently cooled to solid nonwoven scaffolds by removing the residual liquid during the deposition of fibres. The viscous and non-conductive characteristics of the molten polymers makes it suitable for producing ES jets without electrical instability (Muerza-Cascante et al. 2015). The modified version of this technique is the melt electrospinning writing, which allows to manufacture small- to large-volume 3D scaffolds with an accurate and precise topographical structure, relatively high mechanical strength, and appropriate geometry following a layer-by-layer approach. These methods have been investigated recently keeping in view of manufaturing 3D scaffolds bone and cartilage tissue engineering application (Zaiss et al. 2016).

Multiaxial Electrospinning

Multiaxial electrospun set-up offers distinct benefits over solid fibre in the area of bone and cartilage regeneration. Coaxial ES is a modified version of normal electrospinning process where solution is used. This method uses a capillary tube that is internally fixed along a spinneret to protect the internal polymer solution from the external environment for a longer time period (Moghe and Gupta 2008). This technique allows the production of fibres along with the core structures in the internal side of the evolved fibres and was successfully demonstrated in generating nanofibre (Huang et al. 2006; Yu et al. 2011) for bone and related tissue diseases. A number of proteins and hydrophilic polymers such as bovine serum albumin, poly(ethylene glycol), and collagen have extensively been employed as the most frequent core materials (Cui, Zhou and Chang 2010; Su et al. 2012).

ADDITIVE MANUFACTURING (AM)

In tissue engineering techniques, particularly for bone and bone-related tissue regeneration, the fabrication and design of 3D engineered matrix, the so-called scaffold, with desired internal nano-architecture is the essential feature, and this is the most challenging task. The conventional scaffold fabrication techniques cannot fabricate the scaffold with these features. The control of scaffold architecture, biomaterial composition, and scaffold porosity which are the critical factors—can be achieved through appropriate design and fabrication. In this context, AM, the so-called "rapid prototyping", or solid free-form fabrication (SFF), is the most promising technique for producing intricate porous polymeric 3D structures with irregular geometry. These porous structures or scaffolds can be used as suitable substrates for treating complicated tissue defects such as joint defects which consists of bone, cartilage, and other adjoining tissues like tendon, ligament. This technique is thus suitable for fabricating 3D structure that resembles the complexity of native biological tissues (Wong and Hernandez 2012). The technique is based on a computer-controlled process that is used to fabricate 3D solid objects or entities from 3D model data in layered form. Each layer is realized as a thinly sliced horizontal cross-section of the ultimate object. Figure 4.9 shows

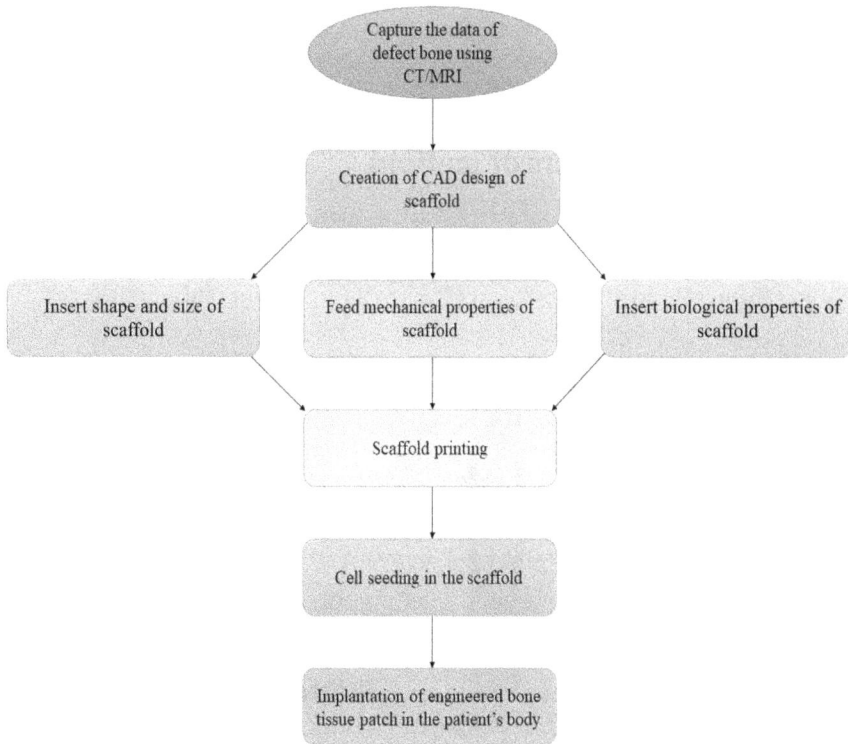

FIGURE 4.9 Steps involved in additive manufacturing of scaffold for bone and cartilage tissue engineering application.

the various steps involved in the AM technique. Many of the issues encountered with the conventional fabrication techniques can be addressed by the AM methodologies through the creation of scaffold design with precise spatial control over the polymer structure. These methods offer to fabricate the customized and patient-specific scaffold structures that are appropriate for regeneration of tissues and organs. Stereolithography, fused deposition modelling (FDM), selective laser sintering (SLS), and 3D printing (3DP) are the four primary rapid prototyping techniques (Wong and Hernandez 2012).

Stereolithography Technology (SLA)

SLA is an AM technique that is used to create a 3D object using liquid photopolymers. The method involves heating of a plastic material to make it a semi-liquid form. Then, a pre-designed 3D model is exposed once over the resin surface coated over the build platform, thereby forming a first layer. The platform moves down according to the layer height, and the resin is then again coated over the platform by the recoating bar following the exposure of a 3D model for the second layer. The print cycle continues this way until the 3D object is complete, following the bottom-up approach.

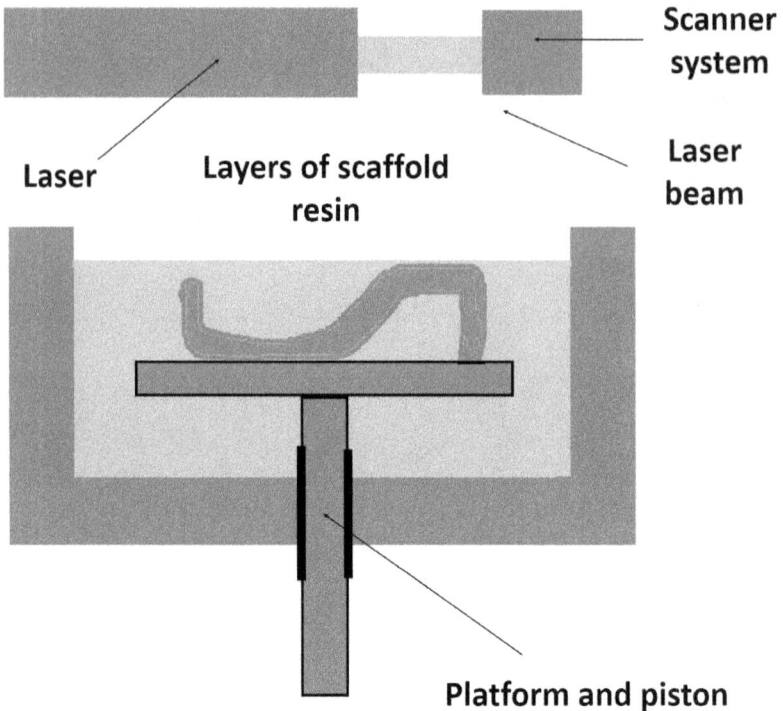

FIGURE 4.10   Showing the Stereolithography Technique (SLA).

The printing is continued in a layer-by layer fashion until the 3D object is completely built following the bottom- up approach by utilizing an ultraviolet laser that is guided by X and Y scanning mirrors (Skoog et al. 2014). Figure 4.10 represents the SLA technique.

Fused Deposition Modelling

Fused deposition modelling technique is one of the old techniques that involves the melting of thermoplastic materials to print its 3D objects and material deposition over a platform according to the pre-designed 3D computer-aided design (CAD) model. Figure 4.11 shows a typical FDM method of fabricating scaffold. Before the printing starts, the 3D CAD data are sliced into multiple layers using a special software and the sliced CAD data are sent to the printer whose movement in the X, Y, and Z directions is controlled by a driving software. The material is melted in a heating chamber, which extrudes through the nozzle in molten form, deposits over the platform, and then solidified. After completion of one layer, either dispenser or platform moves upwards or downwards according to the height of one layer. Like other AM techniques, this process repeats until the 3D object is complete (Vyavahare et al. 2020).

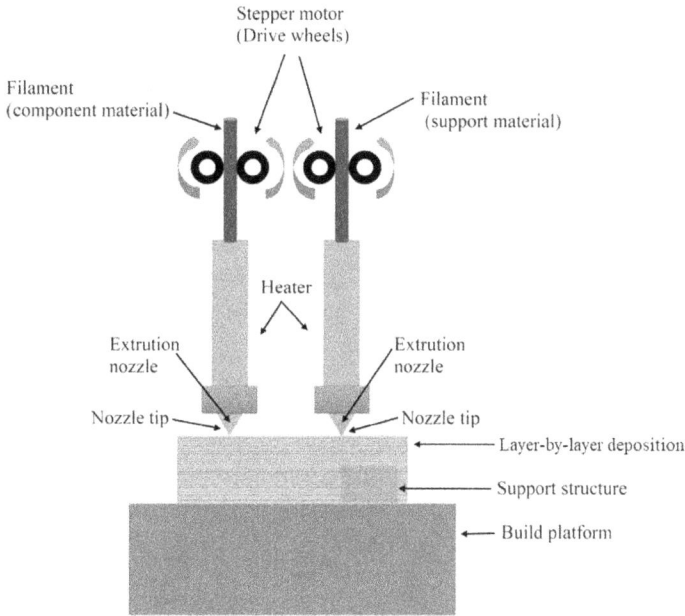

FIGURE 4.11 Fused deposition modelling technique.

Selective Laser Sintering Technology

This technique involves the fusion of glass, ceramic, metal, and plastic powders into 3D shapes by exposing them to a high-power laser light. According to the pre-designed 3D model, the laser light scans the powder bed, and due to the application of high-power laser, the powder material is fused over the bed to create a layer of the model. After completion of one layer, the powder bed moves down, and a new layer of powder is deposited over the bed and re-exposed to the laser light. Thus, the process of powder deposition is repeated until the complete 3D object with the required height is formed as per the CAD model. The set up of a selective laser sintering process is shown in Figure 4.12. It is quite a fast process, with printing taking only a few minutes. This method is different from other methods in a way that it uses material in powder form in place of liquid form for the printing process (Mazzoli 2013).

Three-Dimensional Printing Technique

Three-dimensional printing, the so-called 3DP technique, is an additive manufacturing method employed to create tools and functioning prototype features through the direct use of computer aided design (CAD) models. The 3D printers were invented by Hideo Kodama of Nagoya Municipal Industrial Research Institute with the aim of fabricating 3D plastic models using photo-hardening thermoset polymer in 1981; since then some advanced technology of 3D printing has come up. This technique offers many advantages, including the fabrication of patient-specific scaffold with complex

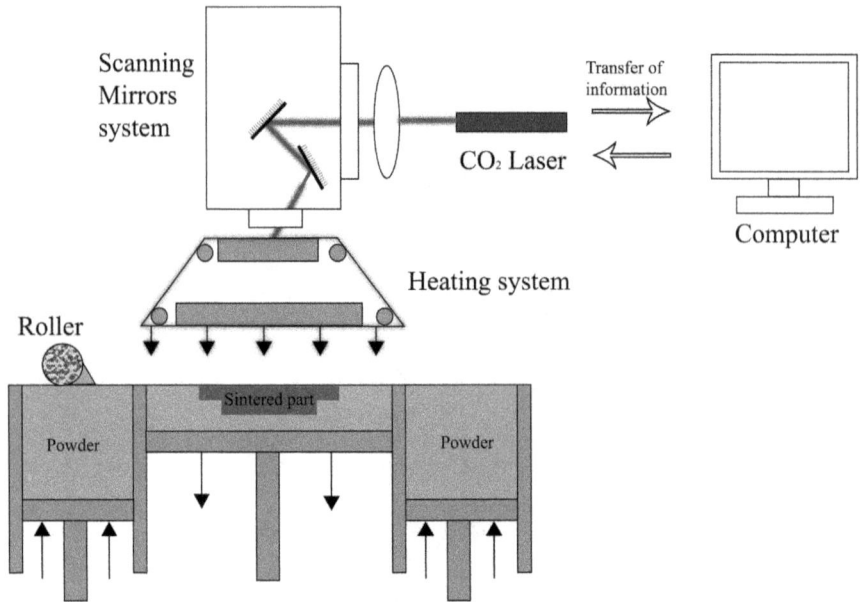

FIGURE 4.12   Schematic of selective laser sintering technique.

structure from a wide spectrum of materials and design flexibility, low cost, and rapid manufacturing compared to the subtractive manufacturing techniques and is therefore gaining in importance (Du, Fu and Zhu 2018; Ngo et al. 2018; Haleem et al. 2020). 3DP technique is utilized to precisely control scaffold structure down to the micron scale. The scaffolds are built following layer-by-layer deposition in this process with continuous supply of little quantity of biomaterial based upon the developed CAD model. Medical image-based modelling combined with 3D printing is very much effective to fabricate a complex customized 3D structure, which closely matches the defect shape and dimension (Bahraminasab 2020) and the mechanical properties. The steps involved in a 3DP process are (i) imaging the defect site using X-ray/ computed tomography (CT) or magnetic resonance imaging (MRI); (ii) conversion of the obtained image data into 3D CAD form and importing of the CAD file; (software packages such as 3D slicer, mimics, 3D doctors, and magics may be useful for the conversion; (iii) conversion of a CAD file to Standard Triangulate Language (STL) file format; (iv) setting up of the created files for printing with appropriate alignment of the part in 3D print software; and (v) printing of the biomaterial. However, the 3D-printed scaffolds have a limitation in mimicking the nanoscale ECM properties of the tissue aimed to replace (Eshkalak et al. 2020).

3DP is a useful technique to fabricate customized porous scaffolds critical for bone tissue regeneration and orthopaedic surgery (Cox et al. 2015; Kelly et al. 2018). Therefore, this technique has been widely used for fabricating scaffold for various BTE applications (Gregor et al. 2017; Tang et al. 2019; Hung et al. 2022). 3DP technology also enables to fabricate scaffold with delicate structures and on multiple scales for various cartilage and their associated complex tissue engineering applications. (Rosenzweig et al. 2015; Schoonraad et al. 2021; Wang et al. 2021; Yang et al. 2022).

Digital Light Processing (DLP) Technology

Digital Light Processing (DLP) technique is the oldest 3D printing technology used way back in the 1980s. In this technique, liquid plastic resins as photopolymers and traditional light sources like arc lamps are used (Webber and Pashuck 2021) and the liquid polymer bed is exposed to light as shown in Figure 4.13. The steps of this technique include 3D printing, and 3D CAD model design by taking and processing the image data from the defect site and transferring it to the printer, which is exposed to the liquid polymer bed through the DLP projector. The light solidifies the liquid polymer according to the 3D design, the bed moves down one layer, and again the liquid polymer comes over the bed, and this process continues. This process is repeated according to the desired number of layers, and finally, the 3D object is created. High-speed printing is the main advantage of this technique due to its exposure to entire polymer layers at once. The robustness and production of high-resolution models are other advantages of this method (Hornbeck). A number of scaffolds have been fabricated by DLP techniques for bone (Zhang et al. 2019), cartilage (Hong et al. 2020; Tao et al. 2022), and osteochondral (Gong et al. 2020; Schoonraad et al. 2021) tissue engineering applications.

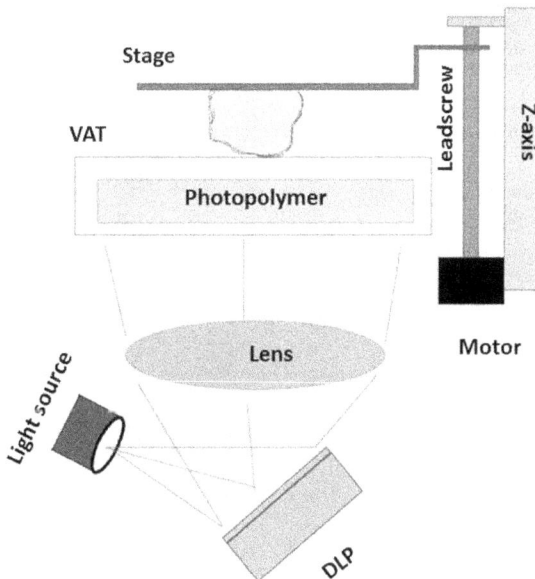

FIGURE 4.13   Digital light processing technology.

Binder Jetting Technology

Binder jetting is basically a powder-based 3DP technique. It has been most widely used to manufacture scaffolds for BTE application. A powdered substance, for example, gypsum and an appropriate liquid-binding agent are interacted to generate 3D objects using this type of 3DP technology known as "binder jetting". The bonding agent works as a strong adhesive to bind the powder layers together, as its name implies (Brunello et al. 2016; Kumar et al. 2016). Some of the binding agents are (5–30%) H_3PO_4, and 10% PVA. After forming one layer, like a conventional 2D inkjet printer, the printer nozzles extrude the binder as a liquid. The build plate lowers a little when each layer is finished to make room for the next layer. In this approach, the powder is dispersed over the platform using a recoating blade. An inkjet nozzle-equipped cartridge is then used to travel across the platform by tossing a binding agent (glue) over the powder, which binds the powder particles into a single layer. Then, the bed moves down, the powder spreads over the platform again, and the process repeats until the desired 3D model is built. The details of the stages of this method are reported elsewhere (Zhou et al. 2014). The popular materials used in this printing technology are ceramics, metals, sand, and plastic (Gungor-Ozkerim et al. 2018). A schematic of the binder jetting technique is shown in Figure 4.14. This method was used in a number of studies related to BTE (Zhou et al. 2014; Shakir et al. 2015). The major disadvantage of this technique is its slow process (Wubneh et al. 2018).

Bioprinting

Bioprinting is an innovative and unique 3DP technique that creates actual or natural tissue-like 3D structures with specific biological activities by combining living cells and other chemicals, such as growth factors, with bio-inks made of organic or synthetic biodegradable materials. This method uses 3D digital computer models created by CAD software to produce complex, layered structures with required

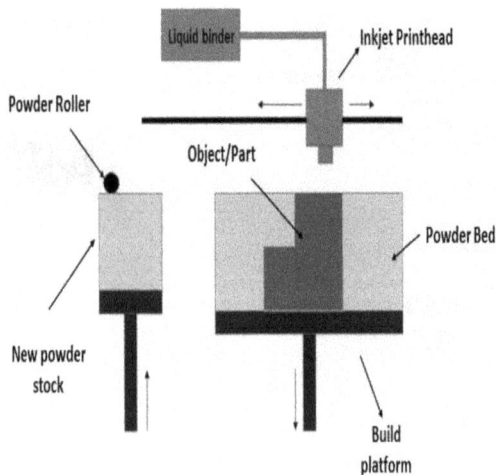

FIGURE 4.14 Schematic of binder jetting technology.

3D architecture, porosity, and tunable structural and mechanical properties. This method is also cost-effective. Additionally, adding cells and bioactive chemicals/molecules to the structures enhance the cellular response. Aqueous-based technologies without solvents have made it possible to directly print biomaterials onto 3D scaffolds for transplantation with or without using cells. Based on the later characteristics, the technique is referred to as acellular and cellular constructs. The acellular bioprinting allows direct printing of the scaffold biomaterial without cells during the printing process. In the cellular method, the biomaterial and cells are printed simultaneously, thereby making a cell-seeded scaffold, also known as construct. In comparison, higher precision and greater shape complexity of the defect tissue or organ can be achieved by acellular bioprinting as it involves less restrictive condition than the cellular bioprinting which involves the issue of maintaining cell viability (Murphy and Atala 2014).

Bioprinting comprises three steps including, pre-bioprinting, bioprinting, and post-bioprinting. Like any other 3DP, in pre-processing or pre-bioprinting step, the anatomic structure of the defect tissue or organ site is obtained by computed tomography (CT) or magnetic resonance imaging (MRI) techniques and then a 3D model is developed by tomographic reconstruction of the images using CAD/computer-aided manufacturing (CAM) software, followed by slicing it into 2D layers with appropriate thickness followed by feeding it into the bioprinter. This step also includes the biomaterial or bio-ink selection. In bioprinting step, the layer-by-layer printing using bio-ink is done by using the obtained CAD model for the fabrication of scaffold and the cell-laden constructs by dispensing cells onto the scaffold structure. Post-processing refers to creating a stable printed tissue by culturing and growing the cell-seeded scaffold in a suitable culture vessel, usually a bioreactor, resulting in a suitable construct or tissue graft by cell differentiation that is ideal for *in vivo* application. During this stage, necessary mechanical and chemical stimulations are applied and signals are transmitted to the cells to control the remodelling and growth of regenerated tissues. The 3D model file is then sent to a slicer, a specialized type of computer application that analyses the geometry and produces several thin layers, or slices, which when arranged in layers vertically form the shape of the original model. Examples of standard slicers used in bioprinting are Cura and Slic3r (Pakhomova, C et al. 2020). Numerous investigations done using the bioprinting method to fabricate scaffolds and constructs for bone and cartilage tissue defect repair have been reported (Leberfinger et al. 2017; Trombetta et al. 2017).

A bioprinted bone scaffold fabricated by multi-bio-ink and printing in different layers and gradients provides engineered tissues with desired physico-chemical and mechanical properties. For instance, cancellous bone-like printable implants with robust mechanical properties encapsulating stem cells into the microparticles of PLGA and controlled-release programming factors aid in creating innovative localized delivery systems for bone repairing. Poly (dopamine) coatings on 3D-printed PLA scaffolds promoted cell adhesion, proliferation, and osteogenesis. Yang and Vaezi created a low-cost production process for 3DP bioactive Polyetheretherketone/hydroxyapatite (PEEK/HA) composite scaffolds and compression moulds for BTE (Li, Chen et al. 2016). 3D bioprinting has many advantages such as it enables imitation of the desired tissue and organs. It has a simple structure, can be used to develop patient- and organ-specific tissue grafts and can coexist with human cells and tissues, intricate procedures can be automated, and it is reliable, and features fewer human errors. However, this technique also possesses a number of disadvantages, such as it is a high-end technology, complexity, challenges to maintain the cell environment, and ethical anxieties.

Decellularization

Decellularization is the process of removing cells and their constituents (especially nucleic acids like DNA and RNA) from the extracellular matrix (ECM) in order to produce a natural matrix with preserved mechanical integrity. Since ECM is vital in tissue formation, decellularized extracellular matrix (dECM) is proven to be an appropriate scaffold for tissue engineering (Gilbert et al. 2006). To date, several decellularization strategies for reconstructing various types of biological organs have been established. The underlying premise in all approaches is to eliminate the cellular based material while unaltering the ECM ultrastructure of the tissue. Decellularization procedures range in terms of the materials utilised (combination of reagents) and the paths to administer the main component, namely airway, vascular, or both (Badylak, Taylor et al. 2011, Crapo, Gilbert et al. 2011, Daryabari, Kajbafzadeh et al. 2019). Decellularization methods are broadly classified into three categories *namely* chemical methods using acids or alkali, detergents, surfactants like ethylenediaminetetraacetic acid with sodium dodecyl sulphate or trypsin with Triton X-100, ammonium hydroxide and sodium deoxycholate, and alcohols; physical methods like sonication, pressurisation, electroporation; and biological methods that use enzymes like nucleases or proteases (Badylak, Taylor et al. 2011, Gilpin and Yang 2017). The enzymatic method is advantageous of avoiding hazardous chemicals and minimizing protein denaturation, resulting in a high degree of ECM content (Gilbert, Sellaro et al. 2006). Decellularized bone matrix-based biomaterials have been widely used as bio-scaffolds in bone tissue engineering because they possess 3D structures, good mechanical characteristics, and osteo-inductivity similar to a natural bone (Chen and Lv 2018). These biomaterials are critical in establishing the physical and mechanical microenvironment required for cell proliferation and survival. Growth factor, chondroitin sulphate, fibronectin, hyaluronic acid, and heparin sulphate, are the components of decellularized bone matrix (DBM), which drives MSCs (mesenchymal stem cells) development into osteoblast (Amirazad, Dadashpour et al. 2022). Furthermore, the porous structure of the bone, which influences differentiation, is conserved. Spongy bone is better suited for decellularization than cortical bone because of its unique architecture, such as spongy construction and porosity. Moreover, spongy bone has a larger surface-to-volume ratio than cortical bone. DBM-based scaffolds are fabricated using DBM solely or in mixing with appropriate bioceramics and polymers to improve mechanical characteristics, osteogenesis, and vascularization (Gilbert, Sellaro et al. 2006). Different types of decellularized scaffolds obtained from human and animal sources have been clinically utilized, primarily for healing of wound and in surgical mesh related devices; however, their application is still restricted, and more research is required before decellularized scaffolds can be used commercially for disease treatment (Damodaran and Vermette 2018).

COMBINED FABRICATION TECHNIQUES

There has been a great interest in fabricating 3D fibrous scaffolds, especially nanofibrous scaffold that can mimic the targeted ECM structure and control the essential biological activities, such as cell adhesion, differentiation, and ECM deposition. The production of electrospun 3D nanofibrous porous ECM mimetic scaffolds with appropriate forms and desired pores have been attempted through a number of approaches. These advances are discussed in this section.

A number of approaches that have been proposed in recent advancement, especially in the electrospinning technology, for fabricating 3D nanofibrous structure are: (i) template-assisted electrospinning; (ii) self-assembly electrospinning; (iii) liquid-assisted or wet electrospinning; (iv) electrospinning writing, and (v) layer-by-layer electrospinning (Figure 4.15) (Soliman et al. 2010; Wu et al. 2014; Su et al. 2021). However, fabricating 3D structures with accurate complex shapes and controllable pore structure using these approaches are difficult to achieve (Naghieh et al. 2017). In several other studies, electrospinning and freeze-shaping techniques have been combined to convert the fabricated electrospun fibres into 3D porous nanofibrous scaffolds (Chen et al. 2019; Ye et al. 2019), success has eluded in obtaining scaffolds with accurate geometry and pore structure. Chen et al. for the first combined 3D printing, freeze-drying, and electrospun fibre-based bio-inks (gelatin/poly (lactic-*co*-glycolic acid) to produce 3D-printed scaffolds with precisely controlled geometry, large pores, and surface morphologies mimicking the native ECM (Chen et al. 2019). ES, dehydrating, homogenizing, and drying by evaporation have been first used to transform the electrospun fibre membranes into the single fibre powder, which was blended with HA, and PEO solution and used as 3D printing ink. The mechanical strength of the resulting 3D-printed scaffolds was then improved while maintaining stable structure by freeze-drying and cross-linking. Figure 4.16 shows different 3D scaffolds resulting from the combination of electrospinning and other fabrication techniques.

Vyas et al. (2020) developed a dual-scale scaffold by coupling 3D-printed microfibres directly with electrospun nanofibres throughout the scaffold. A screw-assisted extrusion 3D printer and ES system were employed to create polycaprolactone dual-scale scaffolds (Vyas et al. 2020). Kim and his team developed a novel fabrication process of manufacturing a hierarchical 3D polymeric scaffold made of melt-plotted PCL strands and PCL micro/nanofibres by combining a rapid prototyping and ES with continuous dispensing systems (Kim et al. 2008). This scaffold overcomes the drawbacks of conventional 3D electrospun dispensed structures by providing appropriate pore size matching with the cell size, promoting initial cell attachment, and high mechanical properties. A schematic of the dual-scale and hierarchical 3D scaffolds manufacturing techniques are depicted in Figure 4.17.

Bosworth et al. (2013) combined electrospun nanofibres with hydrogels and obtained an innovative 3D nanofiber/hydrogel composite scaffold (Figure 4.18). Consequently, the amalgamation of electrospun fibres and hydrogels offers the potential for the development of superior composite scaffolds, which combine the advantages of both structures and also overcome their disadvantages, thereby developing a truly 3D

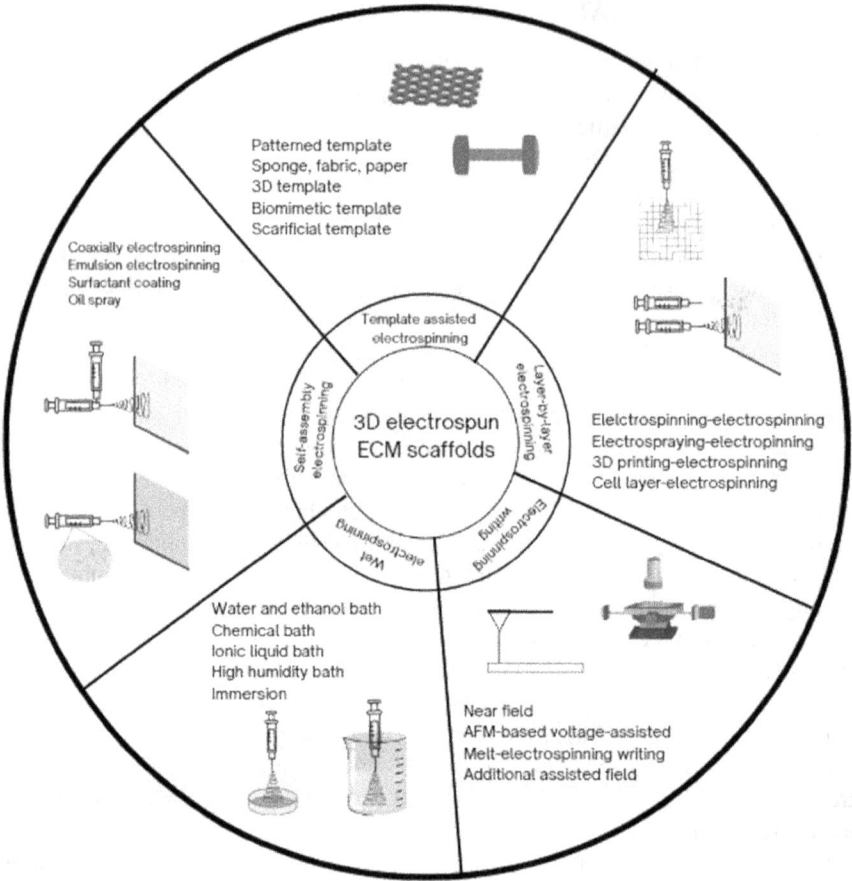

FIGURE 4.15 Different strategies for fabricating nanofibrous 3D scaffold through the advanced electrospinning technology.

environment with enhanced mechanical properties and cell penetration (Bosworth, Turner and Cartmell 2013).

EXERCISE

1. What are scaffolds and what are their functions in bone and cartilage tissue engineering?
2. Why are nanostructured scaffolds preferred for tissue engineering applications? State various methods for making nanofibrous scaffolds.
3. What should be the ideal porosity of a tissue scaffold?
4. What are the essential criteria for selecting a scaffold for tissue reconstruction?
5. Explain the importance of the mechanical properties of the scaffolds when implanted in the human body.

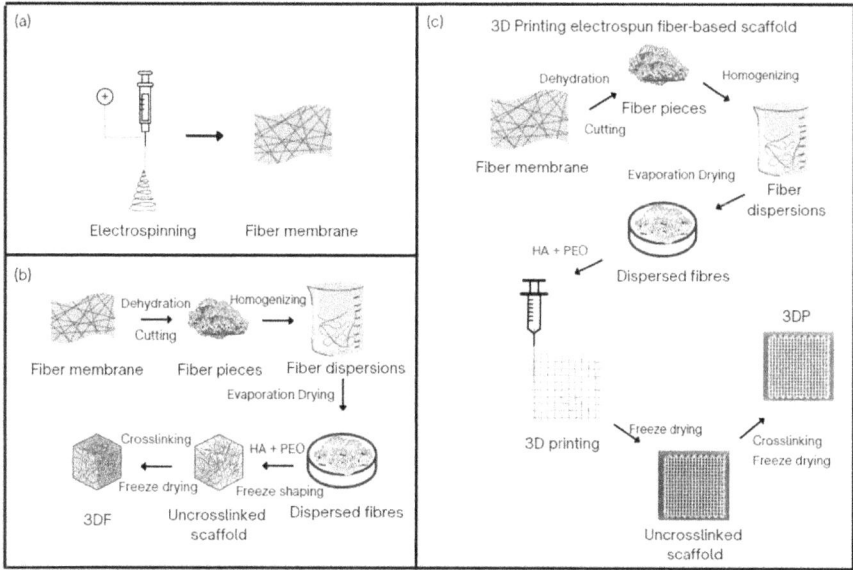

FIGURE 4.16 Showing the different 3D scaffolds resulting from electrospining in combination with other fabrication techniques.

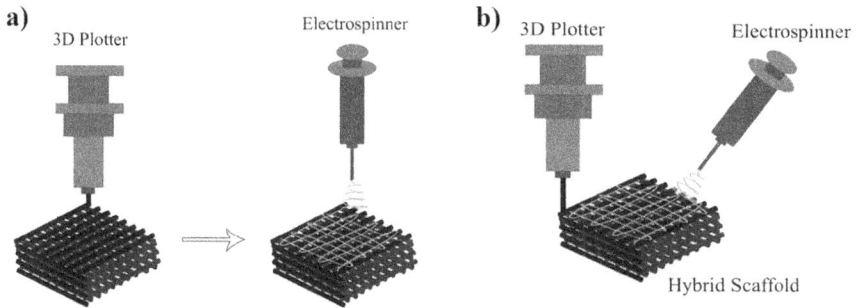

FIGURE 4.17 Schematic representation of a dual-scale scaffold constructed by combining extrusion-based 3D printing and electrospinning and fabrication of a hierarchical 3D scaffold by combining 3D plotter (rapid prototyping) and electrospinning techniques.

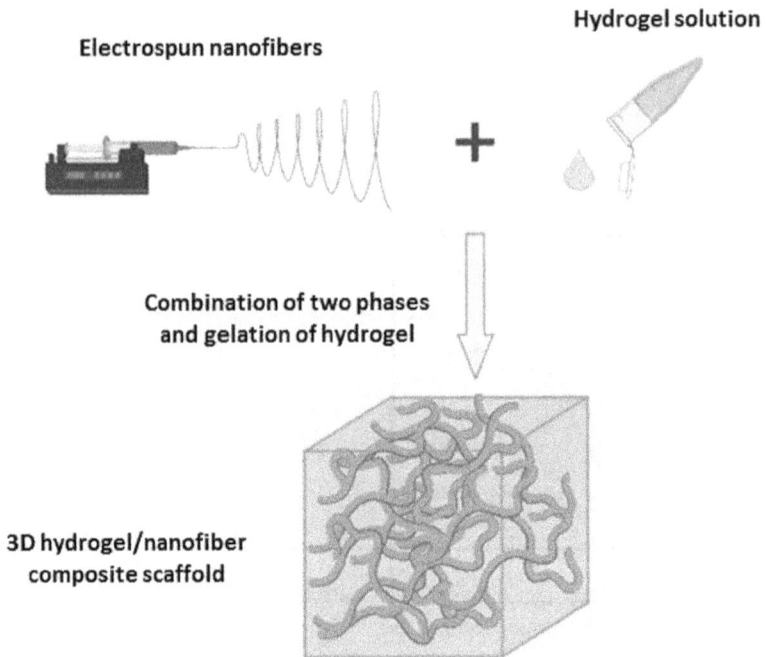

FIGURE 4.18   Fabrication of a 3D composite scaffold by combining hydrogel and electrospun nanofibers.

6. Write the working principle and explain the influencing parameters involved in the electrospinning technique.
7. Explain the various steps involved in 3D bioprinting with a diagram. Explain its advantages and disadvantages over other scaffold fabrication techniques.
8. Explain the importance of fabrication technique on surface morphology, porosity and degradation properties of the scaffold in bone tissue engineering?
9. Describe the FDM method for fabricating 3D object with a neat diagram and leveling its various parts. What is the major drawback for which it is not suitable for tissue engineering scaffold fabrication and how to overcome?
10. What do you mean by rapid prototyping? Explain the various steps involved in this technique?
11. Imagine a person meets with an accident and suffers a knee injury. What type of technique could you suggest for fabricating three-dimensional (3D) polymeric composite structures to treat the patient? Explain the method in detail.
12. What is the principle of free liquid surface electrospinning method? Explain this method with a neat diagram.
13. Explain the phase separation technique for fabricating 3D porous scaffold. Write the advantages of the freeze gelation technique over the freeze-drying technique.

14. What is the function of porogen in scaffold fabrication? In which fabrication technique are porogens used? what are the different types of porogens are used in scaffold fabrication?
15. What are bi-phasic scaffolds? Write the importance of this type of scaffold. Give a few examples of bi-phasic scaffolds that are potential for osteochondral defects.
16. Give a brief account of advancement in electrospinning technique for fabricating bone scaffold.
17. Describe self-assembly and decellularization methods and justify their suitability for the fabrication of bone and cartilage tissue scaffolds.

REFERENCES

Akbarzadeh, R. and A. M. Yousefi. 2014. "Effects of processing parameters in thermally induced phase separation technique on porous architecture of scaffolds for bone tissue engineering". *Journal of Biomedical Materials Research Part B: Applied Biomaterials* 102 (6): 1304–1315.

Amirazad, H., Dadashpour, M. and Zarghami, N. 2022. Application of decellularized bone matrix as a bioscaffold in bone tissue engineering. *Journal of Biological Engineering* 16: 1–18.

Aranaz, I., M. C. Gutiérrez, M. L. Ferrer and F. Del Monte. 2014. "Preparation of chitosan nanocomposites with a macroporous structure by unidirectional freezing and subsequent freeze-drying". *Marine Drugs* 12 (11): 5619–5642.

Asran, A. S., S. Henning and G. H. Michler. 2010. "Polyvinyl alcohol–collagen–hydroxyapatite biocomposite nanofibrous scaffold: Mimicking the key features of natural bone at the nanoscale level". *Polymer* 51 (4): 868–876.

Badylak, S. F., Taylor, D., and Uygun, K. 2011. Whole-organ Tissue Engineering: Decellularization and Recellularization of Three-Dimensional Matrix Scaffolds. *Annual Review of Biomedical Engineering* 13: 27–53. doi:10.1146/annurev-bioeng-071910-124743

Bahraminasab, M. 2020. "Challenges on optimization of 3D-printed bone scaffolds". *BioMedical Engineering OnLine* 19 (1): 1–33.

Beachley, V. and X. J. Wen. 2009. "Effect of electrospinning parameters on the nanofiber diameter and length". *Materials Science & Engineering C-Biomimetic and Supramolecular Systems* 29 (3): 663–668.

Bosworth, L. A., L. A. Turner and S. H. Cartmell. 2013. "State of the art composites comprising electrospun fibres coupled with hydrogels: A review". *Nanomedicine-Nanotechnology Biology and Medicine* 9 (3): 322–335.

Brunello, G., S. Sivolella, R. Meneghello, L. Ferroni, C. Gardin, A. Piattelli, B. Zavan and E. Bressan. 2016. "Powder-based 3D printing for bone tissue engineering". *Biotechnology Advances* 34 (5): 740–753.

Chen, G. and Y. Lv. 2015. "Immobilization and application of electrospun nanofiber scaffold-based growth factor in bone tissue engineering". *Current Pharmaceutical Design* 21 (15): 1967–1978.

Chen, G. and Y. Lv. 2017. Decellularized bone matrix scaffold for bone regeneration, in *Decellularized Scaffolds and Organogenesis*, Springer, 239–254.

Chen, S., Gil, C. J., Ning, L., Jin, L., Perez, L., Kabboul, G., ... and Serpooshan, V. 2021. "Adhesive tissue engineered scaffolds: mechanisms and applications." *Frontiers in Bioengineering and Biotechnology*, 19: 683079, 1–22.

Chen, W., Y. Xu, Y. Liu, Z. Wang, Y. Li, G. Jiang, X. Mo and G. Zhou. 2019. "Three-dimensional printed electrospun fiber-based scaffold for cartilage regeneration". *Materials & Design* 179: 107886.

Costantini, M. and A. Barbetta. 2018. Gas foaming technologies for 3D scaffold engineering. *Functional 3D Tissue Engineering Scaffolds*, Elsevier, 127–149.

Cox, S. C., J. A. Thornby, G. J. Gibbons, M. A. Williams and K. K. Mallick. 2015. "3D printing of porous hydroxyapatite scaffolds intended for use in bone tissue engineering applications". *Materials Science and Engineering: C* 47: 237–247.

Crapo, P. M., Gilbert, T. W., and Badylak, S. F. 2011. An Overview of Tissue and Whole Organ Decellularization Processes. *Biomaterials* 32 (12): 3233–3243. doi:10.1016/j.biomaterials.2011.01.057

Cui, W., Y. Zhou and J. Chang. 2010. "Electrospun nanofibrous materials for tissue engineering and drug delivery", *Science and Technology of Advanced Materials* 11: 1–11.

Damodaran, R., and Vermette, P. 2018. Tissue and Organ Decellularization in Regenerative Medicine. *Biotechnology Progress* 34 (6): 1494–1505. doi:10.1002/btpr.26997

Daryabari, S. S., Kajbafzadeh, A.-M., Fendereski, K., Ghorbani, F., Dehnavi, M., Rostami, M., et al. 2019. Development of an Efficient Perfusion-Based Protocol for Whole-Organ Decellularization of the Ovine Uterus as a Human-Sized Model and In Vivo Application of the Bioscaffolds. *Journal of Assisted Reproduction and Genetics* 36 (6): 1211–1223. doi:10.1007/s10815-019-01463-4

Deitzel, J., W. Kosik, S. McKnight, N. B. Tan, J. DeSimone and S. Crette. 2002. "Electrospinning of polymer nanofibers with specific surface chemistry". *Polymer* 43 (3): 1025–1029.

Ding, B., C. R. Li, Y. Miyauchi, O. Kuwaki and S. Shiratori. 2006. "Formation of novel 2D polymer nanowebs via electrospinning". *Nanotechnology* 17 (15): 3685–3691.

Doshi, J. and D. H. Reneker. 1995. "Electrospinning process and applications of electrospun fibers". *Journal of Electrostatics* 35(2–3): 151–160.

Du, X., S. Fu and Y. Zhu. 2018. "3D printing of ceramic-based scaffolds for bone tissue engineering: An overview". *Journal of Materials Chemistry B* 6(27): 4397–4412.

Duan, J., Z. Zhou, T. Huang, W. Liu, Y. Zhao, W. Wu, X. Li and J. Fang. 2019. "Biocompatibility properties of composite scaffolds based on 1, 4-butanediamine modified poly (lactide-co-glycolide) and nanobioceramics". *International Journal of Polymer Analysis and Characterization* 24 (5): 428–438.

Erkal, T. S. 2012. *Self-Assembly of Peptide Nanofibers and Their Mechanical Properties*, Bilkent Universitesi (Turkey).

Eshkalak, S. K., E. R. Ghomi, Y. Q. Dai, D. Choudhury and S. Ramakrishna. 2020. "The role of three-dimensional printing in healthcare and medicine". *Materials & Design* 194: 1–15.

Farzamfar, S., M. Salehi, S. M. Tavangar, J. Verdi, K. Mansouri, A. Ai, Z. V. Malekshahi and J. Ai. 2019. "A novel polycaprolactone/carbon nanofiber composite as a conductive neural guidance channel: An in vitro and in vivo study". *Progress in Biomaterials* 8 (4): 239–248.

Formhals, A. 1934. "Process and apparatus for preparing artificial threads US patent specification, 1975504".

Gilbert, T. W., T. L. Sellaro and S. F. Badylak. 2006. "Decellularization of tissues and organs". *Biomaterials* 27 (19): 3675–3683.

Gilpin, A., and Yang, Y. 2017. Decellularization Strategies for Regenerative Medicine: from Processing Techniques to Applications. *BioMed Research International*: 9831534. doi:10.1155/2017/9831534

Gong, L., J. Li, J. Zhang, Z. Pan, Y. Liu, F. Zhou, Y. Hong, Y. Hu, Y. Gu and H. Ouyang. 2020. "An interleukin-4-loaded bi-layer 3D printed scaffold promotes osteochondral regeneration". *Acta Biomaterialia* 117: 246–260.

Gregor, A., E. Filová, M. Novák, J. Kronek, H. Chlup, M. Buzgo, V. Blahnová, V. Lukášová, M. Bartoš and A. Nečas. 2017. "Designing of PLA scaffolds for bone tissue replacement fabricated by ordinary commercial 3D printer". *Journal of Biological Engineering* 11 (1): 1–21.

Gungor-Ozkerim, P. S., I. Inci, Y. S. Zhang, A. Khademhosseini and M. R. Dokmeci. 2018. "Bioinks for 3D bioprinting: An overview". *Biomaterials Science* 6 (5): 915–946.

Haleem, A., M. Javaid, R. H. Khan and R. Suman. 2020. "3D printing applications in bone tissue engineering". *Journal of Clinical Orthopaedics and Trauma* 11: S118–S124.

He, J. H. and Y. Q. Wane. 2004. "Allometric scaling for voltage and current in electrospinning". *Polymer* 45 (19): 6731–6734.

Hong, H., Y. B. Seo, J. S. Lee, Y. J. Lee, H. Lee, O. Ajiteru, M. T. Sultan, O. J. Lee, S. H. Kim and C. H. Park. 2020. "Digital light processing 3D printed silk fibroin hydrogel for cartilage tissue engineering". *Biomaterials* 232: 119679.

Huang, Y. C., D. Kaigler, K. G. Rice, P. H. Krebsbach and D. J. Mooney. 2005. "Combined angiogenic and osteogenic factor delivery enhances bone marrow stromal cell-driven bone regeneration". *Journal of Bone and Mineral Research* 20 (5): 848–857.

Huang, Z.-M., Y.-Z. Zhang, M. Kotaki and S. Ramakrishna. 2003. "A review on polymer nanofibers by electrospinning and their applications in nanocomposites". *Composites Science and Technology* 63 (15): 2223–2253.

Huang, Z. M., C. L. He, A. Yang, Y. Zhang, X. J. Han, J. Yin and Q. Wu. 2006. "Encapsulating drugs in biodegradable ultrafine fibers through co-axial electrospinning". *Journal of Biomedical Materials Research Part A: An Official Journal of the Society for Biomaterials, the Japanese Society for Biomaterials, and the Australian Society for Biomaterials and the Korean Society for Biomaterials* 77 (1): 169–179.

Hung, K. S., M. S. Chen, W. C. Lan, Y. C. Cho, T. Saito, B. H. Huang, H. Y. Tsai, C.-C. Hsieh, K. L. Ou and H. Y. Lin. 2022. "Three-dimensional printing of a hybrid bioceramic and biopolymer porous scaffold for promoting bone regeneration potential". *Materials* 15 (5): 1971.

Hutmacher, D. W. 2001. "Scaffold design and fabrication technologies for engineering tissues--state of the art and future perspectives". *Journal of Biomaterials Science, Polymer Edition* 12 (1): 107–124.

Ji, Y., K. Ghosh, X. Z. Shu, B. Li, J. C. Sokolov, G. D. Prestwich, R. A. Clark and M. H. Rafailovich. 2006. "Electrospun three-dimensional hyaluronic acid nanofibrous scaffolds". *Biomaterials* 27 (20): 3782–3792.

Jirsak, O., F. Sanetrnik, D. Lukas, et al. 2005. A method of nanofibres production from a polymer solution using electrostatic spinning and a device for carrying out the method, WO 2005/024101 A1.

Kasoju, N., D. Kubies, T. Sedlačík, O. Janoušková, J. Koubková, M. M. Kumorek and F. Rypáček. 2016. "Polymer scaffolds with no skin-effect for tissue engineering applications fabricated by thermally induced phase separation". *Biomedical Materials* 11 (1): 015002.

Kelly, C. N., A. T. Miller, S. J. Hollister, R. E. Guldberg and K. Gall. 2018. "Design and structure–function characterization of 3D printed synthetic porous biomaterials for tissue engineering". *Advanced Healthcare Materials* 7 (7): 1701095.

Khalf, A. and S. V. Madihally. 2017. "Recent advances in multiaxial electrospinning for drug delivery". *European Journal of Pharmaceutics and Biopharmaceutics* 112: 1–17.

Khorshidi, S., A. Solouk, H. Mirzadeh, S. Mazinani, J. M. Lagaron, S. Sharifi and S. Ramakrishna. 2016. "A review of key challenges of electrospun scaffolds for tissue-engineering applications". *Journal of Tissue Engineering and Regenerative Medicine* 10 (9): 715–738.

Kim, G., J. Son, S. Park and W. Kim. 2008. "Hybrid process for fabricating 3D hierarchical scaffolds combining rapid prototyping and electrospinning". *Macromolecular Rapid Communications* 29 (19): 1577–1581.

Kim, J. F., J. H. Kim, Y. M. Lee and E. Drioli. 2016. "Thermally induced phase separation and electrospinning methods for emerging membrane applications: A review". *Aiche Journal* 62 (2): 461–490.

Kishan, A. P. and E. M. Cosgriff-Hernandez. 2017. "Recent advancements in electrospinning design for tissue engineering applications: A review". *Journal of Biomedical Materials Research Part A* 105 (10): 2892–2905.

Kishan, A. P., A. B. Robbins, S. F. Mohiuddin, M. Jiang, M. R. Moreno and E. M. Cosgriff-Hernandez. 2017. "Fabrication of macromolecular gradients in aligned fiber scaffolds using a combination of in-line blending and air-gap electrospinning". *Acta Biomaterialia* 56: 118–128.

Kumar, A., S. Mandal, S. Barui, R. Vasireddi, U. Gbureck, M. Gelinsky and B. Basu. 2016. "Low temperature additive manufacturing of three dimensional scaffolds for bone-tissue engineering applications: Processing related challenges and property assessment". *Materials Science and Engineering: R: Reports* 103: 1–39.

La Carrubba, V., F. C. Pavia, S. Brucato and S. Piccarolo. 2008. "PLLA/PLA scaffolds prepared via thermally induced phase separation (TIPS): Tuning of properties and biodegradability". *International Journal of Material Forming* 1 (1): 619–622.

Leberfinger, A. N., D. J. Ravnic, A. Dhawan and I. T. Ozbolat. 2017. "Concise review: Bioprinting of stem cells for transplantable tissue fabrication". *Stem Cells Translational Medicine* 6 (10): 1940–1948.

Li, C., C. Vepari, H.-J. Jin, H. J. Kim and D. L. Kaplan. 2006. "Electrospun silk-BMP-2 scaffolds for bone tissue engineering". *Biomaterials* 27 (16): 3115–3124.

Li, J., M. Chen, X. Fan and H. Zhou. 2016. "Recent advances in bioprinting techniques: Approaches, applications and future prospects". *Journal of Translational Medicine* 14 (1): 1–15.

Li, Z., M.-B. Xie, Y. Li, Y. Ma, J.-S. Li and F.-Y. Dai. 2016. "Recent progress in tissue engineering and regenerative medicine". *Journal of Biomaterials and Tissue Engineering* 6 (10): 755–766.

Liu, D., S. D. Feyter, U. M. Cotlet, U. M. Wiesler, T. Weil, A. Herrmann, K. Müllen and F. C. De Schryver. 2003. "Fluorescent self-assembled polyphenylene dendrimer nanofibers". *Macromolecules* 36 (22): 8489–8498.

Liu, D., H. Zhang, P. Grim, S. De Feyter, U. M. Wiesler, A. Berresheim, K. Müllen and F. De Schryver. 2002. "Self-assembly of polyphenylene dendrimers into micrometer long nanofibers: An atomic force microscopy study". *Langmuir* 18 (6): 2385–2391.

Lombardo, M. E., F. C. Pavia, I. Vitrano, G. Ghersi, V. Brucato, F. Rosei and V. La Carrubba. 2019. "PLLA scaffolds with controlled architecture as potential microenvironment for in vitro tumor model". *Tissue and Cell* 58: 33–41.

Lou, T., X. Wang, X. Yan, Y. Miao, Y. Z. Long, H. L. Yin, B. Sun and G. Song. 2016. "Fabrication and biocompatibility of poly (l-lactic acid) and chitosan composite scaffolds with hierarchical microstructures". *Materials Science and Engineering: C* 64: 341–345.

Lozinsky, V. I. and O. Okay. 2014. "Basic principles of cryotropic gelation". *Polymeric Cryogels: Macroporous Gels with Remarkable Properties* 263: 49–101.

Lu, L., J. Temenoff, J. Teßmar and A. G. Mikos. 2004. "Synthetic bioresorbable polymer scaffold". University of Regensburg: 735.

Lu, T., Y. Li and T. Chen. 2013. "Techniques for fabrication and construction of three-dimensional scaffolds for tissue engineering". *International Journal of Nanomedicine* 8: 337.

Lukas, D., A. Sarkar and P. Pokorny. 2008. "Self-organization of jets in electrospinning from free liquid surface: A generalized approach". *Journal of Applied Physics* 103 (8).

Ma, P. X. 2008. "Biomimetic materials for tissue engineering". *Advanced Drug Delivery Reviews* 60 (2): 184–198.

Maghdouri-White, Y., S. Petrova, N. Sori, S. Polk, H. Wriggers, R. Ogle, R. Ogle and M. Francis. 2018. "Electrospun silk–collagen scaffolds and BMP-13 for ligament and tendon repair and regeneration". *Biomedical Physics & Engineering Express* 4 (2): 025013.

Manavitehrani, I., T. Y. Le, S. Daly, Y. Wang, P. K. Maitz, A. Schindeler and F. Dehghani. 2019. "Formation of porous biodegradable scaffolds based on poly (propylene carbonate) using gas foaming technology". *Materials Science and Engineering: C* 96: 824–830.

Matthews, J. A., G. E. Wnek, D. G. Simpson and G. L. Bowlin. 2002. "Electrospinning of collagen nanofibers". *Biomacromolecules* 3 (2): 232–238.

Mazzoli, A. 2013. "Selective laser sintering in biomedical engineering". *Medical & Biological Engineering & Computing* 51 (3): 245–256.

Mikos, A. G., Y. Bao, L. G. Cima, D. E. Ingber, J. P. Vacanti and R. Langer. 1993. "Preparation of poly (glycolic acid) bonded fiber structures for cell attachment and transplantation". *Journal of Biomedical Materials Research* 27 (2): 183–189.

Mikos, A. G., G. Sarakinos, S. M. Leite, J. P. Vacant and R. Langer. 1993. "Laminated three-dimensional biodegradable foams for use in tissue engineering". *Biomaterials* 14 (5): 323–330.

Mishra, R., R. Varshney, N. Das, D. Sircar and P. Roy. 2019. "Synthesis and characterization of gelatin-PVP polymer composite scaffold for potential application in bone tissue engineering". *European Polymer Journal* 119: 155–168.

Mitchell, G. R. 2015. *Electrospinning: Principles, Practice and Possibilities*, Royal Society of Chemistry.

Moghe, A. and B. Gupta. 2008. Co-axial electrospinning for nanofiber structures: Preparation and applications. *Polymer Reviews* 48: 353–377.

Molladavoodi, S., M. Gorbet, J. Medley and H. J. Kwon. 2013. "Investigation of microstructure, mechanical properties and cellular viability of poly (L-lactic acid) tissue engineering scaffolds prepared by different thermally induced phase separation protocols". *Journal of the Mechanical Behavior of Biomedical Materials* 17: 186–197.

Morton, W. 1902. *"Method of dispersing fluids US Patent Specification 705691"*.

Muerza-Cascante, M. L., D. Haylock, D. W. Hutmacher and P. D. Dalton. 2015. "Melt electrospinning and its technologization in tissue engineering". *Tissue Engineering Part B: Reviews* 21 (2): 187–202.

Murphy, S. V. and A. Atala. 2014. "3D bioprinting of tissues and organs". *Nature Biotechnology* 32 (8): 773–785.

Naghieh, S., E. Foroozmehr, M. Badrossamay and M. Kharaziha. 2017. "Combinational processing of 3D printing and electrospinning of hierarchical poly (lactic acid)/gelatin-forsterite scaffolds as a biocomposite: Mechanical and biological assessment". *Materials & Design* 133: 128–135.

Nail, S. L., S. Jiang, S. Chongprasert and S. A. Knopp. 2002. "Fundamentals of freeze-drying". *Development and Manufacture of Protein Pharmaceuticals*: 281–360.

Pakhomova, C., Popov, D., Maltsev, E., Akhatov, I., and Pasko, A. 2020. "Software for bioprinting." *International Journal of Bioprinting* 6(3): 279, 41–61.

Nasiri, B. and S. Mashayekhan. 2017. "Fabrication of porous scaffolds with decellularized cartilage matrix for tissue engineering application". *Biologicals* 48: 39–46.

Ngo, T. D., A. Kashani, G. Imbalzano, K. T. Nguyen and D. Hui. 2018. "Additive manufacturing (3D printing): A review of materials, methods, applications and challenges". *Composites Part B: Engineering* 143: 172–196.

Niu, H., X. Wang and T. Lin. 2011. "Needleless electrospinning: Developments and performances". *Nanofibers-Production, Properties and Functional Applications*, 17–36.

Pavia, F. C., F. S. Palumbo, V. La Carrubba, F. Bongiovì, V. Brucato, G. Pitarresi and G. Giammona. 2016. "Modulation of physical and biological properties of a composite PLLA and polyaspartamide derivative obtained via thermally induced phase separation (TIPS) technique". *Materials Science and Engineering: C* 67: 561–569.

Plikk, P., S. Målberg and A. C. Albertsson. 2009. "Design of resorbable porous tubular copolyester scaffolds for use in nerve regeneration". *Biomacromolecules* 10 (5): 1259–1264.

Ranganathan, S., K. Balagangadharan and N. Selvamurugan. 2019. "Chitosan and gelatin-based electrospun fibers for bone tissue engineering". *International Journal of Biological Macromolecules* 133: 354–364.

Reneker, D. H., A. L. Yarin, H. Fong and S. Koombhongse. 2000. "Bending instability of electrically charged liquid jets of polymer solutions in electrospinning". *Journal of Applied Physics* 87 (9): 4531–4547.

Rim, N. G., C. S. Shin and H. Shin. 2013. "Current approaches to electrospun nanofibers for tissue engineering". *Biomedical Materials* 8 (1): 1–15.

Rosenzweig, D. H., E. Carelli, T. Steffen, P. Jarzem and L. Haglund. 2015. "3D-printed ABS and PLA scaffolds for cartilage and nucleus pulposus tissue regeneration". *International Journal of Molecular Sciences* 16 (7): 15118–15135.

Roseti, L., V. Parisi, M. Petretta, C. Cavallo, G. Desando, I. Bartolotti and B. Grigolo. 2017. "Scaffolds for bone tissue engineering: State of the art and new perspectives". *Materials Science and Engineering: C* 78: 1246–1262.

Schoonraad, S. A., K. M. Fischenich, K. N. Eckstein, V. Crespo-Cuevas, L. M. Savard, A. Muralidharan, A. A. Tomaschke, A. C. Uzcategui, M. A. Randolph and R. R. McLeod. 2021. "Biomimetic and mechanically supportive 3D printed scaffolds for cartilage and osteochondral tissue engineering using photopolymers and digital light processing". *Biofabrication* 13 (4): 044106.

Schugens, C., V. Maquet, C. Grandfils, R. Jérôme and P. Teyssie. 1996. "Biodegradable and macroporous polylactide implants for cell transplantation: 1. Preparation of macroporous polylactide supports by solid-liquid phase separation". *Polymer* 37 (6): 1027–1038.

Semino, C. 2008. "Self-assembling peptides: From bio-inspired materials to bone regeneration". *Journal of Dental Research* 87 (7): 606–616.

Shakir, M., R. Jolly, M. S. Khan, N. e. Iram, T. K. Sharma and S. I. Al-Resayes. 2015. "Synthesis and characterization of a nano-hydroxyapatite/chitosan/polyethylene glycol nanocomposite for bone tissue engineering". *Polymers for Advanced Technologies* 26 (1): 41–48.

Shi, X. M., W. P. Zhou, D. L. Ma, Q. Ma, D. Bridges, Y. Ma and A. M. Hu. 2015. "Electrospinning of nanofibers and their applications for energy devices". *Journal of Nanomaterials* 16(1): 122–122.

Siddiqui Ma, N. 2014. *Development of Chitosan Based Composite Matrices for Bone Tissue Engineering*. Doctoral dissertation.

Singh, B. N. 2017. "Development of novel silk fibroin/carboxymethyl cellulose based electrospun nanofibrous scaffolds for bone tissue engineering application". Doctoral dissertation.

Skoog, S. A., P. L. Goering and R. J. Narayan. 2014. "Stereolithography in tissue engineering". *Journal of Materials Science: Materials in Medicine* 25 (3): 845–856.

Soliman, S., S. Pagliari, A. Rinaldi, G. Forte, R. Fiaccavento, F. Pagliari, O. Franzese, M. Minieri, P. Di Nardo and S. Licoccia. 2010. "Multiscale three-dimensional scaffolds for soft tissue engineering via multimodal electrospinning". *Acta Biomaterialia* 6 (4): 1227–1237.

Su, Y., Q. Su, W. Liu, M. Lim, J. R. Venugopal, X. Mo, S. Ramakrishna, S. S. Al-Deyab and M. El-Newehy. 2012. "Controlled release of bone morphogenetic protein 2 and dexamethasone loaded in core–shell PLLACL–collagen fibers for use in bone tissue engineering". *Acta Biomaterialia* 8 (2): 763–771.

Su, Y., M. S. Toftdal, A. Le Friec, M. Dong, X. Han and M. Chen. 2021. "3D electrospun synthetic extracellular matrix for tissue regeneration". *Small Science* 1 (7): 2100003.

Subia, B., J. Kundu and S. Kundu. 2010. "Biomaterial scaffold fabrication techniques for potential tissue engineering applications". *Tissue Engineering* 141: 13–18.

Sultana, N. and M. Wang. 2008. "Fabrication of HA/PHBV composite scaffolds through the emulsion freezing/freeze-drying process and characterisation of the scaffolds". *Journal of Materials Science-Materials in Medicine* 19 (7): 2555–2561.

Szustakiewicz, K., M. Gazińska, B. Kryszak, M. Grzymajło, J. Pigłowski, R. J. Wiglusz and M. Okamoto. 2019. "The influence of hydroxyapatite content on properties of poly (L-lactide)/hydroxyapatite porous scaffolds obtained using thermal induced phase separation technique". *European Polymer Journal* 113: 313–320.

Tang, X., Y. Qin, X. Xu, D. Guo, W. Ye, W. Wu and R. Li. 2019. "Fabrication and in vitro evaluation of 3D printed porous polyetherimide scaffolds for bone tissue engineering". *BioMed Research International*: 1–8.

Tao, J., S. Zhu, N. Zhou, Y. Wang, H. Wan, L. Zhang, Y. Tang, Y. Pan, Y. Yang and J. Zhang. 2022. "Nanoparticle-stabilized emulsion bioink for digital light processing based 3D bioprinting of porous tissue constructs". *Advanced Healthcare Materials*: 2102810.

Teo, W., M. Kotaki, X. Mo and S. Ramakrishna. 2005. "Porous tubular structures with controlled fibre orientation using a modified electrospinning method". *Nanotechnology* 16 (6): 918.

Teo, W. E. and S. Ramakrishna. 2006. "A review on electrospinning design and nanofibre assemblies". *Nanotechnology* 17 (14): R89–R106.

Theron, A., E. Zussman and A. Yarin. 2001. "Electrostatic field-assisted alignment of electrospun nanofibres". *Nanotechnology* 12 (3): 384.

Theron, S., A. L. Yarin, E. Zussman and E. Kroll. 2005. "Multiple jets in electrospinning: Experiment and modeling". *Polymer* 46 (9): 2889–2899.

Tomihata, K. and Y. Ikada. 1997. "In vitro and in vivo degradation of films of chitin and its deacetylated derivatives". *Biomaterials* 18 (7): 567–575.

Trombetta, R., J. A. Inzana, E. M. Schwarz, S. L. Kates and H. A. Awad. 2017. "3D printing of calcium phosphate ceramics for bone tissue engineering and drug delivery". *Annals of Biomedical Engineering* 45 (1): 23–44.

Udomluck, N., W.-G. Koh, D.-J. Lim and H. Park. 2019. "Recent developments in nanofiber fabrication and modification for bone tissue engineering". *International Journal of Molecular Sciences* 21 (1): 99.

Varesano, A., F. Rombaldoni, G. Mazzuchetti, C. Tonin and R. Comotto. 2010. "Multi-jet nozzle electrospinning on textile substrates: Observations on process and nanofibre mat deposition". *Polymer International* 59 (12): 1606–1615.

Venkatesan, J., I. Bhatnagar and S.-K. Kim. 2014. "Chitosan-alginate biocomposite containing fucoidan for bone tissue engineering". *Marine Drugs* 12 (1): 300–316.

Vyas, C., G. Ates, E. Aslan, J. Hart, B. Huang and P. Barto. 2020. "Three-dimensional printing and electrospinning dual-scale polycaprolactone scaffolds with low-density and oriented fibers to promote cell alignment". *3D Printing and Additive Manufacturing* 7 (3): 105–113.

Vyavahare, S., S. Teraiya, D. Panghal and S. Kumar. 2020. "Fused deposition modelling: A review". *Rapid Prototyping Journal* 26 (1): 176–201.

Wahid, F., T. Khan, Z. Hussain and H. Ullah. 2018. Nanocomposite scaffolds for tissue engineering; properties, preparation and applications. *Applications of Nanocomposite Materials in Drug Delivery*, Elsevier, 701–735.

Wang, H., Z. Wang, H. Liu, J. Liu, R. Li, X. Zhu, M. Ren, M. Wang, Y. Liu and Y. Li. 2021. "Three-dimensional printing strategies for irregularly shaped cartilage tissue engineering: Current state and challenges". *Frontiers in Bioengineering and Biotechnology* 9: 1–21.

Webber, M. J. and E. T. Pashuck. 2021. "(Macro)molecular self-assembly for hydrogel drug delivery". *Advanced Drug Delivery Reviews* 172: 275–295.

Wong, K. V. and A. Hernandez. 2012. "A review of additive manufacturing". *International Scholarly Research Notices* 2012.

Wu, J., C. Huang, W. Liu, A. Yin, W. Chen, C. He, H. Wang, S. Liu, C. Fan and G. L. Bowlin. 2014. "Cell infiltration and vascularization in porous nanoyarn scaffolds prepared by dynamic liquid electrospinning". *Journal of Biomedical Nanotechnology* 10 (4): 603–614.

Wubneh, A., E. K. Tsekoura, C. Ayranci and H. Uludağ. 2018. "Current state of fabrication technologies and materials for bone tissue engineering". *Acta Biomaterialia* 80: 1–30.

Yang, X., S. Li, Y. Ren, L. Qiang, Y. Liu, J. Wang and K. Dai. 2022. "3D printed hydrogel for articular cartilage regeneration". *Composites Part B: Engineering*: 109863.

Yao, Q., K. E. Fuglsby, X. Zheng and H. Sun. 2020. "Nanoclay-functionalized 3D nanofibrous scaffolds promote bone regeneration". *Journal of Materials Chemistry B* 8 (17): 3842–3851.

Yarin, A. L., S. Koombhongse and D. H. Reneker. 2001. "Taylor cone and jetting from liquid droplets in electrospinning of nanofibers". *Journal of Applied Physics* 90 (9): 4836–4846.

Ye, K., D. Liu, H. Kuang, J. Cai, W. Chen, B. Sun, L. Xia, B. Fang, Y. Morsi and X. Mo. 2019. "Three-dimensional electrospun nanofibrous scaffolds displaying bone morphogenetic protein-2-derived peptides for the promotion of osteogenic differentiation of stem cells and bone regeneration". *Journal of Colloid and Interface Science* 534: 625–636.

Yoshimoto, H., Y. Shin, H. Terai and J. Vacanti. 2003. "A biodegradable nanofiber scaffold by electrospinning and its potential for bone tissue engineering". *Biomaterials* 24 (12): 2077–2082.

Yousefi, A.-M., J. Liu, R. Sheppard, S. Koo, J. Silverstein, J. Zhang and P. F. James. 2018. "I-optimal design of hierarchical 3D scaffolds produced by combining additive manufacturing and thermally induced phase separation". *ACS Applied Bio Materials* 2 (2): 685–696.

Yu, D. G., C. Branford-White, S. A. Bligh, K. White, N. P. Chatterton and L. M. Zhu. 2011. "Improving polymer nanofiber quality using a modified co-axial electrospinning process". *Macromolecular Rapid Communications* 32 (9–10): 744–750.

Yu, Y., S. Ren, Y. Yao, H. Zhang, C. Liu, J. Yang, W. Yang and L. Miao. 2017. "Electrospun fibrous scaffolds with iron-doped hydroxyapatite exhibit osteogenic potential with static magnetic field exposure". *Journal of Biomedical Nanotechnology* 13 (7): 835–847.

Zaiss, S., T. D. Brown, J. C. Reichert and A. Berner. 2016. "Poly (ε-caprolactone) scaffolds fabricated by melt electrospinning for bone tissue engineering". *Materials* 9 (4): 232.

Zeinali, R., M. T. Khorasani, A. Behnamghader, M. Atai, L. d. Valle and J. Puiggalí. 2020. "Poly (hydroxybutyrate-co-hydroxyvalerate) porous matrices from thermally induced phase separation". *Polymers* 12 (12): 2787.

Zhang, J., D. Huang, S. Liu, X. Dong, Y. Li, H. Zhang, Z. Yang, Q. Su, W. Huang and W. Zheng. 2019. "Zirconia toughened hydroxyapatite biocomposite formed by a DLP 3D printing process for potential bone tissue engineering". *Materials Science and Engineering: C* 105: 110054.

Zhang, Q., Z. Zhou, C. Peng, T. Huang, Q. Liu, H. Zhou, W. Wang and H. Yan. 2017. "Preparation and properties of novel maleated poly (D, L-lactide-co-glycolide) porous scaffolds for tissue engineering". *Journal of Macromolecular Science, Part B* 56 (7): 505–515.

Zhao, P., H. Gu, H. Mi, C. Rao, J. Fu and L.-s. Turng. 2018. "Fabrication of scaffolds in tissue engineering: A review". *Frontiers of Mechanical Engineering* 13 (1): 107–119.

Zhou, Z., F. Buchanan, C. Mitchell and N. Dunne. 2014. "Printability of calcium phosphate: Calcium sulfate powders for the application of tissue engineered bone scaffolds using the 3D printing technique". *Materials Science and Engineering: C* 38: 1–10.

Zhu, L., S. Chen, K. Liu, W. Wen, L. Lu, S. Ding, C. Zhou and B. Luo. 2020. "3D poly (L-lactide)/chitosan micro/nano fibrous scaffolds functionalized with quercetin-polydopamine for enhanced osteogenic and anti-inflammatory activities". *Chemical Engineering Journal* 391: 123524.

5 Scaffold Properties and Characterization

INTRODUCTION

In tissue engineering (TE), scaffold is the main backbone for the cell and tissue structure and plays an important role in tissue regeneration (Chan and Leong 2008; Morra and Cassinelli 2006). Scaffold offers essential physical, biochemical, and bioactive cues for the cells to respond to the microenvironment that promotes cellular growth and proliferation, guides cell differentiation, and helps in the remoulding process of the damaged bone and cartilage, thereby repairing the lost tissues and maintaining their functions (Spector 2006; Chan and Leong 2008). Tissue engineering scaffold has to perform these multiple tasks while regenerating bone, cartilage, and related tissues to repair the defect and, therefore, must possess a set of desired properties. These properties are classified into different categories such as physico-chemical, mechanical, and biological. These scaffold properties can easily be engineered in order to mimic the properties of native extracellular matrix (ECM). For this, diversified biomaterials are combined to make scaffold by bringing the desired characteristics of the biomaterials in a single platform, achieving the required properties of the scaffold, thereby making them potential for regenerating the targeted tissue. Based on this concept, a lot of scientific research has been directed towards the development of a scaffold with optimized properties in the last three decades. Before *in vitro* and *in vivo* applications, ensuring desired properties of the scaffold and hence their suitability is of utmost importance for successful tissue regeneration activity at a desired level. These important properties are scaffold architecture including the interconnected pore structure, pore dimension and pore distribution, surface morphology, porosity, surface chemistry, surface roughness, hydrophilicity, swelling and water uptake capacity, degradation, sterilizability without losing any desired characteristics and contamination during the tissue regeneration process mechanical, structural, and biological properties like biocompatibility or tissue compatibility, bioactivity, etc. Besides these properties, scaffold must be designed appropriately to recruit and accommodate the cells and provide necessary biochemical and mechanical cues for promoting cellular interactions within it. Nonetheless the selection and adoption of appropriate methods for characterizing the various properties of the scaffolds are also important of immense importance. This chapter describes the various essential properties of the scaffold that make it a potential platform for bone, cartilage and their complex forms,

DOI: 10.1201/9781003245353-5

like osteochondral tissue regeneration. The various techniques and strategies for characterizing the scaffold properties are also the focus of this chapter.

PHYSICOCHEMICAL PROPERTIES

The various physicochemical properties of the scaffold are discussed in the following sections.

SCAFFOLD ARCHITECTURE

The architecture of scaffold is of critical importance in TE. Scaffold must have interconnected pore structure, adequate porosity, and desired pore dimension and pore distribution. Initially, cells interact with the scaffolds via the functional groups or ligands present on the surface of the scaffold biomaterial having Arg-Gly-Asp (RGD) sequences, so that cells adhere to the surface. The density of these ligands depends on the specific surface area within the pores and the mean pore size of the scaffold (O'Brien 2011). The pore size of the scaffolds should be higher than the actual cell size for permitting the cells to penetrate into the scaffold matrix, for binding to the ligands, but should be small enough to provide high surface area with minimum ligand density that binds a critical number of cells to the scaffold surface (O'Brien 2011). The scaffolds, therefore, should possess critical pore size range depending on the cell type and the target tissue, which is to be regenerated (Murphy and O'Brien 2010; Murphy, Haugh, and O'Brien 2010; O'Brien 2011). The pores are essential features of the scaffold helping in counting the cell movement, and also the transport of nutrients, gas, and harmful waste products. The pore size has a positive relationship with the fibre diameter of a fibrous scaffold. For example, the normal osteoblast and chondrocyte cell size is 10 µm. So, the pore size lower than the cell size prevents cell penetration to the scaffold (Wei et al. 2009). Notwithstanding, bigger pore size cells restrict the cell migration as they are lacking ties to create foothold (Yildirim et al. 2010). The interconnectivity among the pores facilitates the necessary cell migration and cell signalling. Pore shape also plays an important role in cell proliferation and differentiation.

Porosity, a significant variable for cell movement in the pores, is the level of void volume in the scaffold. Like pore size, the scaffold should also have adequate porosity to facilitate cell migration, nutrient and oxygen diffusion to the cells within the cell-seed scaffold (construct) as well as to the extra-cellular matrix, and removal of metabolic waste product, which are important for the survival of engineered tissue constructs (Lowery, Datta, and Rutledge 2010). It also provides void space for cell recruitment and cell aggregation, cell migration for tissue vascularization, and differentiation of cells for forming a new tissue and remodelling, thereby promoting host tissue integration (Holzapfel et al. 2013; Causa, Netti, and Ambrosio 2007; Hollister 2005). Inconsistent scaffold porosity may cause prompt misguided cell distribution and cell infiltration. The development of bone cells can be expanded by an increase in porosity. The porosity range of 60–90% is favourable for cell penetration into the scaffold (Curtis and Wilkinson 1997). The optimal porosity of the scaffold helps in nutrient diffusion to rejuvenate the cells, which depends on the types of cell and types of targeted tissue to be regenerated. Besides cell and tissue types, pore size and porosity of scaffolds may vary depending on their application. Porosity may also affect the mechanical properties of the scaffolds (Curtis and Wilkinson 1997; Lowery, Datta, and Rutledge 2010) and other properties such as adsorption, permeability, and mechanical strength. Ideally, the porosity of a tissue engineering scaffold should be ≥ 70% (Chong et al. 2007). A porous scaffold surface has also been reported to enable mechanical interlocking between the scaffolds and the tissue surrounding the defect site, thereby producing a mechanically stable structure (Karageorgiou and Kaplan 2005). The porous interconnected structure and high porosity of scaffold also allow the scaffold to remove the degraded products from the body without affecting the surrounding tissue or organ.

SURFACE CHEMISTRY

The surface chemistry of a scaffold can either promote or prevent protein adsorption and cell attachment through chemical and electrochemical interactions that occur at the scaffold surface. The surface charge of the scaffold plays an important role in mediating protein–cell interactions, protein adsorption, and cell attachment and often promotes cell-scaffold binding as well as imparts antibacterial properties to the scaffold. For example, it was found that fibroblast and osteoblast cells experienced enhanced cell attachment and spreading on hydrogels that possessed positive charge as compared to those were neutral, negatively charged, or contained the RGD ligand (Dave and Gomes 2019). Poly(styrene) scaffolds combined with plasma polymerized acrylic acid were found to exhibit antibacterial behaviour towards bacteria containing a negatively charged cell wall due to charge repulsion between the scaffold surface and the bacteria (Dave and Gomes 2019). Surface charge has also been shown to influence cell differentiation, as demonstrated by Yaszemski's group. They observed that there was a greater extent of chondrocyte differentiation when grown on negatively charged oligo (PEG) fumarate hydrogels as compared to cells grown on neutral or negatively charged hydrogels (Hsin and Yiwei 2011).

The surface properties of the scaffold are often improved by chemical modification using chemical grafting, wherein a protein or monomer is bound to the scaffold surface covalently. This is achieved by the reactive group activation on the scaffold surface using ultraviolet (UV), radiation, plasma, and ozone exposure. The main advantage of chemical modification of the scaffold surface is the long-term stability of the conjugated compounds while its disadvantages include the loss of protein mobility, appearance of proteins on the surface in unusual conformations, and presence of toxic monomer residues on scaffold surface (Dave and Gomes 2019).

SURFACE MORPHOLOGY

The geometry and morphological characteristics of the scaffold have a pivotal role in the cell growth, proliferation, and differentiation into a targeted tissue (O'Brien 2011). Surface morphology mainly includes factors such as the texture and arrangement of

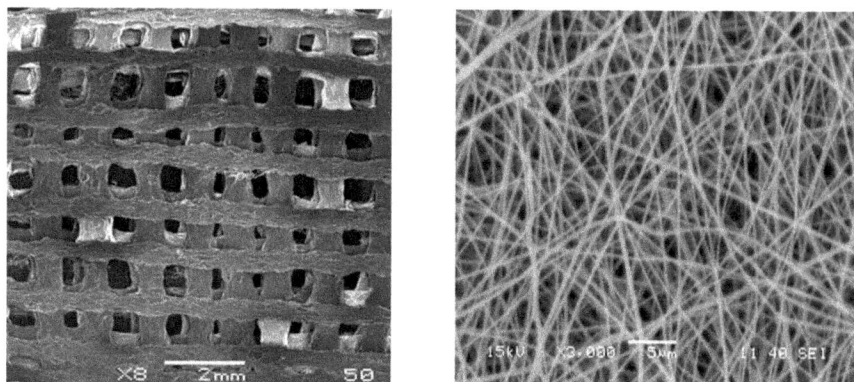

FIGURE 5.1   SEM images showing the morphology of the various scaffolds: (a)(a) sodium alginate/chitosan microfibrous scaffold fabricated by 3D printing technique (magnification 8X). (b) Silk fibroin/gelatin nanofibrous scaffold fabricated by electrospinning at 20 kV with a flow rate of 0.5 ml/hr (10,000X magnification).

various materials at the scaffold surface. The morphology of some scaffolds is shown in Figure 5.1.

Cells make use of special structures called filopodia to sense topographical variations and it is seen that in the presence of aligned topographical structures, of the nanoscale, the cells rearrange themselves to orient the cell body along these features (Denchai, Tartarini, and Mele 2018). This behaviour is often taken advantage of when creating patterned cellular structures. In the case of electrospun nanofibrous scaffolds, fibre diameter also has an influence on the promotion of adhesion and differentiation of specific cell types. For example, nanofibres with a diameter of < 1 μm promoted the growth of endothelial cells and are thus commonly employed in the engineering of vasculature (Łopianiak et al. 2021).

HYDROPHILICITY

Hydrophilicity is a surface property of tissue scaffold and it is referred to as the affinity of the scaffold to water (Law 2014). Hydrophilicity is a vital property for the adherence of cells to the scaffold surface, which in turn significantly influences cell–biomaterial interaction thereby facilitating tissue regeneration. It can also be represented as the ability of wetting biomaterial when contacted with water, thereby playing a key role in regulating cellular interactions in terms of cell adhesion, cell growth, and cell proliferation. Scaffold matrices having higher hydrophilic surfaces enhance the interaction of cells with the scaffold, resulting in an improved cell attachment and proliferation as evident from several studies (Goddard and Hotchkiss 2007; Wei et al. 2009; Yildirim et al. 2010), whereas relatively hydrophobic surfaces (surface lacks affinity to water) are necessary for improved protein adsorption. The wettability of a scaffold surface is usually assessed by contact angle measurement as shown in Figure 5.2. The surface becomes hydrophilic when the value of contact angle (θ) is < 90° and hydrophobic when the value is greater than 90° (Law 2014).

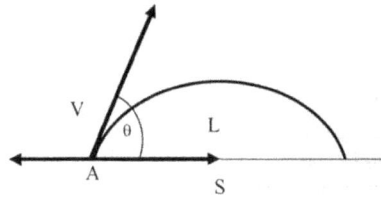

FIGURE 5.2   Sessile drop technique for contact angle measurement.

Source: Ponomar et al. 2022.

The hydrophilicity of the scaffold biomaterial can be improved by mixing it with other biomaterials that have higher hydrophilicity and through chemical treatment. The improvement in hydrophilicity favours cell attachment and proliferation (Kouhi et al. 2018). The alkali treatment proved to be a straightforward way to improve the surface hydrophilicity of the TE scaffold that resulted in enhanced osteoblast adhesion and proliferation (Yeo et al. 2010). In an *in vivo* animal study, the incorporation of bioglass into poly (hydroxybutyrate-co-hydroxyvalerate) enhanced the hydrophilicity of the polymer matrix and thereby promoted the attachment of the rabbit articular chondrocytes and cellular migration and subsequently formed higher cartilage-like ECM with superior mechanical properties than the pure polymer used as the control (Wu et al. 2013).

SURFACE ROUGHNESS OR SURFACE TOPOGRAPHY

The surface topography or surface roughness is an important property of the scaffold. This property influences cellular behaviour such as cell adhesion and cell proliferation on the TE scaffold surface and improves cytocompatibility of the scaffold, thereby facilitating successful tissue regeneration (Ponsonnet et al. 2002). The improvement in surface topology of TE scaffold can be achieved by surface coating. Chemical vapour deposition is a promising technique, which offers proper substrate topology and can penetrate into the complex porous structures of scaffold, thereby coating them completely. In a study, poly ((4-amino-p-xylylene)-co-(p-xylylene)) deposited on the PCL surface by this method demonstrated high cell survival rates and continuous cell proliferation on the coated PCL surface (Hu et al. 2009). The average roughness of 0.387–0.438 µm of 3D nanofibrous scaffold is reported to be highly favourable for cyto-compatibility and protein adsorption, thereby offering successful tissue regeneration (Ranjan and Webster 2009; Curtis and Wilkinson 1997). Surface topography induces cell adhesion as well as tissue integration through mechanical and cell integrin-mediated interlocking. The surface roughness of a scaffold can be classified into three different types: (i) macro-roughness (range: 100 µm to 1 millimeter; (ii) micro-roughness (range:100 nm to 100 µm); and (iii) nano-roughness (<100 nm). In the interim, various cells react adversely to surface roughness. The neurite development and axonal length expansion were demonstrated to be upheld on the rough surface at nanoscale range (6.26–49.38 nm). The human vein endothelial cells, with

10–102 nm rough surface, have been shown to improve cell attachment and tissue development (Hutmacher 2000). For example, surface roughness was accounted for further development of osteoblast growth, and cell behaviour was reliant upon the existence of surface roughness (Liu, Slamovich, and Webster 2006). In a study, the surface roughness of PCL/TCP scaffolds was improved by treating with sodium hydroxide (NaOH) and the scaffolds remarkably influenced the early stage new bone formation (Yeo et al. 2010). In an *in vitro* study, a novel porous PCL polymer surface with a high degree of nanoscale roughness promoted cartilage-producing cells (chondrocyte) proliferation and functions and produced higher intracellular protein and collagen secretion by the chondrocytes in comparison to that observed on pure PCL when used as a control. This modified PCL polymer was demonstrated as a suitable substrate for cartilage tissue-engineering applications (Balasundaram, Storey, and Webster 2014). Yet in another study, NaOH-treated 2D PLGA scaffold enhanced the functions of osteoblasts and chondrocytes. Furthermore, NaOH-treated PLGA 3D scaffolds showed a higher degree of hydrophilicity as well as surface roughness at nanoscale, thereby resulting in an enhanced articular cartilage tissue repair by chondrocyte differentiation *in vitro* (Park et al. 2005). The immobilization of hyaluronic acid on the surface of a biodegradable PLGA macroporous scaffold exhibited an enhanced chondrocyte cell attachment, proliferation, and differentiation, thereby promoting cartilage tissue regeneration (Yoo et al. 2005).

SWELLING AND WATER UPTAKE CAPACITY

The swelling behaviour and the water uptake are crucial factors of the TE scaffold. These properties have a great influence on the hydrolytic degradation of the scaffold, transport of water and nutrients to the scaffold, and removal of harmful waste material from the scaffold (Sultana and Khan 2012; Diermann et al. 2019; Zhu et al. 2010). Therefore, the scaffold should have adequate swelling and water uptake properties. These scaffold properties may be influenced by adding other biomaterials, by morphology of the scaffold etc. In a study, the water uptake capacity of poly (3-hydroxybutyrate-*co*-3-hydroxyvalerate) scaffold was enhanced by adding α-wollastonite which resulted in an increased cell viability of the scaffold (Ribas et al. 2019). The addition of water-soluble polymers like PVA and polyethylene oxide, improved the properties of hydrogel including swelling behaviour and gel strength. (Tranquilan-Aranilla et al. 1999; Maolin et al. 2000). In another study, carrageenan/poly(vinyl pyrrolidone) hydrogel prepared using different electron beam dose exposures revealed that the morphology of the developed hydrogel affects the swelling properties. Hydrogel with a lower pore size decreases its water uptake capacity because of the formation of dense inter-polymeric network. Increased water uptake capacity of the poly(vinyl pyrrolidone) scaffolds was achieved upon incorporation of functionalized cellulose nanocrystals in it (do Amaral Montanheiro et al. 2019).

STERILIZABILITY

Sterilizability of the scaffolds is a prerequisite in tissue engineering. This property is important for *in vitro* cell culture and also *in vivo* applications including clinical trials for maintaining aseptic conditions. This is also crucial for any scaffold biomaterial to tolerate sterilization for getting approval from regulatory bodies before proceeding with clinical trials and sterility assurance minimizes the risk of infections, which is a major health care concern (Galante et al. 2018; Hofmann et al. 2014). Commonly used techniques to sterilize scaffolds include irradiation, plasma sterilization, and chemical sterilization. Irradiation techniques are of three types: γ-irradiation, electron beam irradiation, and UV irradiation. Electron beam radiation is a simple technique that sterilizes the scaffold over a short duration of time. However, it is limited by its in ability to penetrate the scaffold. For greater penetration power, the intensity of the electron beam must be increased; however, this may cause damage to the scaffold; thus this method is not suitable for the sterilization of thicker scaffold structures. UV sterilization makes use of UV light in the range of 200–280 nm to sterilize the scaffolds and has also been found to be effective over short periods of time. The two most important factors affecting UV sterilization are the duration of radiation exposure and the wavelength of UV radiation. γ-irradiation, on the other hand, has excellent penetration power but it often changes the chemical and mechanical properties of the scaffold post-sterilization and so is less preferred compared to electron beam irradiation (Dai et al. 2016).

Plasma sterilization is comparatively a recent technique that uses reactive species present in gas plasma to sterilize the scaffolds. It is carried out at low-temperature conditions and improves the cell–material interactions post-sterilization, although the exact mechanism of this phenomenon is not yet clear. The sterilization effect of this technique is influenced by a number of factors, including the O_2 content, flow rate of gas, plasma excitation frequency, operating pressure and temperature. This method has also been known to alter the mechanical properties of the scaffold owing to inducing material cross-linking or degradation as well as induce a toxic effect if persisting after post-sterilization (Dai et al. 2016). Common chemicals used for sterilization include ethylene oxide, peroxyacetic acid, and ethanol. While all three chemicals have a good sterilization effect, they may cause side effects such as degradation of scaffold and chemical modification of the scaffold structure depending on the scaffold material. Thus, it is important to first evaluate the interactions of the used chemical agent with the scaffold material before use. Newer techniques used for sterilization include supercritical carbon-di-oxide (sCO_2), antibiotics, and freeze-drying. However, enough studies have not employed these techniques to fully determine their mechanisms of action, efficiency, and possible side effects; so, these techniques need to be further studied before they can be used for large-scale sterilization processes. Sterilization may adversely affect material properties. For example, the mechanical properties of porous 3-D SF scaffolds have been significantly decreased upon sterilizing by different sterilization methods except dry autoclaving (Hofmann et al. 2014).

BIODEGRADATION

The degradation of scaffold is an indispensable aspect in bone and cartilage TE. When a scaffold is placed inside the defective area of the body, it encounters body fluids and a variety of enzymes that degrade scaffold with time, creating void space, thereby to accommodate the new tissue formed. This process is called biodegradation and it is a vital process because the generated void space allows the ingrowth of the neotissue, remodelling of the engineered ECM formed and matches the new tissue formation. The biodegradation of the scaffold should also be accompanied by the removal of the degraded products through normal body function and without producing any harmful or toxic effect on the surrounding tissues, thereby avoiding an immune response (Echeverria Molina, Malollari, and Komvopoulos 2021). The appropriate rate of degradation of the TE scaffolds is therefore of prime importance in mimicking the cell or tissue growth in *in vitro* or *in vivo* conditions (Kumbar et al. 2008; Lee et al. 2009). In the ideal case, the degradation rate of scaffold should conform to the rate of generation of neotissue or ECM synthesis without producing harmful toxic by-products and, furthermore, it should be solubilized during the process of tissue regeneration. Besides affecting the mass of the scaffold, biodegradation often affects the crystallinity, geometry, and topology (Zhang, Zhou, and Zhang 2014; Milošev et al. 2017).

The scaffold should not degrade too rapidly or degrade slowly. If the degradation is faster than the formation of new tissue, the cells would not be able to form the required level of ECM-like structure, making the tissue formation infeasible, and also there will be difficulty for the produced byproducts to be removed from the body so quickly (Pucino et al. 2019). Whereas if the degradation is too slow, it may have a negative impact on the tissue regeneration process (Sanz-Herrera, García-Aznar, and Doblaré 2009; Holloway et al. 2014). The degradation rate of the TE scaffolds is influenced by various factors such as composition of the scaffold biomaterial, culture environment like pH and types of enzymes, and scaffold structures like porous, hydrogels, or film, surface modification methods, mechanical environment, and external interference like heat, and radiation. Many other factors that may have an adverse effect on the degradation rate include the implant location, age, gender, and comorbidities. (Roman et al. 2017). The variation in self-repairing capability of the orthopaedic tissues, *viz.,* bone, tendon, ligament, and blood vessel, represents that the scaffold should have appropriate degradation rates to facilitate the generation of neotissue *in vitro* and *in vivo*. Therefore, achieving controlled degradation rates of different scaffolds is still the major objective of TE research. As for example, degradation posed a critical issue when silk-based biomaterial was used for TE application (Cao and Wang 2009). Furthermore, it is extremely important that the engineered ECM maintain the required mechanical strength during the tissue regeneration process in spite of undergoing degradation. The properties such as molecular weight, composition, and crystallinity of the scaffold biomaterial can be modified to achieve the desired controlled degradation rate.

MECHANICAL AND STRUCTURAL PROPERTIES

Mechanical properties are essential factors that maintain the scaffold integrity during the process of tissue regeneration and shape stability of the damaged tissue, which become more critical in bone and related tissue regeneration (Song, Rane, and Christman 2012). The scaffold must match the mechanical properties of the host tissue, and be able to avoid possible adverse effects that result from the stress-shielding mechanism such as shear stress, formation of fibrotic encapsulation, unstable angiogenesis, tensile and compression stress, and other forces at the defect site (Zahedi et al. 2010; Elsner, Shefy-Peleg, and Zilberman 2010) and this property can be fine-tuned based on lineage-specific differentiation (Harley et al. 2007). A scaffold with a high tensile strength can withstand *in vitro* cellular growth and organization of the new tissue formed. A scaffold with the desired elastic modulus promotes osteogenic differentiation of cells. The mechanical strength also makes the scaffold stable, thereby enabling it to endure the compressive behaviour *in vivo* (Holzapfel et al. 2013; O'Brien 2011).

The study of mechanobiology has emphasized the importance of impact of mechanical strength of the scaffold on the cells seeded over it. When traction forces were exerted on the scaffolding matrix, many mature cell types were shown to be influenced by the scaffold stiffness showing different morphology and cell adhesion characteristics (Chan and Leong 2008). The desired mechanical strength of bone can be achieved by devising a composite model by taking into account the bone as a composite at the nanometer scale. The weak apatite in the bone can act as a hardening stage through flexible collagen giving an intense network (Grad et al. 2004). The open cells with lower density are usually delivered by an organization of poles, whereas the shut cells are delivered when the poles are dynamically spread and level due to an increase in the thickness of the bars or plates of the cancellous bone. The scaffold should maintain a linear elasticity at low stress under compression, following a long plateau of collapsing cell wall and thereafter a regime showing a steep rise in stress (Kumbar et al. 2008). The mechanical properties of the polymeric scaffold can also be improved by coating and cross-linking with suitable polymers and other cross-linking agents, by modifying scaffold structures (e.g. fibrous scaffold) and reinforcement using various nanoparticles (Zhao et al. 2021; Li et al. 2021; Bas et al. 2019).

The structural properties of the scaffold refer to phases, crystallinity, molecular composition, and functional groups. In any TE process, scaffolds serve as cell career systems or as delivery vehicles for drugs for tissue regeneration. Therefore, the cellular material should be able to colonize the host cell sufficiently for the targeted tissue regeneration. Alternatively, the scaffolds combine with the suitable cells and thereby promote osteogenic lineage formation or release some soluble molecules for the lineage formation *in vivo*. Sequentially, these cells are expanded by culturing *in vitro* and seeded on the scaffold resulting in cell-seeded scaffold (construct) that is implanted into the defect site of the body (Lowery, Datta, and Rutledge 2010). The properties of the tissue scaffold vary depending on the type of targeted tissues to be repaired, which may be hard (e.g. bone) or soft (e.g. muscle). For example, in bone TE, the bone defect area is filled with a biologically functionalized scaffold that should be able to withstand the load of the regenerated bone ECM. The scaffold properties including its size, shape, wall thickness, surface chemistry and morphology, pore size and pore interconnectivity, the rate of resorption and degradation, porosity, mechanical strength, and stability influence bone tissue regeneration and healing (Chan and Leong 2008; Chong et al. 2007). All the properties of the scaffold must be designed for a specific application of TE, that depends on a number of factors, like body location, age, and severity of tissue damage. The mechanical strength must be adequate enough to enable the scaffold to bear the physiological stress and to decrease the stress shielding.

Semi-crystalline polymers are usually chosen as a material because they increase the mechanical performance of the end product because of the augmentation in stiffness and strength of the material by the crystalline phase, whereas the amorphous phase possesses good absorbing impact energy (Hutmacher 2000; Liu, Slamovich, and Webster 2006; Chan and Leong 2008; Lowery, Datta, and Rutledge 2010), which mostly occurs above the glass transition temperature. At this temperature, the conformational and translational motions become more dynamic and the modulus is mostly affected by the crystalline fraction (Chong et al. 2007).

Functional groups are referred to as the structural units that govern the chemical reactivity of a molecule or substance under a specified condition. The functional groups play a critical role in the functionality of TE scaffold because they form the interface between the scaffolds and the cells, thereby facilitating cell–scaffold interaction. Functionalization of the scaffold biomaterials possessing specific functional groups is one of the most unique approaches to enhance and regulate various cellular events like cell adhesion, cell growth, migration, differentiation, and ECM deposition (Zhao et al. 2015). Numerous approaches, such as physico-chemical, mechanical, and biological approaches, have been evolved for functionalizing a scaffold biomaterial (Tallawi et al. 2015), thereby enhancing cell attachment and cell–biomaterial interaction. For an example, bone morphogenetic protein 2 (BMP-2) of composite electrospun silk/PEO fibres, functionalized with hydroxyapatite (HAp) nanoparticles, supported the osteogenic differentiation of human bone marrow-derived mesenchymal stem cell (hBMSCs) (Niu et al. 2017). Electrospun scaffolds with nanofibrous architecture with a gradient of functional groups was developed by adding PEG as additives to the polymer solution (Zonderland et al. 2020). In a study, prepared thiol-functionalized mesoporous bioactive glass and amino-functionalized mesoporous bioglass scaffolds stimulated adhesion, proliferation, and differentiation of hBMSCs (Zonderland et al. 2020).

Biological Properties

The biological properties of the scaffolds in bone and cartilage tissue engineering are very important. An ideal scaffold gives a structure that is compatible with cell adhesion, attachment, proliferation, and differentiation, support normal cellular activity and thereby can finally organizes into form the extracellular matrix (ECM) structure. During the culture, cells interact with the scaffold by attachment, and protein adsorption through the cell receptor (e.g. integrin) to give binding sites to the cells, in this manner interceding cell attachment. Thus, cell bond works with the arrival of dynamic mixtures that give signals for cell expansion and also separation. Nevertheless, the cell behaviour on the scaffold is enormously impacted by factors including the surface topography, surface chemistry, and scaffold architecture scaffold (Sultana and Wang 2008). The important biological properties of the scaffolds are described in the following section.

Biocompatibility or Tissue Compatibility

Biocompatibility or tissue compatibility is the foremost criterion of any tissue engineering scaffold. The scaffold should be recognized by the cells or their components, thereby facilitating cells to attach, proliferate, migrate onto the surface and interior of the scaffold, and differentiate into the targeted tissue during *in vitro* culturing and *in vivo* transplantation without eliciting any severe immunological or inflammatory response such as cytotoxicity, genotoxicity, immunogenicity, mutagenicity, and thrombogenicity to the host that might cause the hindrance of tissue healing or implant rejection by the body.

Bioactivity

The scaffold biomaterial should have intrinsic properties to induce necessary interaction with the cellular components and regulate their activities during neotissue synthesis. For these events, the scaffold must possess biological cues like cell-adhesive ligands to support cell attachment and physical cues, for example, topography that influences the morphology of the cell and alignment. Ligands, like arginine-glycine-aspartic (RGD) and tyrosine-isoleucine-glycine-serine-arginine (YIGSR), improve the bioactive property of the scaffold. The bioactivity of a 3D nanofibrous scaffold is shown to have the ability to form bone-like apatite representing the bone binding potential of the scaffold (Davies and Baldan 1997; Marcolongo et al. 1998a). This property advances the healing process by accelerating the regeneration process of bone tissue and deposition of hydroxy apatite. The scaffold also acts as a delivery vehicle for providing growth factors (growth-stimulating signals) to enhance the tissue regeneration for which the scaffold must be compatible with the various bioactive molecules and also act like an encapsulation method for the controlled release of the biomolecules without affecting bioactivity. Given an example, the hydrogels prepared through covalent or ionic cross-linking can entrap proteins and subsequently release them by a mechanism governed by swelling characteristics of the hydrogel scaffold (Berger et al. 2004).

Specific Tissue-Inducing Properties

The scaffold should have the capacity to support cell adhesion, proliferation, migration, and differentiation with specific phenotypic tissue, like osteo-conductivity and osteo-inductivity properties in bone TE (Yang et al. 2001). This has been described elaborately in Chapter 8 and 9.

CHARACTERIZATION OF THE SCAFFOLD

A comprehensive assessment of the scaffold propeties is essential to understand its performance for successful bone and cartilage tissue regeneration. A wide range of methods for characterizing the physico-chemical, mechanical, structural and biological properties of the scaffolds are described below.

MORPHOLOGICAL CHARACTERIZATION

Scanning Electron Microscopic Analysis

The study of the surface detail including the morphology of a scaffold is of immense importance, as the surface properties have great influence on its *in vivo* performance, such as cell adhesion and biocompatibility, and this should be carried out at high magnification and with a high level of resolution. Furthermore, the study of the cells and tissue behaviour at the interface of the scaffold biomaterials is also important. In this context, the use of an advanced surface imaging technique like scanning electron microscope (SEM) is an important tool to assess the surface characteristics of the scaffold and has been widely used in the TE field. The analysis of SEM provides high-quality images of the scaffold with spatial resolution. SEM images provides information about the various scaffold surface characteristics such as morphology that reveals the shape and size of the pores as well as the pore network, topography that discloses the surface features like texture, smoothness or roughness, chemical composition of the material, and crystallographic information related to the atomic arrangement in the materials.

SEM utilizes an accelerated electron beam emitted from a filament carrying a high amount of kinetic energy. The emitted electron beam is focused onto the surface of the solid sample to be characterized using a set of lenses present in the electron column. The incident electron beam interacts with the sample surface, penetrates the surface, and interacts inside the surface, and, finally, the beam is decelerated by the solid surface. This interaction of the electron beams with the atoms of the samples results in a variety of signals. These signals are comprised of secondary electrons that result in SEM images, backscattered electrons, and characteristic X-rays, which are collected as signals to form the images of the topography or relative atomic number for understanding the composition of the sample surface. The generated high-resolution SEM images are analyzed to reveal the shapes of the objects by allowing the measurement of very small features and objects precisely, spatial variations in chemical compositions, and the pattern and dimensions of pores and fibres (Akhtar et al. 2018). Figure 5.3 presents a typical Scanning Electro Microscope with its differents parts.

SEM has been widely used to observe and assess the morphology of porous scaffold, and fibre size in the case of fibrous scaffold (both micro- and nanofibres) as shown in Figure 5.4. In this method, scaffolds are subjected to a vacuum drier for complete removal of moisture present in it and cut into small pieces. The dried scaffolds are coated with platinum using sputter coater prior to the imaging. The pore size is determined by an image analysis software such as Image J. Usually, the average pore size is calculated by considering about 20–25 pores that are randomly selected by graphical measurement on SEM images (Bhardwaj and Kundu 2011). The chemical composition of the scaffold is determined from SEM images using energy dispersion X-ray spectrometer (EDX).

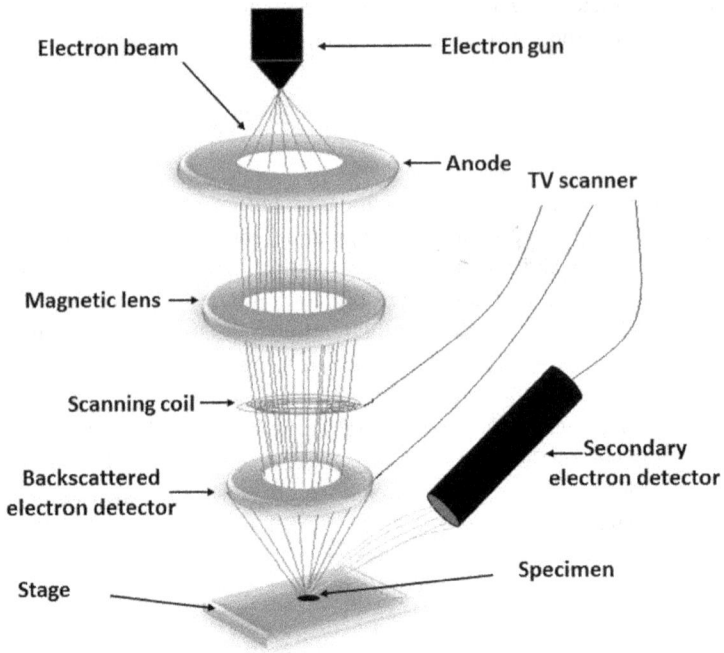

FIGURE 5.3 Diagram of a scanning electron microscope (SEM) with different parts.

Atomic Force Microscope (AFM)

AFM is a powerful non-optical imaging technique that can be used for analysing almost all types of surfaces of rigid materials, such as polymers, glass and ceramics, composites, and biological samples at the atomic level. It was developed by IBM scientists Binnig, Quate, and Gerber in 1985 (Binnig, Quate, and Gerber 1986). AFM allows to assess the topography or roughness of the scaffold surface in an accurate and non-destructive means with very high resolution in the order of fractions of a nanometer in different conditions including in air, liquids, or ultrahigh vacuum with the help of a scanning probe microscope (Marti, Drake, and Hansma 1987). The diagram of an atomic force microscope is shown in Figure 5.5. It consists of a flexible micro-fabricated cantilever typically made of silicon or silicon nitride integrated with a sharp tip (the radius of curvature of the tip is in the order of nanometre) called probe at its free end forming a spring. The probe scans the surface. When the tip comes in contact with the specimen surface, the deflection of cantilever occurs due to the forces acting between the tip and the specimen, which is detected by an optical method normally using a laser beam reflected from the back side of the cantilever and directed towards a split photodetector. A piezoelectric ceramic scanner controls the tip movement relative to the sample surface. The reflected light beam is then focused to a specific position by the movement of the specimen surface to maintain a constant force between the sample surfaces, thereby generating 3D topographical images as indicated in Figure 5.6.

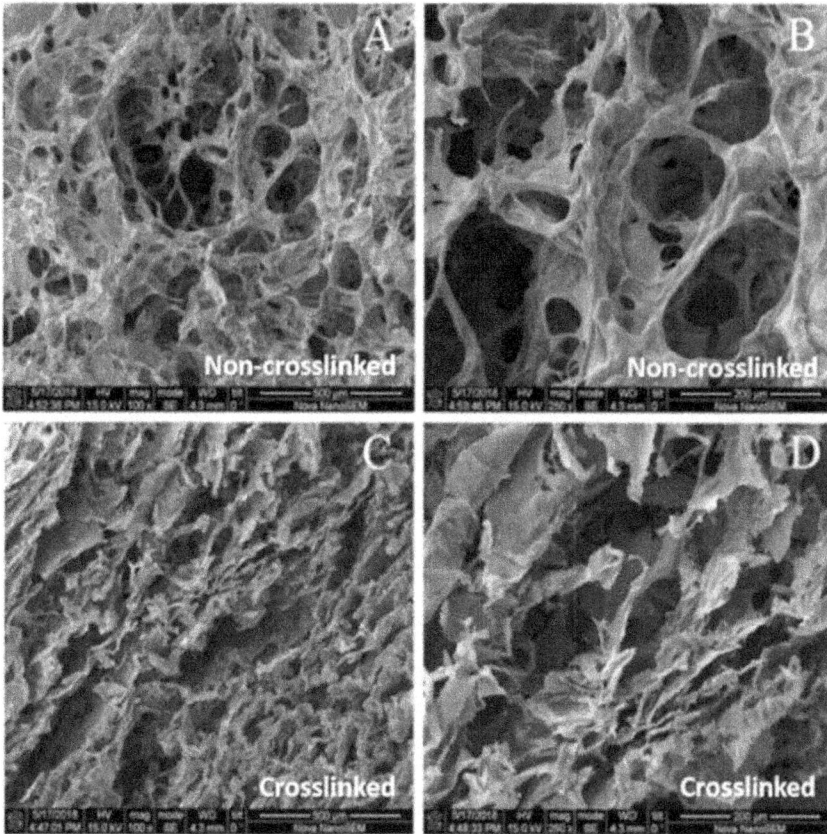

FIGURE 5.4 Illustrating the SEM micrographs of porous (top) and nanofibrous (bottom) scaffolds.

Source: Campos et al. 2022; Lim 2022.

The advantages of AFM are (i) generating a 3D surface profile; (ii) not needing any special treatment like metal or carbon coating of the specimen that modify or damage the sample irreversibly; and (iii) obtaining the final image devoid of charging artefacts. Besides air, AFM modes are able to work well in a liquid environment, thereby enabling it to characterize the biological samples including the biomacromolecules and living organisms.

Transmission Electron Microscope

Transmission Electron Microscope (TEM) is a microscopic method that works on the same basic principles of the light microscope, except that it utilizes electrons in place of photons or light. However, the difference lies in the wavelength of light. Although TEMs use electron as "light source" but it can produce images with lower wavelength and thousand times higher resolution than that obtained with a light microscope. This

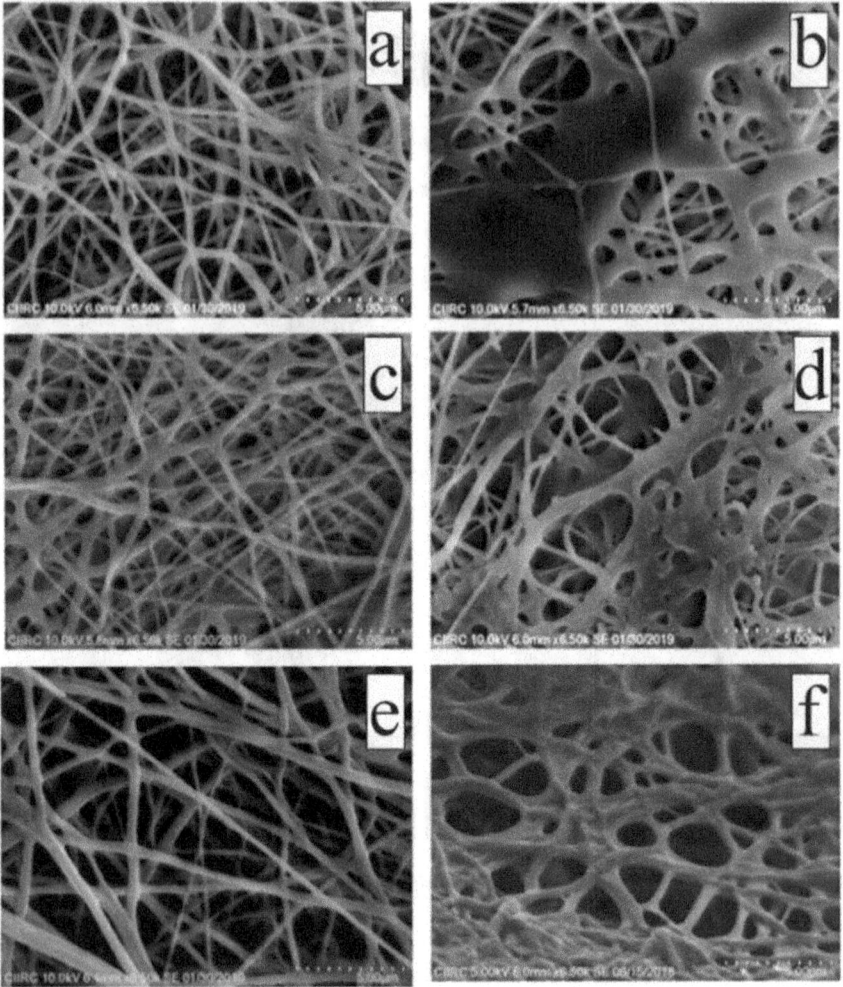

FIGURE 5.4   (Continued)

technique characterizes the microstructure of the scaffold biomaterials with very high spatial resolution because of easily achievable small de Broglie wavelengths and offering negligible differences in functionality (Lopez Marquez et al. 2022; Buseck, Cowley, and Eyring 1989). TEM can assess the morphology, crystal structure, phases, etc., of polymeric structures. However, the method can only handle the specimen with very low optimal thickness, that is, in the nanometer range (Mayer et al. 2007; Lopez Marquez et al. 2022), which limits its application for a wide variety of scaffolds. This technique is particularly useful to characterize nanoparticles and individual fibres, with an exceptional resolution (Lopez Marquez et al. 2022; Smith, Smallwood, and Macneil 2010).

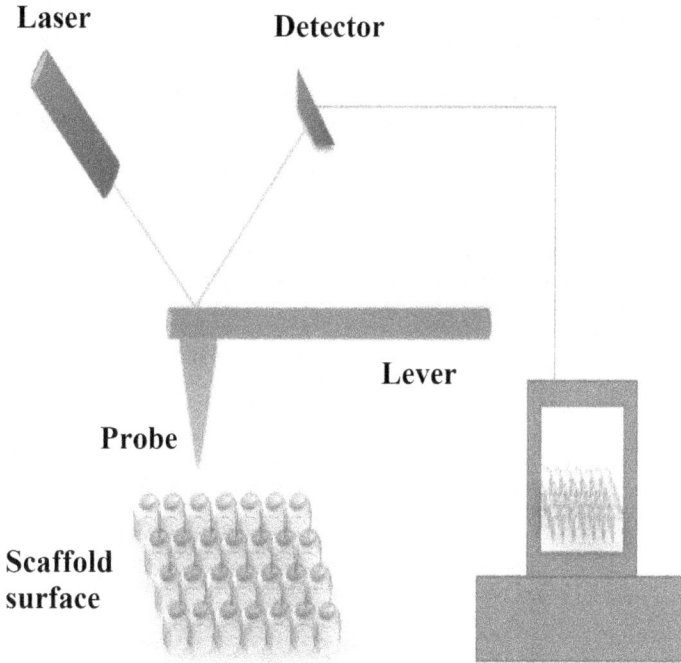

FIGURE 5.5 Diagram of an atomic force microscope.

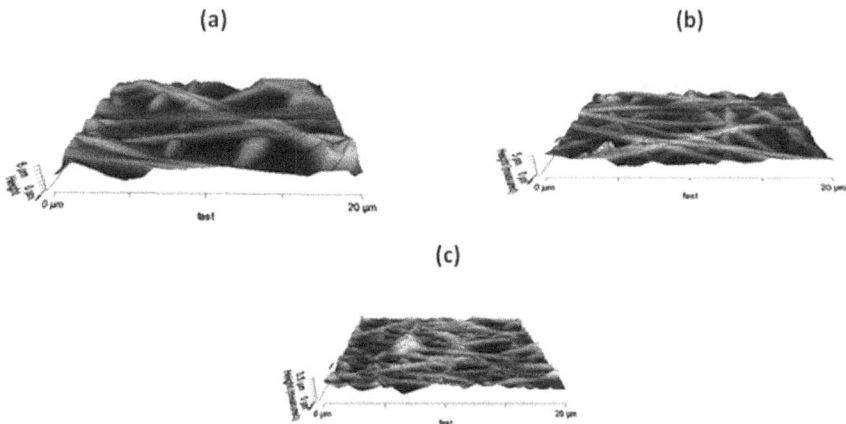

(a) (b)

(c)

FIGURE 5.6 Illustrating the atomic force microscopic images of the nanocomposite scaffolds.

Source: Mani, Jaganathan, and Supriyanto 2019.

TEM images have been widely used in determining the size and morphology of nanoparticles in TE applications (Miyauchi et al. 2010; Jurczyk et al. 2011). HAp particularly in nano sizes widely used for repairing bone and related hard tissues has been widely characterized by TEM as shown in Figure 5.7 (Considine, Holzwarth,

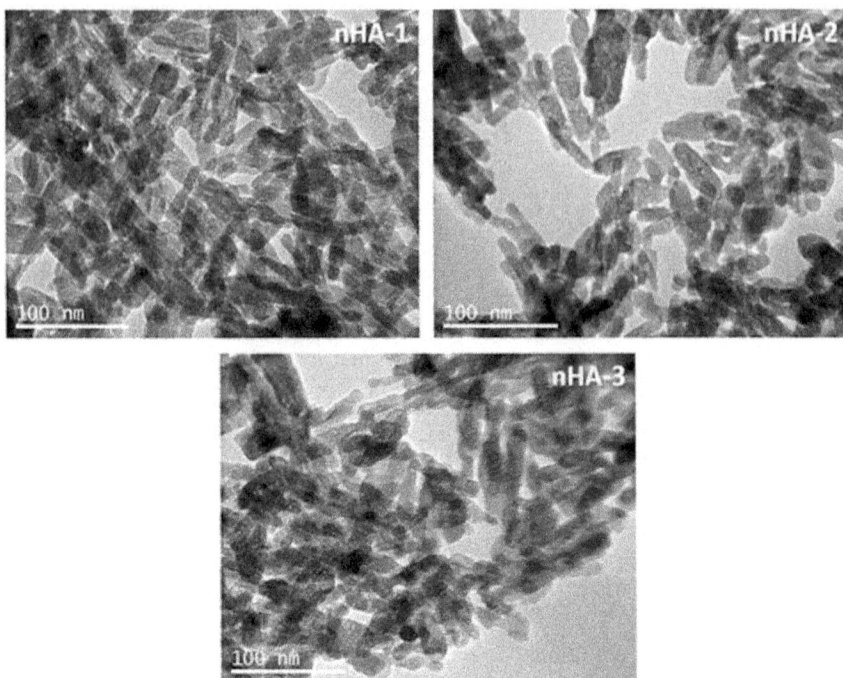

FIGURE 5.7   Transmission electron microscopy images of nanohydroxyapatite materials.

Source: Kavasi et al 2021.

and Ma 2011). It has also been applied for characterizing individual fibres, specifically fibers containing nanomaterials (Zhang and Chen 2010). TEM confirmed the increase in size and growth of nano-HAp crystals, as well as their crystallinity when PEG was added to it (Min et al. 2004). The enhancement of nano-HAp growth with an increase of PEG molecular weight was also revealed by TEM images. However, high-resolution transmission electron microscopy has allowed for characterizing the crystallographic structure at an atomic scale.

Porosity

As already explained, the scaffolds should possess optimal porosity for successful tissue regeneration. A number of techniques are used to measure the porosity of the scaffolds; some of the important techniques are presented as follows.

(i) Gravimetric method: This is the simplest and rapid, but not so accurate method. In this method the total porosity representing the total volume of pore space within the scaffolds from the bulk and true density of the biomaterial is measured.

$$Total\ Porosity = 1 - \frac{\rho_{scaffold}}{\rho_{material}}$$

where $\rho_{scaffold}$ and $\rho_{material}$ denote the apparent density of the scaffold and the material, respectively (Maspero et al. 2002; Guarino et al. 2008).

(ii) Mercury porosimetry: In this method, the mercury intrusion porosimeter is used to measure the total pore volume fraction and average pore diameter (Guarino et al. 2008; Mayer and Stowe 1965). The scaffold porosity is calculated from intrusion data based on the correlation between the applied pressure and pore size or pore diameter, using the so-called Washburn equation $D = (1 / P)4\gamma(\cos\varphi)$ (Rockwood et al. 2011), in which, D, γ, and P are the pore diameter, surface tension, and applied pressure, respectively, and φ is the contact angle measured between mercury and the pore wall. In a study, the pore size distribution, pore volume, and porosity of the fabricated silk fibroin nanofibrous mats by electrospinning method have been determined using this method under a pressure gradient of 0.5–2000 psi and with prior degassing of the system at about 30 μm of Hg (Min et al. 2004; Lowery 2009). However, this method suffers from drawbacks such as requiring high pressure that results in the collapse of soft biomaterials like hydrogel, toxicity, and cost of mercury which limits its use for determining porosity of many tissue scaffold types (y Leon 1998).

(iii) Liquid displacement method: This is another simple, but an indirect method of measuring scaffold porosity by using a displacement liquid like ethanol, which can easily penetrate into the pores without influencing the important scaffold properties like shrinkage in size or swelling of the material tested (Shi et al. 2002). The porosity is calculated using the following equation:

$$Porosity = \frac{V_1 - V_3}{V_2 - V_3}$$

where V_1, V_2, and V_3 denote, respectively, the volume of liquid used to submerge the scaffold, the volume of the liquid plus liquid-impregnated scaffold, and the liquid volume remaining after the removal of liquid-impregnated scaffold. This is a widely used method for the development of scaffold for bone and cartilage tissue regeneration (Zhao et al. 2002; Zhang and Ma 1999; Vishwanath, Pramanik, and Biswas 2016)
(iv) CAD models: It is used for the designing of scaffold with appropriate 3D structure, pore size, and porosity (Sun et al. 2004). The porosity of the scaffold matrix is calculated using the following equation (Lee et al. 2006):

$$Porosity = 1 - \frac{V_{solid}}{V_{total}} x\ 100\%$$

where V_{solid} and V_{total} represent the volume of the solid and the total volume of the scaffold, respectively.

STRUCTURAL PROPERTIES

X-Ray Diffraction

X-ray diffraction analysis is a non-destructive characterization technique used for analysing the microstructure and phase identification, thereby determining the chemical composition of the scaffolds. This method follows the Bragg's law of diffraction which states that when a crystal is visualized as a set of reflecting planes that are equally spaced at a distance d and an X-ray beam with wavelength λ collimated to the crystal at an angle θ, the reinforcement of reflected waves relates to $\sin\theta = n\lambda/2d$, where n denotes an integer known as the order of reflection. Thus, the Bragg's law of diffraction is defined by the equation: $n\lambda = 2d\sin\theta$

Actually, when an X-ray strikes the sample, the diffracted rays are produced because of the interaction of the incident rays with the sample, which are detected, processed, and analysed. The intensity of these diffracted rays scattered at different angles of the sample is plotted to exhibit the diffraction pattern as displayed in Figure 5.8.

X-ray diffraction (XRD) technique is routinely used for phase analysis of bone and cartilage TE scaffolds. For example, the phase analysis of a 3D electrospun silk fibroin nanofibrous composite bone scaffold was done by an X-ray diffractometer using Cu-Kα radiation of 0.1542Å wavelength with a step-scan mode at 2θ range of 10–80°, 2°/min scanning speed, voltage of 30 kV and current of 30 mA. The crystallinity of the nanofibrous scaffold and the % β-crystalline content caused by enzymatic degradation has been measured by analysing XRD data using X'pert high score, Origin Pro 8, and Joint Committee on Powder Diffraction Studies (JCPDS) softwares.

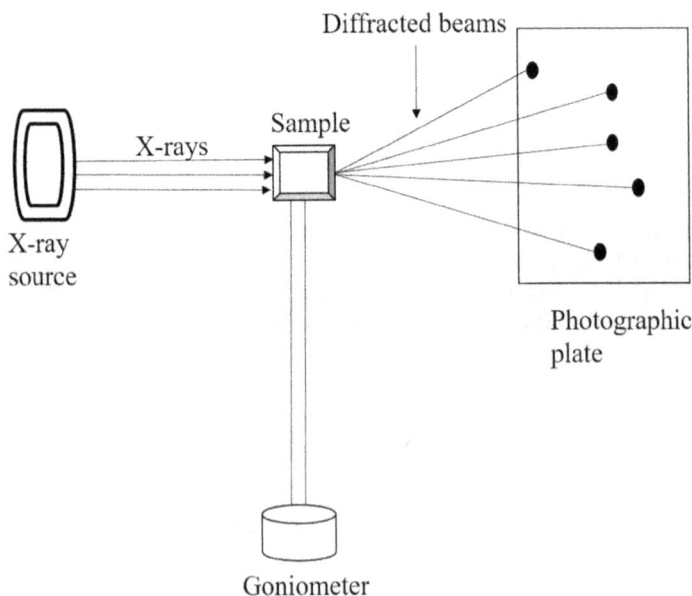

FIGURE 5.8 Principle of X-ray diffraction technique.

In an another study, XRD was performed on the developed cross-linked chitosan scaffolds with porous structure for cartilage TE application (Shamekhi et al. 2017; Vishwanath, Pramanik, and Biswas 2016; Agrawal and Pramanik 2016).

Fourier Transform Infrared Spectroscopy

Fourier Transform Infrared Spectroscopy (FTIR) is used for identifying organic and inorganic compounds, and determining as well as quantifying the molecular composition and the different functional groups existing in the biomaterial. The method involves the mixing of scaffold samples with the KBr powder followed by palletization into transparent disks using a hydraulic press before performing FTIR analysis. FTIR can operate in a transmittance mode at a scanning range of 500–4000 cm^{-1} with a 8 cm^{-1} resolution (Lowery, Datta, and Rutledge 2010). FTIR was used to analyse the molecular composition and functional groups present in the silk fibroin blend by operating with a scanning range of 4000 cm^{-1} to 400 cm^{-1}, 8 cm^{-1} resolution, and scan numbers of 60. The infrared absorption spectrum, emission, and photoconductivity of the material including solid, gas, or liquid are used to detect different functional groups present in the sample through the obtained spectrum data in an automated software of spectroscopy. Like XRD, FTIR has also been used routinely for determining the specific functional groups present in the scaffolds that were used for several *in vitro* and *in vivo* tissue regeneration applications for bone, cartilage, and more complex situations like osteochondral or osteoporosis (Nouri-Felekori et al. 2021; Huang et al. 2018; Zakhireh et al. 2021; Pacheco et al. 2021; Hafezi et al. 2012; Filová et al. 2020).

Mechanical Strength

It is of utmost importance to have adequate mechanical strength to support the cellular growth over the implanted scaffolds. Different types of mechanical properties of the scaffolds are involved depending on their applications and, hence, different testing methods are used. For example, compression test is normally used for bone scaffolds (Balagangadharan, Dhivya, and Selvamurugan 2017), whereas tensile test is useful for cartilage scaffolds. The testing methods may also depend on the scaffold geometry and types: for example, mechanical strength of 3D porous and 2D fibrous scaffolds is determined by compression and tensile strength tests respectively. The various mechanical properties that are important for the tissue engineering scaffold include the following:

(i)   the ultimate tensile strength of the structure is the maximum stress that a material can bear while being stretched before breaking, beyond which the scaffold may permanently be deformed.

(ii)   the tensile strength is the strength upto which a scaffold or material can be elongated before it breaks; this test is especially necessary for fibrous scaffold.

(iii)   the compression test determines the compressive strength in terms of degree of compression of a scaffold. In this test the sample is compressed and deformed at varying loads which is recorded.

(iv)   the Young's modulus, also referred to as the modulus of elasticity, relates to the slope of the linear part of the generated stress–strain curve as shown in

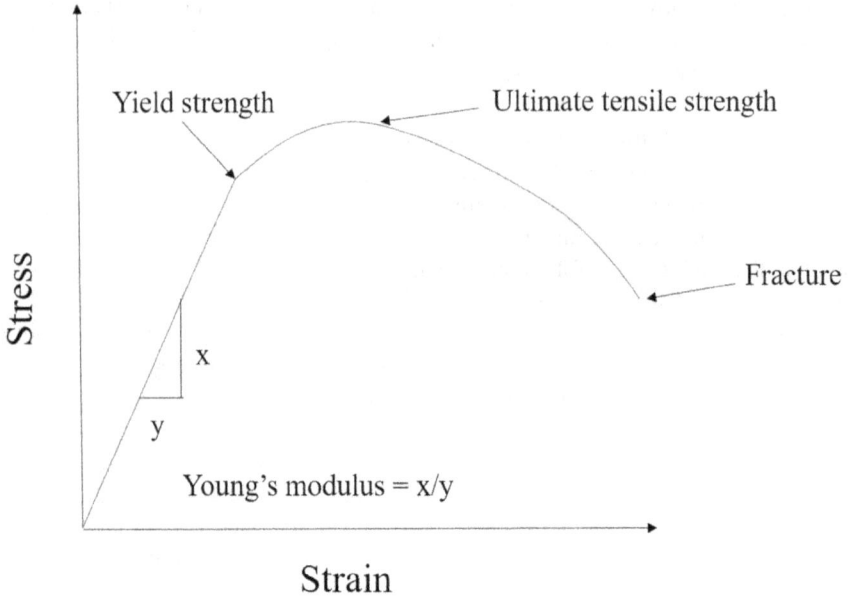

FIGURE 5.9 A typical Stress–strain curve of a material.

Figure 5.9. This is also used to measure scaffold stiffness from the force versus extension graph.

(v) The elastic limit is the maximum stress that can be withstood by a material without any permanent deformation. Scaffold structure fabricated from brittle biomaterials tends to break at or beyond their elastic limit; however, ductile materials deform at stress above their elastic limit tested for porous scaffold. A typical stress–strain curve of a material is presented in Figure 5.9.

The ultimate tensile strength of an electrospun silk scaffold with nanofibrous architecture was measured by a universal testing machine with 1 KN load cell under ambient conditions and 65% relative humidity. The scaffold with 50 mm × 12 mm rectangular shapes and 0.30 mm ± 0.01 mm thickness was fixed with a double-sided glue tape. The strength of the scaffold was determined at crosshead speed and gauge length of 20 mm/min and 30 mm, respectively. The breaking stress and the % strain were determined from the generated stress–strain plot. In another study, the compressive strengths of the silk fibroin/chitosan-based 3D porous scaffolds were obtained using a 1 KN load cell and 1 mm/min crosshead speed at room temperature. The compressive strength of the scaffold was calculated by the equation $S = F_{max} / A$, where F_{max} and A are the applied force and cross-sectional area of the scaffold, respectively. For an *in vivo* experiment with New Zealand white rabbit, a 3D-printed polycaprolactone (PCL)–hydrosxyapatite (HAp) scaffold designed based on the CT 3D reconstruction data was subjected to mechanical testing and thereby recording the loading force, deformation, and maximum affordable pressure (Yao et al. 2015).

Swelling Behaviour and Water Uptake Capacity

The swelling behaviour or water uptake capacity of the scaffold is measured by the conventional gravimetric method. This property is often expressed as equilibrium swelling ratio (E_s), percent swelling (% swelling), or percent water uptake (% water uptake). In this method, the scaffolds are usually exposed to simulated body fluid (SBF), which can be prepared in the laboratory by dissolving 7.995 g NaCl, 0.224 g KCl, 0.368 g $CaCl_2 \cdot 2H_2O$, 0.305 g $MgCl_2 \cdot 6H_2O$, 0.174 g K_2HPO_4, 0.349 g $NaHCO_3$, and 0.161 g $Na_2SO_4 \cdot 10H_2O$ in 1 L of distilled water and by maintaining the pH of the solution at 7.4 by adding Tris/HCl. Phosphate buffer saline (PBS) can also be used in place of SBF solution. The dried scaffold samples (W_d) are immersed in SBF and the wet weight (W_w) of the scaffold is recorded at a predetermined time interval till equilibrium or saturation is reached. After the stipulated time period, scaffolds are taken out from the solution followed by removing trace amount of surface adsorbed water with a filter paper and then wet weight is recorded. The equilibrium swelling ratio is defined as the ratio of increased weight ($W_w - W_d$) to the initial dry weight (W_d) of the scaffold, and is calculated by the equation: $E_s = (W_w - W_d)/W_d$. The % water uptake (W_u) is calculated by the equation: $W_u = (W_w - W_d)/W_w \times 100$ and % swelling is calculated by the equation: $(W_w - W_d)/W_d \times 100$ (Hofmann et al. 2006). For an example, the swelling behaviour of the nanofibrous scaffolds for BTE applications was studied by treating the sample in PBS solution at pH 7.4 and 37°C for 96 hours (Andiappan et al. 2013).

Contact Angle Measurement (Hydrophilicity)

The wetting property, or hydrophilicity, of scaffold is important for cell attachment and cell survival. This property is evaluated by measuring the contact angle, the angle at which the liquid–vapour interface meets the surface of the scaffold. This measurement basically quantifies the wettability of a solid surface when it contacts a liquid. The equilibrium contact angle represents the relative strength of the molecular interaction of the liquid, solid, and vapour. In TE, it measures the capacity of a scaffold to hold liquid or water when it is implanted into the defect site of the body, thereby making it come in contact with the body fluids. The wetting properties of a nanofibrous scaffold have been measured by a dynamic contact angle measurement system, using goniometer, by axisymmetric drop shape analysis-no apex (ADSA-NA) (Skinner, Rotenberg, and Neumann 1989).

Biodegradation

Biodegradation is studied by incubating the scaffolds in either PBS or SBF solution for a specific time period and measuring the change in weight in the presence of an enzyme like lysozyme, or protease. In this method, the dried sample with an initial weight (W_0) is treated in SBF for a specific time period. The sample is taken from the SBF solution at a regular interval and is freeze-dried. Then the final weight (W_t) is measured (Peter et al. 2010). The remaining weight % (W_R) is calculated by the formula: $\% \: Weight \: remaining = 100 - [(W_0 - W_t)/W_0 \times 100]$. In a study, silk fibroin was shown to be degraded in the presence of protease enzyme (Wongnarat and Srihanam 2013).

TABLE 5.1
List of Techniques for Characterization of Scaffold

Characterization Type	Specific Property	Techniques
Physicochemical	Morphology Porosity Hydrophillicity Biodegradation Swelling behaviour and water uptake capacity	Microscopy analysis such as SEM, AFM, and TEM Gravimetric method/mercury intrusion porosimetry/ liquid displacement method/ CAD model Contact angle Treatment in SBF/PBS solution Treatment in SBF/PBS solution
Structural	Crystallinity, microstructure analysis and phase identification molecular composition and functional groups	XRD FTIR
Mechanical	Stress–strain correlation, compressive strength for porous scaffold, tensile strength for fibrous scaffold, stiffness, Young's modulus, elastic limit	Mechanical tester
Biological	Biocompatibility	*In vitro* cell study and *in vivo* animal study

Bioactivity

The bioactivity of a scaffold representing the formation of bone-like apatite reflects its bone-binding potential (Davies and Baldan 1997; Marcolongo et al. 1998b). Bioactivity improves healing through an accelerated bone tissue regeneration and hydroxyapatite deposition. The bioactive potential of a scaffold is measured by SEM and EDX analysis. The list of the various characterisation techniques that are used for evaluating the properties of the TE scaffold is given in Table 5.1.

EXERCISE

1. Explain the principle of SEM for characterizing scaffold with a schematic diagram.
2. Explain the principle of AFM for characterizing scaffold. What are its advantages and disadvantages?
3. Explain the principle and applications of TEM.
4. Define the term "biodegradability" and explain its importance in tissue regeneration.

5. Describe how swelling behaviour has a substantial impact on the characteristics of scaffolds.
6. Explain the importance of sterilization in tissue engineering? Mention some of the commonly used techniques to sterilize tissue scaffolds.
7. Explain how surface properties of scaffold are important in tissue engineering.
8. Explain how porosity and biodegradability of scaffolds play important role in tissue engineering.
9. Explain the importance of XRD in scaffold characterization.
10. Explain Braggs' law of diffraction.
11. Explain the importance of FTIR in scaffold characterization. Write about the sample preparation method for FTIR.
12. Mention and explain the different methods of porosity measurement.
13. What is the importance of contact angle? How can it be measured?
14. How surface roughness is important in bone tissue engineering?
15. Write about the various mechanical properties which are important for the scaffold and describe their methods of determination..
16. Define: (a) Biocompatibility and (b) Bioactivity.
17. A porous scaffold was developed and tested for swelling behaviour in PBS. The data for swelling is given in the table.

Time	Weight of the scaffold
0	0.046
4	0.642
8	0.764
16	0.952
24	0.985

Find the swelling percentage and plot the graph for swelling behaviour and explain.

18. A chitosan porous scaffold was developed for cartilage tissue regeneration. To assess the degradation pattern, the scaffolds was cut into small pieces and immersed into the SBF. After degradation the scaffolds samples were dried and degraded scaffolds were weighed at 7th, 10th, 14th, and 28th day. The recorded values are given in the below table.

Days	Dry weight	Degraded weight
7th	0.068	0.051
10th	0.073	0.047
14th	0.065	0.029
28th	0.084	0.031

i. Find the degradation percentage of the scaffold.

    ii. Draw a graph of time vs. degradation percentage and explain the degradation pattern of the scaffold

19. A chitosan based 3D porous nanocomposite scaffold was developed and subjected to porosity measurement by liquid displacement method using ethanol. Initially 92 mL of ethanol was taken in a measuring flask and then the scaffold was immersed into it due to which the volume of the ethanol increased up to 95 mL. After soaking for particular time period the scaffold was taken out carefully by removing the extra ethanol and then it was found that only 65 ml of ethanol remained in the flask. Find the porosity of the scaffold and justify the suitability of the scaffold for bone tissue engineering scaffold..

20. A PVA film was developed and subjected to tensile strength measurement. The measurement of the film was given as 20 mm length and 0.16 mm² cross-sectional area. The film was broken after 4 mm elongation under the maximum load of 8 N. Find the Young's modulus of the film.

21. Mention any two instruments that can be used for assessing surface characteristics of scaffold. Explain the principle of any one of them.

22. Explain how pore size of scaffold is important for bone and cartilage tissue engineering. How pore size os scaffold is measured?

REFERENCES

Agrawal, P., and K. Pramanik. 2016. "Chitosan-poly (vinyl alcohol) nanofibers by free surface electrospinning for tissue engineering applications". *Tissue Engineering and Regenerative Medicine* 13 (5): 485–497.

Akhtar, K., Khan, S. A., Khan, S. B., & Asiri, A. M. 2018. "Scanning electron microscopy: Principle and applications in nanomaterials characterization". In *Handbook of Materials Characterization*, 113–145. Springer.

Andiappan, M., S. Sundaramoorthy, N. Panda, G. Meiyazhaban, S. B. Winfred, G. Venkataraman, and P. Krishna. 2013. "Electrospun eri silk fibroin scaffold coated with hydroxyapatite for bone tissue engineering applications". *Progress in Biomaterials* 2 (1): 6.

Balagangadharan, K., S. Dhivya, and N. Selvamurugan. 2017. "Chitosan based nanofibers in bone tissue engineering". *International Journal of Biological Macromolecules* 104: 1372–1382.

Balasundaram, G., D. M. Storey, and T. J. Webster. 2014. "Novel nano-rough polymers for cartilage tissue engineering". *International Journal of Nanomedicine* 9: 1845.

Bas, O., F. Hanßke, J. Lim, A. Ravichandran, E. Kemnitz, S.-H. Teoh, D. W. Hutmacher, and H. G. Börner. 2019. "Tuning mechanical reinforcement and bioactivity of 3D printed ternary nanocomposites by interfacial peptide-polymer conjugates". *Biofabrication* 11 (3): 035028.

Berger, J., M. Reist, J. M. Mayer, Olivia Felt, N. A. Peppas, and R. Gurny. 2004. "Structure and interactions in covalently and ionically crosslinked chitosan hydrogels for biomedical applications". *European Journal of Pharmaceutics and Biopharmaceutics* 57 (1): 19–34.

Bhardwaj, N., and S. C. Kundu. 2011. "Silk fibroin protein and chitosan polyelectrolyte complex porous scaffolds for tissue engineering applications". *Carbohydrate Polymers* 85 (2): 325–333.

Binnig, G., C. F. Quate, and C. Gerber. 1986. "Atomic force microscope". *Physical Review Letters* 56 (9): 930.

Buseck, P., J. Cowley, and L. Eyring. 1989. *High-Resolution Transmission Electron Microscopy and Associated Techniques*: Oxford University Press.

Campos, Y., G. Fuentes, A. Almirall, I. Que, T. Schomann, C. K. Chung, C. Jorquera-Cordero, L. Quintanilla, J. C. Rodríguez-Cabello, and A. Chan. 2022. "The Incorporation of etanercept into a porous tri-layer scaffold for restoring and repairing cartilage tissue". *Pharmaceutics* 14 (2): 282.

Cao, Y., and B. Wang. 2009. "Biodegradation of silk biomaterials". *International Journal of Molecular Sciences* 10 (4): 1514–1524.

Causa, F., P. A. Netti, and L. Ambrosio. 2007. "A multi-functional scaffold for tissue regeneration: The need to engineer a tissue analogue". *Biomaterials* 28 (34): 5093–5099.

Chan, B. P., and K. W. Leong. 2008. "Scaffolding in tissue engineering: General approaches and tissue-specific considerations". *European Spine Journal* 17 (4): 467–479.

Chong, E. J., T. T. Phan, Ivor Jiun Lim, Y. Z. Zhang, B. Huat Bay, S. Ramakrishna, and C. Teck Lim. 2007. "Evaluation of electrospun PCL/gelatin nanofibrous scaffold for wound healing and layered dermal reconstitution". *Acta Biomaterialia* 3 (3): 321–330.

Considine, G. D. 2005. "Van Nostrand's encyclopedia of chemistry encyclopedia of chemistry". Chapter 5: 261.

Curtis, A., and C. Wilkinson. 1997. "Topographical control of cells". *Biomaterials* 18 (24): 1573–1583.

Dai, Z., J. Ronholm, Y. Tian, B. Sethi, and X. Cao. 2016. "Sterilization techniques for biodegradable scaffolds in tissue engineering applications". *Journal of Tissue Engineering* 7: 2041731416648810.

Dave, K., and V. G. Gomes. 2019. "Interactions at scaffold interfaces: Effect of surface chemistry, structural attributes and bioaffinity". *Materials Science and Engineering: C* 105: 110078.

Davies, J. E., and N. Baldan. 1997. "Scanning electron microscopy of the bone-bioactive implant interface". *Journal of Biomedical Materials Research* 36 (4): 429–440.

Denchai, A., D. Tartarini, and E. Mele. 2018. "Cellular response to surface morphology: Electrospinning and computational modeling". *Frontiers in Bioengineering and Biotechnology* 6: 155.

Diermann, S. H., M. Lu, G. Edwards, M. Dargusch, and H. Huang. 2019. "In vitro degradation of a unique porous PHBV scaffold manufactured using selective laser sintering". *Journal of Biomedical Materials Research Part A* 107 (1): 154–162.

do Amaral Montanheiro, T. L., L. Stieven Montagna, V. Patrulea, O. Jordan, G. Borchard, R. G. Ribas, T. M. B. Campos, G. P. Thim and A. P. Lemes. 2019. "Enhanced water uptake of PHBV scaffolds with functionalized cellulose nanocrystals". *Polymer Testing* 79: 106079.

Echeverria Molina, M. I., K. G. Malollari, and K. Komvopoulos. 2021. "Design challenges in polymeric scaffolds for tissue engineering". *Frontiers in Bioengineering and Biotechnology*: 231.

Elsner, J. J., A. Shefy-Peleg, and M. Zilberman. 2010. "Novel biodegradable composite wound dressings with controlled release of antibiotics: Microstructure, mechanical and physical properties". *Journal of Biomedical Materials Research Part B: Applied Biomaterials* 93 (2): 425–435.

Filová, E., Z. Tonar, V. Lukášová, M. Buzgo, A. Litvinec, M. Rampichová, J. Beznoska, M. Plencner, A. Staffa, and J. Daňková. 2020. "Hydrogel containing anti-CD44-labeled microparticles, guide bone tissue formation in osteochondral defects in rabbits". *Nanomaterials* 10 (8): 1504.

Galante, R., Terezinha J. P., R. Colaco, and A. P. Serro. 2018. "Sterilization of hydrogels for biomedical applications: A review". *Journal of Biomedical Materials Research Part B: Applied Biomaterials* 106 (6): 2472–2492.

Goddard, J. M., and J. H. Hotchkiss. 2007. "Polymer surface modification for the attachment of bioactive compounds". *Progress in Polymer Science* 32 (7): 698–725.

Grad, S., K. Gorna, S. Gogolewski, and M. Alini. 2004. "Scaffolds for cartilage tissue engineering: Effect of pore size". *European Cells and Materials* 7 (1): 1–3.

Guarino, V., F. Causa, P. Taddei, M. Di Foggia, G. Ciapetti, D. Martini, C. Fagnano, N. Baldini, and L. Ambrosio. 2008. "Polylactic acid fibre-reinforced polycaprolactone scaffolds for bone tissue engineering". *Biomaterials* 29 (27): 3662–3670.

Hafezi, F, F. Hosseinnejad, A. A. I. Fooladi, S. M. Mafi, A. Amiri, and M. R. Nourani. 2012. "Transplantation of nano-bioglass/gelatin scaffold in a non-autogenous setting for bone regeneration in a rabbit ulna". *Journal of Materials Science: Materials in Medicine* 23 (11): 2783–2792.

Harley, B. A., T. M. Freyman, M. Q. Wong, and L. J. Gibson. 2007. "A new technique for calculating individual dermal fibroblast contractile forces generated within collagen-GAG scaffolds". *Biophysical Journal* 93 (8): 2911–2922.

Hofmann, S., C. T. Wong Po Foo, F. Rossetti, M. Textor, G. Vunjak-Novakovic, D. L. Kaplan, H. P. Merkle, and L. Meinel. 2006. "Silk fibroin as an organic polymer for controlled drug delivery". *Journal of Controlled Release* 111 (1–2): 219–227.

Hofmann, S., K. S. Stok, T. Kohler, A. J. Meinel, and R. Müller. 2014. "Effect of sterilization on structural and material properties of 3-D silk fibroin scaffolds". *Acta Biomaterialia* 10 (1): 308–317.

Hollister, S. J. 2005. "Porous scaffold design for tissue engineering". *Nature Materials* 4 (7): 518–524.

Holloway, J. L, H. Ma, R. Rai, and J. A. Burdick. 2014. "Modulating hydrogel crosslink density and degradation to control bone morphogenetic protein delivery and in vivo bone formation". *Journal of Controlled Release* 191: 63–70.

Holzapfel, B. M., J. Christian Reichert, J.-T. Schantz, U. Gbureck, L. Rackwitz, U. Nöth, F. Jakob, M. Rudert, J. Groll, and D. Werner Hutmacher. 2013. "How smart do biomaterials need to be? A translational science and clinical point of view". *Advanced Drug Delivery Reviews* 65 (4): 581–603.

Holzwarth, J. M., and P. X. Ma. 2011. "Biomimetic nanofibrous scaffolds for bone tissue engineering". *Biomaterials* 32 (36): 9622–9629.

Hsin, I. C., and W. Yiwei. 2011. "Cell responses to surface and architecture of tissue engineering scaffolds". *Regenerative Medicine and Tissue Engineering–Cells and Biomaterials*, IntechOpen, 569–588.

Hu, W.-W., Y. Elkasabi, H.-Y. Chen, Y. Zhang, J. Lahann, S. J. Hollister, and P. H. Krebsbach. 2009. "The use of reactive polymer coatings to facilitate gene delivery from poly (ε-caprolactone) scaffolds". *Biomaterials* 30 (29): 5785–5792.

Huang, G. P., A. Molina, N. Tran, G. Collins, and T. L. Arinzeh. 2018. "Investigating cellulose derived glycosaminoglycan mimetic scaffolds for cartilage tissue engineering applications". *Journal of Tissue Engineering and Regenerative Medicine* 12 (1): e592–e603.

Hutmacher, D. W. 2000. "Scaffolds in tissue engineering bone and cartilage". *Biomaterials* 21 (24): 2529–2543.

Jurczyk, M. U., K. Jurczyk, A. Miklaszewski, and M. Jurczyk. 2011. "Nanostructured titanium-45S5 bioglass scaffold composites for medical applications". *Materials & Design* 32 (10): 4882–4889.

Karageorgiou, V., and D. Kaplan. 2005. "Porosity of 3D biomaterial scaffolds and osteogenesis". *Biomaterials* 26 (27): 5474–5491.

Kavasi, R. M., C. C. Coelho, V. Platania, P. A. Quadros, and M. Chatzinikolaidou. 2021. "In vitro biocompatibility assessment of nano-hydroxyapatite". *Nanomaterials* 11(5): 1152.

Kouhi, M., M. Fathi, M. P. Prabhakaran, M. Shamanian, and S. Ramakrishna. 2018. "Enhanced proliferation and mineralization of human fetal osteoblast cells on PHBV-bredigite nanofibrous scaffolds". *Materials Today: Proceedings* 5 (7): 15702–15709.

Kumbar, S. G., S. P. Nukavarapu, R. James, L. S. Nair, and C. T. Laurencin. 2008. "Electrospun poly (lactic acid-co-glycolic acid) scaffolds for skin tissue engineering". *Biomaterials* 29 (30): 4100–4107.

Law, K.-Y.. 2014. *Definitions for Hydrophilicity, Hydrophobicity, and Superhydrophobicity: Getting the Basics Right.* ACS Publications.

Lee, K.-W., S. Wang, L. Lu, E. Jabbari, B. L. Currier, and M. J. Yaszemski. 2006. "Fabrication and characterization of poly (propylene fumarate) scaffolds with controlled pore structures using 3-dimensional printing and injection molding". *Tissue Engineering* 12 (10): 2801–2811.

Lee, S. H., W. Y. Zhou, M. Wang, W. L. Cheung, and W. Y. Ip. 2009. "Selective laser sintering of poly (l-lactide) porous scaffolds for bone tissue engineering". *Journal of Biomimetics, Biomaterials and Tissue Engineering* 1: 81–89.

Li, Y., J. Zhou, S. Hu, J. Wang, K. Wang, and W. Wang. 2021. "Methods of improving the mechanical properties of hydrogels and their research progress in bone tissue engineering". *Zhongguo xiu fu Chong Jian wai ke za zhi= Zhongguo Xiufu Chongjian Waike Zazhi= Chinese Journal of Reparative and Reconstructive Surgery* 35 (12): 1615–1622.

Lim, D-J.. 2022. "Cross-Linking agents for electrospinning-based bone tissue engineering". *International Journal of Molecular Sciences* 23 (10): 5444.

Liu, H., E. B. Slamovich, and T. J. Webster. 2006. "Increased osteoblast functions among nanophase titania/poly (lactide-co-glycolide) composites of the highest nanometer surface roughness". *Journal of Biomedical Materials Research Part A: An Official Journal of the Society for Biomaterials, the Japanese Society for Biomaterials, and the Australian Society for Biomaterials and the Korean Society for Biomaterials* 78 (4): 798–807.

Lopez Marquez, A., I. Emilio Gareis, F. J. Dias, C. Gerhard, and M. F. Lezcano. 2022. "Methods to characterize electrospun scaffold morphology: A critical review". *Polymers* 14 (3): 467.

Łopianiak, I., M. Wojasiński, A. Kuźmińska, P. Trzaskowska, and B. A. Butruk-Raszeja. 2021. "The effect of surface morphology on endothelial and smooth muscle cells growth on blow-spun fibrous scaffolds". *Journal of Biological Engineering* 15 (1): 1–17.

Lowery, J. L.. 2009. "Characterization and modification of porosity in electrospun polymeric materials for tissue engineering applications". Massachusetts Institute of Technology.

Lowery, J. L., N. Datta, and G. C. Rutledge. 2010. "Effect of fiber diameter, pore size and seeding method on growth of human dermal fibroblasts in electrospun poly (ε-caprolactone) fibrous mats". *Biomaterials* 31 (3): 491–504.

MacDonald, A. F., M. E. Harley-Troxell, S. D. Newby, and M. S. Dhar. 2022. "3D-Printing graphene scaffolds for bone tissue engineering". *Pharmaceutics* 14 (9): 1834.

Mani, M. P., S. Kumar Jaganathan, and E. Supriyanto. 2019. "Enriched mechanical strength and bone mineralisation of electrospun biomimetic scaffold laden with ylang oil and zinc nitrate for bone tissue engineering". *Polymers* 11 (8): 1323.

Maolin, Z., H. Hongfei, F. Yoshii, and K. Makuuchi. 2000. "Effect of kappa-carrageenan on the properties of poly (N-vinyl pyrrolidone)/kappa-carrageenan blend hydrogel synthesized by γ-radiation technology". *Radiation Physics and Chemistry* 57 (3–6): 459–464.

Marcolongo, M., P. Ducheyne, J. Garino, and E. Schepers. 1998a. "Bioactive glass fiber/polymeric composites bond to bone tissue". *Journal of Biomedical Materials Research* 39 (1): 161–170.

Marti, O., B. Drake, and P. K. Hansma. 1987. "Atomic force microscopy of liquid-covered surfaces: Atomic resolution images". *Applied Physics Letters* 51 (7): 484–486.

Maspero, F. A., K. Ruffieux, B. Müller, and E. Wintermantel. 2002. "Resorbable defect analog PLGA scaffolds using CO2 as solvent: Structural characterization". *Journal of Biomedical Materials Research: An Official Journal of the Society for Biomaterials, the Japanese Society for Biomaterials, and the Australian Society for Biomaterials and the Korean Society for Biomaterials* 62 (1): 89–98.

Mayer, J., L. A. Giannuzzi, T. Kamino, and J. Michael. 2007. "TEM sample preparation and FIB-induced damage". *MRS Bulletin* 32 (5): 400–407.

Mayer, R. P., and R. A. Stowe. 1965. "Mercury porosimetry—breakthrough pressure for penetration between packed spheres". *Journal of Colloid Science* 20 (8): 893–911.

Milošev, I., V. Levašič, J. Vidmar, S. Kovač, and R. Trebše. 2017. "pH and metal concentration of synovial fluid of osteoarthritic joints and joints with metal replacements". *Journal of Biomedical Materials Research Part B: Applied Biomaterials* 105 (8): 2507–2515.

Min, B.-M., G. Lee, S. H. Kim, Y. S. Nam, T. S. Lee, and W. H. Park. 2004. "Electrospinning of silk fibroin nanofibers and its effect on the adhesion and spreading of normal human keratinocytes and fibroblasts in vitro". *Biomaterials* 25 (7–8): 1289–1297.

Miyauchi, T., M. Yamada, A. Yamamoto, F. Iwasa, T. Suzawa, R. Kamijo, K. Baba, and T. Ogawa. 2010. "The enhanced characteristics of osteoblast adhesion to photofunctionalized nanoscale TiO2 layers on biomaterials surfaces". *Biomaterials* 31 (14): 3827–3839.

Mostofi, F., M. Mostofi, B. Niroomand, S. Hosseini, A. Alipour, S. Homaeigohar, J. Mohammadi, M. A. Shokrgozar, and H. Shahsavarani. 2022. "Crossing phylums: Butterfly wing as a natural perfusable three-dimensional (3D) bioconstruct for bone tissue engineering". *Journal of Functional Biomaterials* 13 (2): 68.

Morra, M., and C. Cassinelli. 2006. Biomaterials surface characterization and modification. *International Journal of Artificial Organs* 29 (9): 824–833.

Murphy, C. M., M. G. Haugh, and F. J. O'Brien. 2010. "The effect of mean pore size on cell attachment, proliferation and migration in collagen–glycosaminoglycan scaffolds for bone tissue engineering". *Biomaterials* 31 (3): 461–466.

Murphy, C. M., and F. J. O'Brien. 2010. "Understanding the effect of mean pore size on cell activity in collagen-glycosaminoglycan scaffolds". *Cell Adhesion & Migration* 4 (3): 377–381.

Niu, B., B. Li, Y. Gu, X. Shen, Y. Liu, and L. Chen. 2017. "In vitro evaluation of electrospun silk fibroin/nano-hydroxyapatite/BMP-2 scaffolds for bone regeneration". *Journal of Biomaterials Science, Polymer Edition* 28 (3): 257–270.

Nouri-Felekori, M., N. Nezafati, M. Moraveji, S. Hesaraki, and T. Ramezani. 2021. "Bioorthogonal hydroxyethyl cellulose-based scaffold crosslinked via click chemistry for cartilage tissue engineering applications". *International Journal of Biological Macromolecules* 183: 2030–2043.

O'Brien, F. J. 2011. "Biomaterials & scaffolds for tissue engineering". *Materials Today* 14 (3): 88–95.

Pacheco, I. K. C., F. Da Silva Reis, C. Ernanda Sousa De Carvalho, J. M. Elias De Matos, N. Martins Argôlo Neto, S. De Araújo França Baeta, K. Rovaris Da Silva, H. Victor Dantas, F. Barbosa De Sousa, and A. Cristina Vasconcelos Fialho. 2021. "Development of castor polyurethane scaffold (*Ricinus communis* L.) and its effect with stem cells for bone repair in an osteoporosis model". *Biomedical Materials* 16 (6): 065006.

Park, G. E., M. A. Pattison, K. Park, and T. J. Webster. 2005. "Accelerated chondrocyte functions on NaOH-treated PLGA scaffolds". *Biomaterials* 26 (16): 3075–3082.

Peter, M., Nitya Ganesh, N. S., S. V. Nair, T. Furuike, H. Tamura, and R. Jayakumar. 2010. "Preparation and characterization of chitosan–gelatin/nanohydroxyapatite composite scaffolds for tissue engineering applications". *Carbohydrate Polymers* 80 (3): 687–694.

Ponomar, M., E. Krasnyuk, D. Butylskii, V. Nikonenko, Y. Wang, C. Jiang, T. Xu, and N. Pismenskaya. 2022. "Sessile drop method: Critical analysis and optimization for measuring the contact angle of an ion-exchange membrane surface". *Membranes* 12 (8): 765.

Ponsonnet, L., V. Comte, A. Othmane, C. Lagneau, M. Charbonnier, M. Lissac, and N. Jaffrezic. 2002. "Effect of surface topography and chemistry on adhesion, orientation and growth of fibroblasts on nickel–titanium substrates". *Materials Science and Engineering*: C 21 (1–2): 157–165.

Pucino, V., M. Certo, V. Bulusu, D. Cucchi, K. Goldmann, E. Pontarini, R. Haas, J. Smith, S. E. Headland, and K. Blighe. 2019. "Lactate buildup at the site of chronic inflammation promotes disease by inducing CD4+ T cell metabolic rewiring". *Cell Metabolism* 30 (6): 1055–1074. e8.

Ranjan, A., and T. J. Webster. 2009. "Increased endothelial cell adhesion and elongation on micron-patterned nano-rough poly (dimethylsiloxane) films". *Nanotechnology* 20 (30): 305102.

Ribas, R. G., T. L.A. Montanheiro, L. S. Montagna, R. Falchete do Prado, A. Paula Lemes, T. M. Bastos Campos, and G. P. Thim. 2019. "Water uptake in PHBV/Wollastonite scaffolds: A kinetics study". *Journal of Composites Science* 3 (3): 74.

Rockwood, D. N., R. C. Preda, T. Yücel, X. Wang, M. L. Lovett, and D. L. Kaplan. 2011. "Materials fabrication from bombyx mori silk fibroin". *Nature Protocols* 6 (10): 1612–1631.

Roman, M. D., R. Sorin Fleaca, A. Boicean, D. Bratu, V. Birlutiu, L. Liviu Rus, C. Tantar, and S. Ioan Cernusca Mitariu. 2017. "Assesment of synovial fluid pH in osteoarthritis of the HIP and knee". *Rev. Chim* 68 (6): 1242–1244.

Sanz-Herrera, J. A., J. M. García-Aznar, and M. Doblaré. 2009. "On scaffold designing for bone regeneration: A computational multiscale approach". *Acta Biomaterialia* 5 (1): 219–229.

Shaban, N. Z., M. Y. Kenawy, N. A. Taha, M. M. Abd El-Latif, and D. A. Ghareeb. 2021. "Cellulose acetate nanofibers: Incorporating hydroxyapatite (HA), HA/berberine or HA/moghat composites, as scaffolds to enhance in vitro osteoporotic bone regeneration". *Polymers* 13 (23): 4140.

Shamekhi, M. A., A. Rabiee, H. Mirzadeh, H. Mahdavi, D. Mohebbi-Kalhori, and M. B. Eslaminejad. 2017. "Fabrication and characterization of hydrothermal cross-linked chitosan porous scaffolds for cartilage tissue engineering applications". *Materials Science and Engineering: C* 80: 532–542.

Shi, G., Q. Cai, C. Wang, N. Lu, S. Wang, and J. Bei. 2002. "Fabrication and biocompatibility of cell scaffolds of poly (l-lactic acid) and poly (l-lactic-co-glycolic acid)". *Polymers for Advanced Technologies* 13 (3–4): 227–232.

Skinner, F. K., Y. Rotenberg, and A. W. Neumann. 1989. "Contact angle measurements from the contact diameter of sessile drops by means of a modified axisymmetric drop shape analysis". *Journal of Colloid and Interface Science* 130 (1): 25–34.

Smith, L. E., R. Smallwood, and S. Macneil. 2010. "A comparison of imaging methodologies for 3D tissue engineering". *Microscopy Research and Technique* 73 (12): 1123–1133.

Spector, M. 2006. Biomaterials-based tissue engineering and regenerative medicine solutions to musculoskeletal problems. *Swiss Medical Weekly* 136 (19–20): 293–301.

Song, A., A. A. Rane, and K. L. Christman. 2012. "Antibacterial and cell-adhesive polypeptide and poly (ethylene glycol) hydrogel as a potential scaffold for wound healing". *Acta Biomaterialia* 8 (1): 41–50.

Sultana, N., and T. H. Khan. 2012. "In vitro degradation of PHBV scaffolds and nHA/PHBV composite scaffolds containing hydroxyapatite nanoparticles for bone tissue engineering". *Journal of Nanomaterials* 2012.

Sultana, N., and M. Wang. 2008. "Fabrication of HA/PHBV composite scaffolds through the emulsion freezing/freeze-drying process and characterisation of the scaffolds". *Journal of Materials Science: Materials in Medicine* 19 (7): 2555–2561.

Sun, W., B. Starly, A. Darling and C. Gomez. 2004. "Computer-aided tissue engineering: Application to biomimetic modelling and design of tissue scaffolds". *Biotechnology and Applied Biochemistry* 39 (1): 49–58.

Tallawi, M., E. Rosellini, N. Barbani, M. G. Cascone, R. Rai, G. Saint-Pierre, and A. R. Boccaccini. 2015. "Strategies for the chemical and biological functionalization of scaffolds for cardiac tissue engineering: A review". *Journal of the Royal Society Interface* 12 (108): 20150254.

Tranquilan-Aranilla, C., F. Yoshii, A. M. Dela Rosa, and K. Makuuchi. 1999. "Kappa-carrageenan–polyethylene oxide hydrogel blends prepared by gamma irradiation". *Radiation Physics and Chemistry* 55 (2): 127–131.

Vishwanath, V., K. Pramanik, and A. Biswas. 2016. "Optimization and evaluation of silk fibroin-chitosan freeze-dried porous scaffolds for cartilage tissue engineering application". *Journal of Biomaterials Science, Polymer Edition* 27 (7): 657–674.

Wei, J., T. Igarashi, N. Okumori, T. Igarashi, T. Maetani, B. Liu, and M. Yoshinari. 2009. "Influence of surface wettability on competitive protein adsorption and initial attachment of osteoblasts". *Biomedical Materials* 4 (4): 045002.

Wongnarat, C., and P. Srihanam. 2013. "Degradation behaviors of Thai bombyx mori silk fibroins exposure to protease enzymes". *Engineering* 05: 61.

Wu, J., K. Xue, H. Li, J. Sun, and K. Liu. 2013. "Improvement of PHBV scaffolds with bioglass for cartilage tissue engineering". *PLoS One* 8 (8): e71563.

y Leon, C. A. L.. 1998. "New perspectives in mercury porosimetry". *Advances in Colloid and Interface Science* 76: 341–372.

Yang, S., K.-F. Leong, Z. Du, and C.-K. Chua. 2001. "The design of scaffolds for use in tissue engineering. Part I. Traditional factors". *Tissue Engineering* 7 (6): 679–689.

Yao, Q., B. Wei, Y. Guo, C. Jin, X. Du, C. Yan, J. Yan, W. Hu, Y. Xu, and Z. Zhou. 2015. "Design, construction and mechanical testing of digital 3D anatomical data-based PCL–HA bone tissue engineering scaffold". *Journal of Materials Science: Materials in Medicine* 26 (1): 1–9.

Yeo, A., W. J. Wong, H. H. Khoo, and S. H. Teoh. 2010. "Surface modification of PCL-TCP scaffolds improve interfacial mechanical interlock and enhance early bone formation: An in vitro and in vivo characterization". *Journal of Biomedical Materials Research Part A: An Official Journal of the Society for Biomaterials, the Japanese Society for Biomaterials, and the Australian Society for Biomaterials and the Korean Society for Biomaterials* 92 (1): 311–321.

Yildirim, E. D., R. Besunder, D. Pappas, F. Allen, S. Güçeri, and W. Sun. 2010. "Accelerated differentiation of osteoblast cells on polycaprolactone scaffolds driven by a combined effect of protein coating and plasma modification". *Biofabrication* 2 (1): 014109.

Yoo, H. Sang, E. Ah Lee, J. Jin Yoon, and T. Gwan Park. 2005. "Hyaluronic acid modified biodegradable scaffolds for cartilage tissue engineering". *Biomaterials* 26 (14): 1925–1933.

Zahedi, P., I. Rezaeian, S.-O. Ranaei-Siadat, S.-H. Jafari, and P. Supaphol. 2010. "A review on wound dressings with an emphasis on electrospun nanofibrous polymeric bandages". *Polymers for Advanced Technologies* 21 (2): 77–95.

Zakhireh, S., K. Adibkia, Y. Beygi-Khosrowshahi, and M. Barzegar-Jalali. 2021. "Osteogenesis promotion of selenium-doped hydroxyapatite for application as bone scaffold". *Biological Trace Element Research* 199 (5): 1802–1811.

Zhang, H., Li Zhou, and W. Zhang. 2014. "Control of scaffold degradation in tissue engineering: A review". *Tissue Engineering Part B: Reviews* 20 (5): 492–502.

Zhang, H., and Z. Chen. 2010. "Fabrication and characterization of electrospun PLGA/MWNTs/hydroxyapatite biocomposite scaffolds for bone tissue engineering". *Journal of Bioactive and Compatible Polymers* 25 (3): 241–259.

Zhang, R., and P. X Ma. 1999. "Poly (α-hydroxyl acids)/hydroxyapatite porous composites for bone-tissue engineering. I. Preparation and morphology". *Journal of Biomedical Materials Research: An Official Journal of the Society for Biomaterials, the Japanese Society for Biomaterials, and the Australian Society for Biomaterials* 44 (4): 446–455.

Zhao, F., Y. Yin, W. W. Lu, J. C. Leong, W. Zhang, J. Zhang, M. Zhang, and K. Yao. 2002. "Preparation and histological evaluation of biomimetic three-dimensional hydroxyapatite/chitosan-gelatin network composite scaffolds". *Biomaterials* 23 (15): 3227–3234.

Zhao, H., J. Liao, F. Wu, and J. Shi. 2021. "Mechanical strength improvement of chitosan/hydroxyapatite scaffolds by coating and cross-linking". *Journal of the Mechanical Behavior of Biomedical Materials* 114: 104169.

Zhao, S., J. Zhang, M. Zhu, Y. Zhang, Z. Liu, Y. Ma, Y. Zhu, and C. Zhang. 2015. "Effects of functional groups on the structure, physicochemical and biological properties of mesoporous bioactive glass scaffolds". *Journal of Materials Chemistry B* 3 (8): 1612–1623.

Zhu, H., J. Shen, X. Feng, H. Zhang, Y. Guo, and J. Chen. 2010. "Fabrication and characterization of bioactive silk fibroin/wollastonite composite scaffolds". *Materials Science and Engineering: C* 30 (1): 132–140.

Zonderland, J., S. Rezzola, P. Wieringa, and L. Moroni. 2020. "Fiber diameter, porosity and functional group gradients in electrospun scaffolds". *Biomedical Materials* 15 (4): 045020.

6 Stem Cells for Cartilage, Bone, and Related Tissue Regeneration

INTRODUCTION

Besides scaffold with appropriate three-dimensional design and nanofibrous architecture, suitable cell source, cell types and their efficient delivery are also crucial factors for producing functionally equivalent tissue in the field of orthopedic tissue engineering. In this context, the self-renewal and commitment to differentiate into specific cell lineages and thereby provide excellent tissue regenerative potential make stem cell as the most promising cell type for tissue regeneration. The development of stem cell technology in combination with tissue engineering technique has opened up innovative and promising ways of producing bone and cartilage tissue substitutes for their repair when they got damaged. Several studies have shown the potentiality of these combined areas to enhance the viability, differentiation, and therapeutic efficacy of the transplanted stem cells. However, delivery of the specific types of cells to the defect tissues or organs for their repair and restoration of function is the main driving force in tissue engineering technique. Therefore, suitable cell types and their sources are of immense importance for the success of this technique. With the advent of tissue engineering in the 1980s, more prominently in the 1990s, mesenchymal stem cells (MSCs) were transformed into the bone, cartilage, and other musculoskeletal tissues through the process of cell differentiation. In the beginning of the 21st century, the MSCs-based clinical therapies have been evolved by adopting different strategies including the 3D scaffold-based tissue-engineering approach to produce functional tissues for the replacement of damaged orthopaedic tissues including the bone, cartilage, and other related tissues like ligament, tendon, etc., transplantation of MSCs, MSCs acting as cytokine or growth factor producers stimulating or triggering the repair or inhibiting the tissue degenerative processes, etc. In tissue engineering, the production of engineered tissue requires cells to populate on the matrices resulting in tissue that resembles the native tissue. The success of the neotissue generation relies on the potential cell source which is one of the vital factors in TE technique. Although the use of primary cells of the patient's own body is ideal, harvesting this cell is a concern, which offers several limitations such as the invasive nature of collection of the cell samples and potentiality of the cells in the diseased state (Daniel Howar et al. 2008). Therefore, much attention has been given in the last two decades to explore the different stem cell sources

DOI: 10.1201/9781003245353-6

and the method of their isolation from potential sources. Moreover, the lack of understanding of the fundamentals of stem cells is another important aspect for the scientists to working with it. Keeping all these in view, a lot of research attention has been directed towards stem cell research and their therapeutic applications in recent decades. This chapter discusses the basics of the stem cells including their types, potential sources, functions, expansion and its controlling factors, characterization, and their differentiation into various tissues with emphasizing on their differentiation into bone, cartilage, and their combined complex tissues. Furthermore, the technical and ethical issues concerning the use of stem cells for tissue regeneration have also been highlighted.

STEM CELLS AND THEIR CHARACTERISTICS

Stem cells are undifferentiated cells, which have the potentiality to renew themselves in the laboratory for a long period and to differentiate into multiple specialized cells through cell division. Stem cells are available in both embryos and adult tissues. These undifferentiated cells are found in some specific areas of the body, known as stem cell niches, and play a crucial role in growth and development during childhood and homeostasis throughout adulthood (Preston et al. 2003). The self-renewal characteristic of the stem cell refers to the ability of dividing and renewing for a longer period of time through cell division. A small group of stem cells can produce even millions of cells in the laboratory and can retain their long term self-renewal activity in appropriate conditions. Stem cells cannot perform specialized functions because they do not possess any tissue-specific structures. Many factors like specific signaling molecules and environmental conditions make stem cells to maintain their unspecialized characteristics. This unspecialized characteristic of stem cells can give rise to many specialized cells including the bone, muscle, blood, nerve cells, cardiac, and many other cell types (Zakrzewski et al. 2019). Once stem cells are derived and maintained in the laboratory, they can be controlled in unspecialized state without spontaneously differentiating into specific cell types. The differentiation property that refers to the ability of transformation of stem cells into specialized cells is sometimes called regeneration ability, as they can be inspired to become tissue- or organ-specific cells with specific functions. During differentiation, stem cells pass through several sub-stages to become specialized cells. The differentiation process is triggered by several signalling molecules (BMP (Bone Morphogenetic protein), TGF-β (transforming growth factor), IgF (Insulin like growth factor), FGF-2 (Fibroblast Growth Factor-2), etc.) that exist inside and outside of the stem cells (Seita and Weissman 2010). The internal signals are regulated by the specific genes of the cells, which are interspersed through long stranded DNA carrying coded instructions for cellular structure and their function. The various external signals, such as the chemicals secreted by other cells and physical contact with the adjacent cells, also have an influence on differentiation of stem cells. In addition, certain signalling molecules like transforming growth factor (β (TGF β)), activin, growth factors, albumins, found in the microenvironment of cells also act as external stimuli for their differentiation (Sánchez Alvarado and Yamanaka 2014). Stem cells with these properties act as an internal repair system in the body. Even after being preserved in an inactive condition for many months, stem cells are able to form replica and specialized cells. Specific growth factors have an important role for their differentiation into specialized cell line in appropriate environmental conditions.

CLASSIFICATION OF STEM CELLS

Stem cells can be classified depending on their ability to regenerate different types of cell lineages or according to their potency or differential potential which is defined as their ability to differentiate into specialized cell types. Stem cells are also classified depending on their sources (Ota 2008).

CLASSIFICATION BASED ON POTENCY

Totipotent Stem Cells

Totipotent stem cells, also referred to as embryonic stem cells have the highest differentiation potential so called potency among all stem cells and they are able to can produce a complete individual or all cells of the body. The fertilized oocyte is an example of totipotent cell. The early stage (1–3 days) of embryonic cells, till eight cells stage, are called the totipotent cells. In later stage, these cells can develop either any of the three germ layers, *viz.* ectoderm, endoderm, and mesoderm, or form a placenta (Figure 6.1). Each germ layer has the capacity to provide specific tissues; for example, ectoderm gives rise to gut, lung, liver, mesoderm gives rise to bone and muscle, whereas endoderm gives rise to brain and skin (Figure 6.1) (Baker and Pera 2018).

Pluripotent Stem Cells (PSCs)

These types of stem cells are basically the successor of totipotent cells. They have the potency to transform into all kinds of specialized cells except the extra-embryonic cells forming three primary germ layers of the body. They have the potential to form any cell or tissue that the body necessitates to repair itself. This property is called pluripotency. PSCs have the unique capability of maintaining self-renewal characteristics for an infinite time period as well as their pluripotent status. Embryonic stem cells (ESCs) are pluripotent and they can form osteogenic cells, chondrogenic cells, smooth muscle cells, and many other cell types (Figure 6.1). Pluripotency is a continuum which starts from complete pluripotent cells like ESCs, induced pluripotent stem cells, and ends with less potency—multi-, oligo-, or unipotent cell types (Dejosez and Zwaka 2012).

Multipotent Stem Cells

These types of stem cells have the ability to differentiate into multiple cell types belonging to a specific cell lineage. Unlike PSCs, these stem cells have less potency. For instance, haematopoietic stem cells (HSCs) can produce various types of blood cells like red blood cells (RBCs), white blood cells (WBCs), and platelets (Figure 6.1) (Sobhani et al. 2017). Although HSC, during differentiation process, may become oligopotent cell which limits their differentiation ability to cells of its lineage, some multipotent cells are able to transform into pluripotent cells.

Oligopotent Stem Cells

These stem cells can differentiate to form very few cells due to restricted differentiation potential. For instance, when HSC, a multipotent stem cell, is differentiated, its differentiation potential decreases and it becomes an oligopotent stem cell. These oligopotent stem cells can be differentiated into lymphoid or myeloid stem cells. They can also divide into WBC or RBC (Bissels, Eckardt, and Bosio 2013).

Unipotent Stem Cells

These stem cells are obtained from multipotent stem cells. Even though these stem cells have self-generating property, they can differentiate to form only one cell type lineage on their own for example dermatocytes. Hence, these cells have the lowest differentiation potential among all other types of stem cells. The unique properties of self-renewal and single-cell differentiation properties make these stem cells favourable therapeutic candidates in regenerative medicine, for example, germline stem cells (producing gametes, sperm, egg) and epidermal stem cells (producing skin) (Figure 6.1) (Bissels, Eckardt, and Bosio 2013).

Classification Based on Sources

Stem cells are also classified based on their sources or origin. Stem cells are broadly categorized into two types, embryonic stem cell and adult or mature stem cell according to their origin. Embryonic germ cells and induced pluripotent stem cells (iPSCs) are the other types of stem cells. These stem cell types are described in the following sections.

Embryonic Stem Cells

As their name suggests, these stem cells are produced from the embryos. The majority of these cells are derived from the blastocyst, which is formed in the early development of life. Blastocyst is basically the five- to six-day-old embryo formed from fertilized eggs. Almost every type of cell in the human body can be formed by these cells. In humans, the development of the blastocyst starts about 5 days after fertilization, when the morula, a ball of a few dozen cells, develops a cavity filled with fluid. After cell division or cleavage, the blastocyst contains around 200–300 cells with a diameter of 0.1–0.2 mm (Wray and Hartmann 2012). It has an inner cell mass (ICM), eventually giving rise to the embryos (Figure 6.1). The ICM has two distinct cell layers, which are known as epiblast and hypoblast. The epiblast forms three germ layers such as amnionic ectoderm, extra embryonic mesoderm, and this process is known as gastrulation. The yolk sac is formed by the cells of hypoblast, which also creates the lining of the blastocoel. The cells present in the outside layer of the blastocyst collectively form the trophoblast, which is also known as trophoectoderm. Trophoblast envelops the ICM and the blastocoel, a fluid-filled space. The trophoblast plays a role in the formation of placenta. Additionally, it is the home of multipotent stem cells. The remaining ICM cells form the epiblast, that gives rise to three germ layers, namely ectoderm, endoderm, and mesoderm. ESCs are generated from the ICM. Different techniques, such as immunosurgery and enzymatic, and physical approaches, are used to isolate the ICM from blastocyst which are discussed below (Tang et al. 2010; Guo et al. 2016).

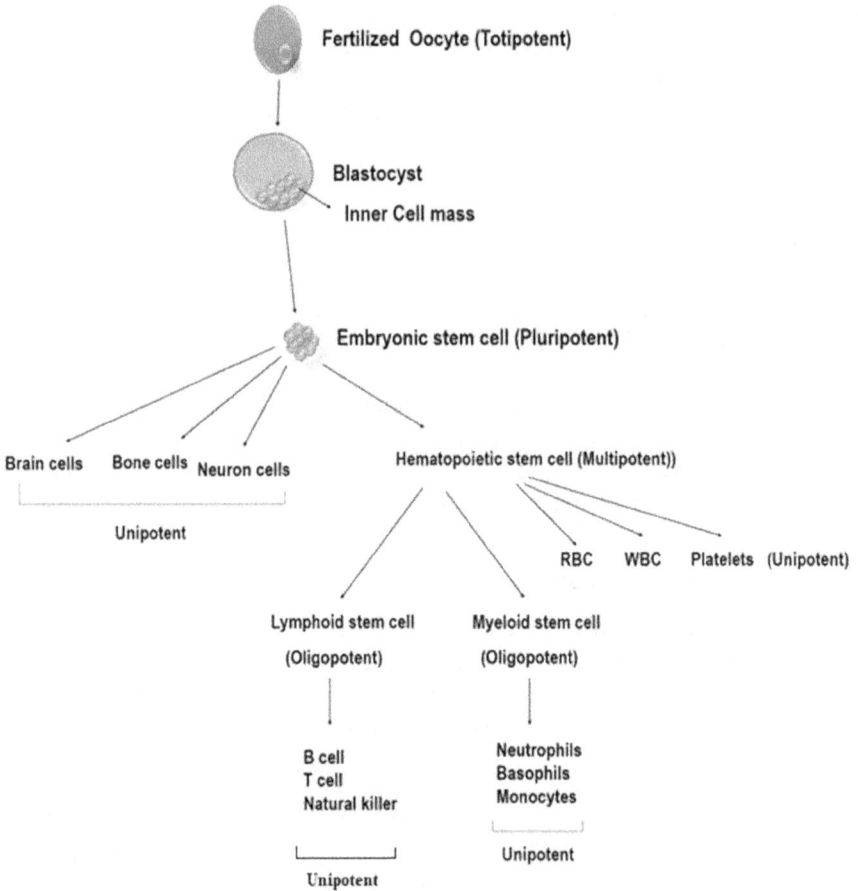

FIGURE 6.1   Classification of stem cells based on potency.

Immunosurgery Method

In this method, enzyme pronase is used to dissolve the zona pellucida in the trophoblast of the blastocyst before being pre-incubated with antiserum (e.g. rabbit anti-mouse serum) followed by being subjected to a supplement like guinea-pig complement serum, which causes cytotoxicity leading to the death of trophoblasts selectively. This technique can isolate enormous number of ICMs at a time, which may harm the ICMs owing to cytotoxicity effect. Only the structural integrity of the blastocyst can protect the ICMs from being susceptible to any kind of immune reaction, because of which, this approach works well with embryos of high quality with intact trophoectoderm (Matahine et al. 2008).

Enzymatic Method

Like the immunosurgery technique, pronase enzyme is also utilized in this procedure to break down the zona pellucida, while trophectoderm is usually digested using trypsin enzyme. Hyaluronidase, collagenase, and dispase are the other enzymes that can also be used for digestion (Matahine et al. 2008).

Physical Method

In this procedure, ICM is collected from the blastocyst by disrupting the trophecto-derm with a pipette or a needle. Laser-aided dissection can also be employed for this purpose. The acid tyrode's solution at pH 3.4 is also used to dissolve the zona pellu-cida. In some methods, whole blastocyst is cultured, and the ICM is isolated through the expansion of the culture (Li et al. 2011). *In vitro* culture is used to grow stem cells that are derived from the ICM. These are pluripotent in nature and involved in the for-mation of all somatic and germ cells due to their pluripotency. However, these stem cells do not have any contribution towards the formation of trophectoderm or extra embryonic layer, so they are not totipotent. ICM is diploid with a lack of G1 phase and remains mostly in the S phase of the cell cycle (Sukoyan et al. 1993).

Adult Stem Cells (ASCs)

ASCs, also referred to as somatic or tissue-specific stem cells, are undifferentiated stem cells that exist in small number among specialized or differentiated cells in an adult tissue or organ throughout the body. These types of stem cells are able to differentiate into many specialized cells or tissue lineages, and thereby having the ability to regenerate the damaged tissue or organ and multiply several times via cell division to replace the dying cells. Unlike ESCs, these cells have compara-tively limited potency for self-renewal and production of various cell types. These cells are more specialized than the ESCs despite being in a non-specific state. Unlike ESCs which are named or recognized by their source, the origin of ASCs in some mature tissues is not clear and hence is currently being researched. ASCs may remain non-dividing for a longer time period unless they are stimulated by a normal requirement of adequate cells for the maintenance of normal tissues, or to repair disease, or damaged tissues.

ASCs are principally responsible for conserving and restoring the tissue in which they are present. They can produce mature cell types with distinct morphologies and specific functions along various lineages (multipotent) (Clevers 2015; Fuente et al. 2005). ASCs can be found in many tissues such as haematopoietic or blood-forming tissues. Numerous organs and tissues, including the adipose or fat tissue, amniotic fluid, brain, bone marrow, deciduous teeth, gut, skin, peripheral blood, liver, ovarian, epithelium, synovium, skeletal muscle, teeth, testis, umbilical cord, and cord blood, have been found to contain ASCs. They are also believed to be found in a particular region of specific tissue known as "stem cell niche". In many tissues, a relatively very small number of stem cells are present, and once they are taken out from the body, their potentiality to divide becomes restricted, which is one of the major challenges being faced in producing significant amount of stem cells. Haematopoietic, endothe-lial, mammary, mesenchymal, neural, neural crest, olfactory, and testicular are some of the examples of the several types of ASCs (Lin, Niparko, and Ferrucci 2014a). Haematopoietic stem cells can provide all types of blood cells including the RBC, B-lymphocytes, T-lymphocytes, natural killer cells, neutrophils, basophils, eosinophils, monocytes, and macrophages (Mordechail et al. 1973). MSCs, the other type of ASCs isolated from the stroma, or connective tissue, that covers the body's organs and other tissues can be used to produce new bone, cartilage, fat, and other tissues of the body (Ogawa 1993). Various health issues can be solved using these stem cells. MSCs can differentiate into multiple varieties of cell types or tissues such as adipose or fat cells, osteogenic cells, and chondrogenic cells. These stem cells are derived from the tissues like adipose tissue Wharton's jelly, bone marrow, and others. Adipose tissue, bone, cartilage, and many other tissues are produced by mesenchymal stromal cells, which are present in bone marrow other than haemopoietic cells (Sousa et al. 2014). To isolate MSCs from bone marrow, various techniques like aspiration, density gradient centrifugation, or sedimentation can be used. MSCs can be isolated from trophoblastic tissues, including the placenta, cord blood, and, Wharton's jell using digestive enzymes. Lipoaspiration and collagenase digestion have been used to isolate multipotent cells like MSCs (Ma et al. 2014). Some of the important methods to isolate adult stem cells are discussed here.

Density Gradient Centrifugation

To recover stem cells from the cord blood, whole blood cells or peripheral blood and bone marrow mononuclear cells are usually enriched by the density gradient centrifugation method. This method relies upon the different densities of cells within a heterogeneous sample. The later is layered on the top of a suitable density gradient medium with low viscosity and low osmotic pressure before being centrifuged. The blood samples are centrifuged at high speeds after the addition of solutions such as Percoll, Ficol, Hipaq, and Sucrose resulting in the separation of cells in different layers according to their density (Figure 6.2). This method is usually applied to separate lymphocytes (Juopperi et al. 2007). Among these techniques, Ficoll-Paque density gradient centrifugation is the most simplest and the most commonly used method. This method can be applied for a small sample size. In this method, the

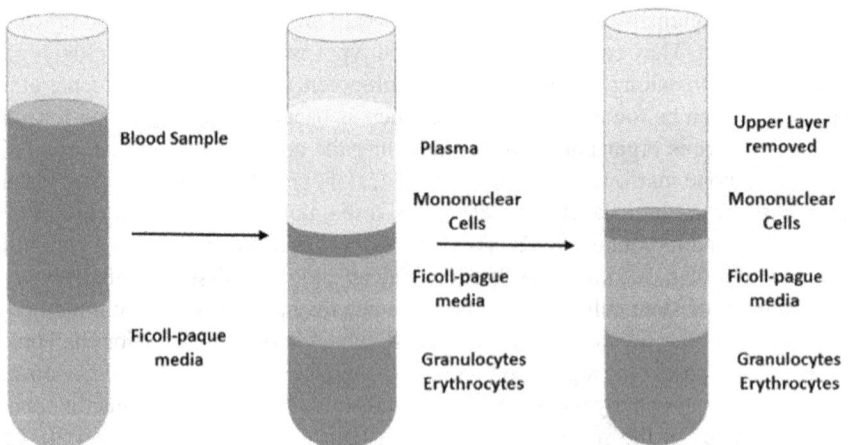

FIGURE 6.2 Density gradient centrifugation method for the separation of mononuclear cells from blood.

collected blood samples are diluted and treated with anticoagulants. Anticoagulants, such as heparin, citrate, EDTA (Ethylene Diamine Tetra-acetic Acid), acid citrate dextrose, and citrate phosphate dextrose can be used. The treated samples are layered on the Ficoll-Paque solution and then centrifuged. After centrifugation, different layers formed including the bottom layer containing the erythrocytes and granulocytes sediment followed by the Ficoll-Plaque layer, the upper layer contains plasma, and the interface layer existing between the plasma and Ficoll-Paque layers consists of lower density lymphocytes, platelets, and monocytes. The upper layer containing plasma is taken out by a sterile pipette, and thereby leaving the mononuclear cell layer undisturbed. The mononuclear cells at the interface are transferred to a sterile centrifuge tube by a sterilized pipette and then centrifuged for its separation (Jaatinen and Laine 2007).

Hoechst Side Population Method

Hoechst side population is a powerful method for identifying and separating or sorting stem cells from various tissues. In this method, Hoechst, a cell permeable DNA-binding dye, is loaded into the interested cell population (e.g. stem cells) and these fluorescent cells are detected by flow cytometry (Goodell 2005; Goodell et al. 1996). stem cells are separated based upon the dye efflux characteristics of the ATP-binding cassette transporters. In flow cytometry, a sub-population of cells which is different from the main cell population on the basis of specific markers is called a side population. All the cells belonging to the side population have certain characteristics, for example, exhibition of stem cell-like characteristics. However, this distinction is dependent on the identifying markers used for the side population. Blue fluorescence is exhibited when Hoechst/bisbenzimide 33342 binds to DNA. The high efflux of the dye observed to occur in the side population, usually consists of stem cells. Molecules belonging to the ATP-binding cassette family, for example, MDR1 (P-glycoprotein) and ABCG2, membrane proteins (transporters) are responsible for this efflux (Mimeault and Batra 2009).

Fluorescence-Activated Cell Sorting (FACS)

FACS, also called fluorescence-assisted cell sorting, is a specialized category of flow cytometry and is an indispensable tool in the field of stem cell technology for the separation of specific cell types, especially rare cell population like stem cells from a mixed population with high purity (Johnson, Dooner, and Quesenberry 2007). The cells are separated based on the principle of the specific light scattering and fluorescent intensity of cells when they pass through a laser beam. In this method, the cells are tagged with fluorescent dyes which are usually attached to antibodies (e.g. PE or FITC-conjugated antibodies which are red and green fluorescent dyes excited by green and blue light, respectively, CY3 and CY5) bind to specific proteins on target cells (cell surface markers). The fluorescent labelled cells are incubated and the cells are then resuspended in phosphate buffered saline to remove the unbound dye. The suspended cells with high flow rate pass through a flow cytometer, in which the individual cell passes the laser beam by liquid droplets by which the fluorescent dyes are excited and detectors are used to measure the intensity of the fluorescence emitted, and the generated forward-scattered, and side-scattered light. The cells are sorted

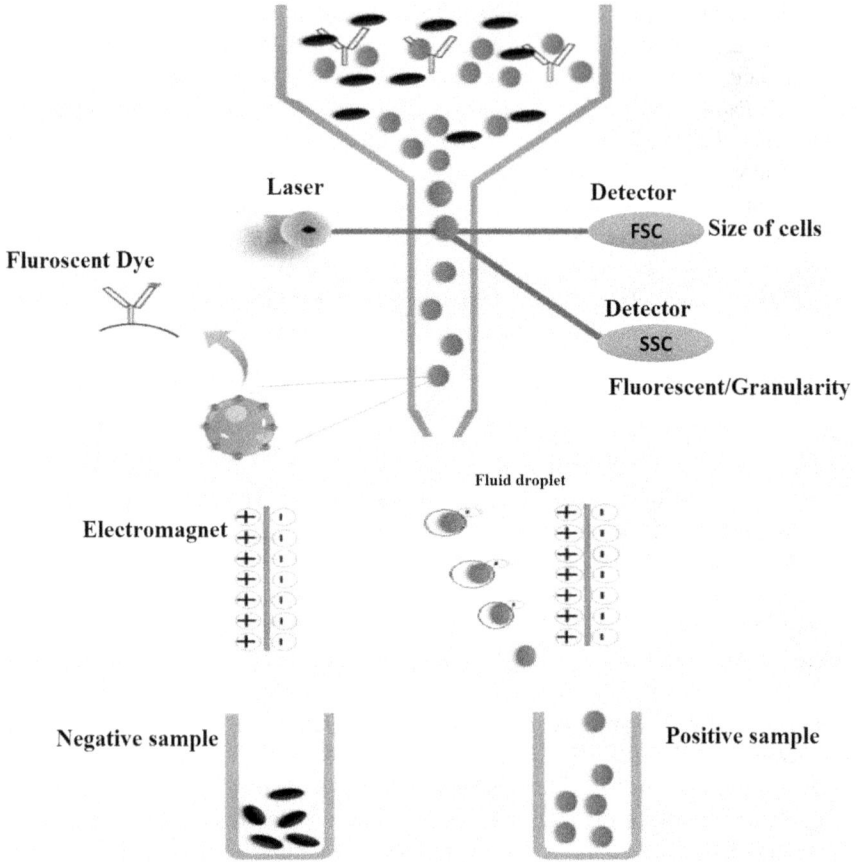

FIGURE 6.3   Isolation of cells by Fluorescence-activated cell sorting (FACS) Technique.

into groups based on electrostatic deflection system (electromagnet) that divides the droplets into containers based upon their fluorescence charge intensity like: cells exhibiting fluorescence are positively charged and cells without showing fluorescence are negatively charged (Figure 6.3). Blood cells can be easily sorted without the help of antibodies based on the forward scatter and side scatter of the laser beam. Cell size is indicated by forward scatter, while cell internal complexity, such as granularity, is indicated by the side scatter (Basu et al. 2010). The sorted cells with specific groups are collected in tubes for further analysis. The purity of the cells is measured by a microscope or by flow cytometry and it is calculated by dividing the number of cells in a group by the total number of cells separated.

Magnetic Activated Cell Sorting (MACS)

MACS, also called immunomagnetic cell separation, sorts specific cells from a mixed cell population based upon their surface protein expression. It involves the targeting cells for separation through the interaction of antibodies with specific cell surface antigens. In this cell sorting technique, the cells to be sorted are incubated with magnetic nanoparticles (magnetic beads) coated with antibodies against stem cell surface antigens. After incubation, the cells are exposed to a magnetic field while the cells passthrough a flow column. Cells that bind to the column are positively selected, while the negatively selected cells flow down (Schmitz, Radbruch et al. 1994). It is a fast and simple method and hence it is one of the most commonly used methods for isolating high-purity populations of specific cell groups.

Embryonic Germ Cells

These cells are produced from that part of the embryo or foetus which ultimately gives rise to gametes (i.e. egg or sperm) and constitutes embryonic germ cells. These cells have the properties similar to those of embryonic stem cells under certain conditions. Like ESCs, the embryonic germ cells are PSCs.

Induced Pluripotent Stem Cells

Induced pluripotent stem cells, also referred to as iPSCs, are adult somatic stem cells that are genetically reprogrammed to ESCs stem cell-like state by being manipulated to express genes and factors, thereby maintaining the specific properties of ESCs. Human iPSCs are capable of expressing stem cell markers and producing cells that are distinct from all the three germ layers. Thus, they can act as a source of cells specific to the donor that can be harnessed for tissue regeneration therapies. Human iPSCs are produced by the transfection of non-pluripotent cells like adult fibroblasts, with specific stem cell-associated genes using viral vectors such as retroviruses. Post-transfection (3–4 weeks), transfected cells start to exhibit PSCs-like morphology and biochemical properties and they are then isolated through morphological selection, doubling time, antibiotic selection, or using a reporter gene (Yamanaka 2012; Trounson and DeWitt 2016). Drug development and screening by toxicological testing, producing patient- or disease-specific PSCs, and the study of the development and function of human tissue and disease models are the important uses of iPSCs in the transplantation and tissue regeneration fields. Usually, viruses are employed in the introduction of reprogramming factors into the adult cells; however, this process needs careful control and testing before its application to humans. iPSC-derived tissues must be closely identical to the donor cells and thereby may evade immune rejection. Adult tissues like bone marrow, muscle, and brain having distinct populations of adult stem cells can regenerate cells lost due to normal wear and tear, accidental injury, and disease. Although it holds great potential, the use of iPSCs is limited due to the oncogenic potential of one of the four genes that induces pluripotency, namely, c-myc. The created cells may also be prone to tumour formation due to the viral transfection systems and pluripotency induction is a slow and gradual process that has a very low efficiency (Inoue and Yamanaka 2011; Rowntree and McNeish 2010). In spite of having much potential for therapeutic application of iPSCs, there are some technical issues involved in using these cells. Unlike ESCs, the iPSCs are widely diversified because of their differences in genetic background, epigenetic memory, and reprogramming. Studies have also shown that the cells of the transitional phase differ significantly from those in the previous and fully reprogrammed phase (Kobold et al. 2015). Induced pluripotent cells possess similar morphology and gene expression, but have issues such as low growth rate due to poor quality of differentiation, DNA methylation, and transcription errors. Furthermore, Krüppel-like factor (KLF4), one of the factors commonly used to reprogram somatic cells, is capable of disrupting the neurogenesis of iPSCs. Therefore, it is necessary to comprehend factor-induced reprogramming more thoroughly (Armstrong et al. 2010).

APPLICATION OF STEM CELLS

In recent decades, the application of stem cells as a promising therapeutic agent has widely been accepted, which has led to the advanced scientific research for the development of a wide spectrum of treatment strategies. The various applications including the developing disease models, drug screening, toxicity testing of newly developed drugs, developing patient- and disease-specific PSCs and in regenerative medicine are discussed below.

In Vitro Research on Disease Models

One of the important applications of stem cells is in disease modelling, which is considered to serve as a potential platform to analyse the biochemical mechanisms associated with the normal and disease phenotypes. Especially, multigenic diseases need extensive molecular studies for better understanding of these diseases as they are complex in nature; therefore, more targeted therapeutic strategy is developed. Molecular investigations, particularly in complex, and multigenic disorders, contribute to a better knowledge of the disease and tailored therapeutic approaches. In this context, stem cells provide an ideal *in vitro* system for studying developmental processes at the molecular and cellular levels. For example, MSCs possessing self-renewal ability has been emerged as attractive stem cells for developing *in vitro* disease modelling because of their excellent differentiation ability into different tissue types including the osteoblasts, chondrocytes, adipocytes, etc., and they are abundantly present in the human body. So, MSCs harvested from the patient can be used as novel human models for many diseases affecting tissues. Similarly, neural stem cells as ideal models were used to study the mechanisms of cell differentiation related to the central nervous system for psychiatric, neurodegenerative, and brain tumour conditions, and stem cell-derived systems were developed as models for cardiovascular disease conditions (Hombach-Klonisch et al. 2008; Dottori et al. 2012).

DRUG SCREENING

In the past several years, numerous pharmaceutical strategies have been adopted to treat various degenerative disorders. Approved pharmacological therapy is the first line of choice for preserving damaged cells and inspiring endogenous tissue regeneration processes, thereby delaying the progression of both degenerative disorders and harmful effects. Stem cells harvested from various tissues, like bone marrow, have recently emerged as a promising cell source in experimental treatment therapies for a number of degenerative diseases (Zuba-Surma et al. 2012). Due to their distinct functional characteristics, stem cells may be an attractive source of new cells to replace the deteriorating indigenous cells in the nervous system, heart, and other organs. A number of *in vivo* experimental studies using animal models for investigating many defect tissues have demonstrated that stem cell-based therapeutic approaches can restore and maintain the function of the damaged tissues. PSCs, like human embryonic stem cells (hESCs) or human induced pluripotent stem cells (hiPSCs) with a disease-linked mutation, can be isolated as hESCs from pre-implantation diagnosed embryos or reprogrammed from patient tissue samples. These PSCs may be differentiated to study the development of the disease phenotype *in vitro* and screen medications for a potential therapeutic molecule that the developed cellular system will validate. These unique cell models have been used the same way they have been used for differentiation and toxicity testing (Maury et al. 2012).

NEW DRUG TOXICITY TESTING

Human stem cells and their derivatives have the potential to provide ample supplies of various types of tissues that can be used for developing toxicity models,. These can be used as alternative tissue models to the conventional animal models with high accuracy, and without sacrificing the animal (Scott, Peters, and Dragan 2013). hESCs have been demonstrated to be used in mechanistic studies, including disease pathway and developmental toxicity assessments, as well as drug toxicity screening. The reprogramming somatic cells like iPSCs resembling hESCs-like cell enable the design of tests or assays, which can be used to determine the impact of the patient's genetic background or history of environmental exposure to toxicity response. Differentiated somatic stem cells and immature PSCs-based *in vitro* model can be used to test the drugs or environmental toxic chemicals causing cell damage involving a battery of assessments such as cytotoxicity, functional, genomic, and proteomic assays. Developmental toxicity tests are used to determine whether test chemicals or drugs have an influence on cell differentiation. The functional alternation in mature cells is readily detectable, such as action potential generation and albumin secretion, which can be used in functional testing in order to ensure changes in the physiological condition of the cells (Mori and Hara 2013).

DEVELOPING PATIENT AND DISEASE-SPECIFIC PLURIPOTENT STEM CELLS

Many patient-specific stem cells may be generated through developing PSCs from adult somatic tissues of human origin. Researchers have recently succeeded in isolating PSCs from individual patients with a variety of primary and complicated genetic abnormalities and differentiating them into the specific cell lineages affected by the diseases. It has been observed that induced human pluripotent stem cells may create functional cardiac myocytes (Amarenco et al. 2011).

REGENERATIVE MEDICINE

The recent advancement in the techniques to isolate and expand ESCs and adult stem cells has opened up their numerous new applications leading to the pre-clinical animal and human clinical trials, and thereby hold great promise in regenerative medicine for the treatment of various diseases (Giachino, Basak, and Taylor 2009). These therapeutic treatments can promote cell viability, proliferation, differentiation, reprogramming, and homing by acting as target cells or their niches (Egashira, Yuasa, and Fukuda 2011).

STEM CELL EXPANSION AND CHARACTERIZATION

The expansion of stem cell presents a significant challenge in cell and tissue-based regenerative therapy. Efficient substrates and techniques are required for their expansion at the various stages of regeneration process. Stem cells can be cultured in different ways depending on their types. A specific stem cell type requires specific culture conditions as well as appropriate growth medium. Stem cells exhibit a wide spectrum of variety and, therefore, they require different media types and culture conditions for their growth, proliferation or expansion. For growing and conserving stem cells, either in their undifferentiated condition or for transforming them into a particular lineage or cell type, a variety of techniques and products are available (Ota 2008). The methods of culturing of stem cells and their property characterisation are highlighted next.

CULTURING OF ESCs

During the culture of hESCs, the maintenance of their ability of self-regeneration and pluripotency requires appropriate conditions to maintain them in an undifferentiated state. Before culturing, the pre-implantation stage of embryo is used to isolate ICM cells, which are then transferred to a culture flask containing the nutrient medium. The inner surface of the culture flask or culture dish acts as a support for the cells to adhere, divide, and spread (Dellatore, Garcia, and Miller 2008). To inhibit the cell division, a feeder layer is coated onto the inner surface or simply the feeder layer acting as a sticky attachment site for the hESCs is used. Besides providing sticky surface, the feeder layer also releases growth factors and nutrients for the cells into the culture medium. Initially, the growth factors and substrate for culturing of ESCs were obtained from feeder cell layers such as inactivated mouse embryonic fibroblasts derived from fibroblasts of foetal mouse. These cells are seeded and propagated for 3 to 4 days before being exposed to ultraviolet irradiation or mitomycin C for the inactivation of mitosis in cells. However, the use of mouse embryonic cells often leads to the risk of transmission of viruses or other macromolecules, such as infectious or foreign proteins and particles present in mouse cells, to the human cells. STO (SIM immortalized cell line with thioguanine and ouabain-resistance), BRL (Buffalo rat liver cells), and SNL (Sub clone of STO) examples of other cell lines, which are derived from mouse fibroblasts can be used as feeder cells to support the growth of hESCs as well as iPSCs (Gerrard et al. 2005; Xiao, Yuan, and Sharkis 2006).

Alternative feeder layers, often known as feeder cell-free layers, have also been established to overcome the limitations of the feeder cell layers. The defined and the conditioned media are the two types of feeder cell-free media, both of which facilitate the growth of stem cells without causing differentiation. The defined medium usually contains various recombinant growth factors as supplement; however, it lacks serum. This media added with leukaemia inhibitory factors and bone morphogenetic protein promotes stem cell proliferation and pluripotency while inhibiting differentiation (Akopian et al. 2010). According to Chen et al. (2010), Y-27632 and thiazovivin are examples of Rho-associated coiled-coil containing protein kinase (ROCK) inhibitors that can improve the viability of the freshly isolated stem cells (Chen et al. 2010). Basic fibroblast growth factors (bFGFs) are generally not supplemented with the most of the stem cell culture media except the hESCs media which contains either bFGF or FGF2. Whereas bovine serum albumin is used in most of the defined culture medium for human cell culture. However, the use of serum-free media suffers from epigenetic modifications in cultured cells including the histone modification, methylation, and inactivation of X-chromosome in female ESCs (McEwen et al. 2013). When serum-free media is used for culturing cells, the expression of the cancer marker CD30 was observed, which was absent in cells cultured with foetal calf serums (Chung et al. 2010). Cells release growth-promoting substances as they divide and grow during the culture process, and the media is replaced with fresh media after a certain time interval. However, there is still a small chance of virus contamination with this medium, but it is less likely than with feeder cells from other species. Conditioned media is more advantageous than defined media since it contains added supplements; however, variability among different batches of media is still a concern (Pereira et al. 2014). For human cell culture human foreskin fibroblasts are mainly used to prepare conditioned media. An extracellular matrix (ECM), such as culture matrix containing different types of ECM proteins, polysaccharides like vitronectin, and proteoglycans to develop stem cells without feeder layers is essential. Various types of stem cells require different culture matrices, each of which has the ability to either maintain pluripotency or promote differentiation (Ireland et al. 2020). In order to grow hESCs, cells in feeder-free culture conditions, extracellular matrix like MatrigelTM or laminin, as well as conditioned media from mouse embryonic fibroblasts or human fibroblasts can be utilized (Bigdeli et al. 2008). The cells on the cultured plates continue to survive, divide, and grow throughout the culture. Then re-plating, also known as subculturing, that involves gentle detachment of the cells from the culture plate is done once they have grown large enough to reach its confluency. The later is defined as the percentage area of the culture dish or culture flask is covered by the cells adhered to it. This process is known as "passaging" or subculturing which is important to avoid the adverse impact of the overcrowding on the cell expansion.. For several months, this technique is performed multiple times. Huge number of ESCs can be produced from the original cells once the cell lines are established. ESCs are a collection of pluripotent stem cells that can be multiplied in cell culture for an infinite time period without undergoing differentiation (Javazon, Beggs, and Flake 2004).

ESCs Characterization

Stem cells often experience phenotypic and genotypic changes as well as mosaicism. After the freshly cultured stem cells have acquired sufficient density, screening for pluripotency, proper gene expression, and a normal karyotype are performed along with frequently checking the stability of the stem cells. In addition, contamination is verified in the cells growing on feeder layers. Scientists evaluate the cells to check if they possess the essential features that define them as ESCs at various stages of their development and this process is known as characterization (MacIntyre et al. 2011). The various laboratory tests which are performed regularly to check the essential properties of the ESCs are the following:

- Growing and subculturing:—growing and subculturing of stem cells for a longer period of time, which may be even for several months, can ensure whether the cells are able to grow and regenerate themselves over time. During this period, the cells are observed under microscope for changes in morphology and healthiness of the growing cells.
- Determination of transcription factors:—different transcription factors are formed by the undifferentiated cells, among which Nanog and Oct4 are the most important. These transcription factors are detected using specialized methods. Cell differentiation and development of an embryo are dependent on the ability of these transcription factors by turning genes on and off at appropriate times. These genes are responsible for retaining the undifferentiated state, and self-renewal characteristic of the stem cells.
- Identification of cell surface marker genes: Identifying the existence of specific cell surface marker genes which are commonly expressed by undifferentiated cells. This is the most versatile method for characterizing stem cells, based on their surface antigen phenotype (Draper et al. 2004).
- Examination of chromosomes: This method involves examining whether the chromosomes are fragmented or the change in chromosomal count which is done by a microscopic observation. However, this method is not able to determine genetic alteration in the cells.
- Evaluation of cell viability: Determining the viability of the frozen cells through subculturing for a longer period of time after freezing, and thawing, followed by replating the cells.
- Deiermination of pluripotency: The pluripotency of hESCs or iPSCs are determined by various methods, *viz.,* alkaline phosphatase activity (ALP), immunohistochemistry study for expression of pluripotency-associated markers such as OCT4, SOX2, TRA-1, etc., production of embryoid bodies together

with the detection of gene expression associated with the three germ layers. The different methods are as follows: (i) cells are allowed to differentiate naturally in cell culture, (ii) cells are induced to differentiate into particular cells that are attributed to the three types of germ layers, (iii) cells are injected into a mouse model having a weak immune system to investigate the benign tumour formation which is known as teratoma. This type of mouse immune system does not reject the human stem cells as its immune system is compromised and this allows the researchers to analyse the human stem cells for growth and differentiation.

The presence of a variety of differentiated or partially differentiated cell types in the teratomas implies that ESCs can be differentiated into a variety of cell types (Stacey 2009). Furthermore, the confirmation of pluripotency is done by the following procedures:

(i) When putative ESCs are cultivated without supplements using the hanging drop method, they form spherical clusters of cells from all the three germ layers (Zhang, Chen et al. 2019).
(ii) The presence of Many marker genes such as AFP and GATA-4,; Flt1 and PAX6, and SOX1 in ectoderm, mesoderm and endoderm respectively are detected.
(iii) Pluripotency in ESCs is also demonstrated by the production of cells from all the three germ layers when they are implanted into nude mice. This study is performed by haematoxylin–eosin staining method.
(iv) Chimera is the formation of an individual made up of diploid cells from two distinct individuals. When albino mouse ESC is injected into a normal mouse blastocyst, the contributions from the ESC show the creation of chimeras (Hong et al. 2013).
(v) ESCs are injected into a tetraploid blastocyst that is produced by electrofusion. The trophectoderm can be produced by a tetraploid blastocyst, but it cannot divide to produce a fetus. By the incorporation of ESCs in tetraploid blastocyst, the development of a foetus occurs, which reveals the pluripotency nature of ESCs (Wen et al. 2014).

CULTURING OF ADULT STEM CELLS

Tissue-specific stem cells are multipotent adult stem cells that are present in various differentiated tissues in the body. MSCs and HSCs are the two major types of adult stem cells that are most frequently used for cell-based therapeutic application. MSCs are more attractive for the tissue repair and regeneration activities owing to their easy availability, self-renewal, immuno-modulating and regenerative potential and they can be derived from various tissue sources, *viz.,* bone marrow, fat tissue, skeletal muscle, trabecular bone, periosteum, synovial membrane, teeth, umbilical cord and cord blood, liver, spleen, and peripheral blood (Haynesworth et al. 1992; Eslaminejad 2014; Zuk et al. 2001; Lee et al. 2004; Rebelatto et al. 2008; Sarugaser et al. 2005; Miura et al. 2003). MSCs derived from the bone marrow have been reported to produce cartilage and bone-like tissue *in vivo*, and have the ability to differentiate along multiple cell lineages, namely, bone, cartilage, and fat or adipose tissue. A massive *in vitro* expansion of MSCs is needed for either transplantation or tissue engineering products development (Martin et al. 2014; Friedenstein, Piatetzky-Shapiro, and Petrakova 1966; Shirasawa et al. 2006).

There is little variation in the procedure for culturing adult stem cells depending on the cell sources. The mononuclear cells (MNCs) are usually isolated from a particular cell source following any isolation technique (e.g. Ficoll-Paque density gradient) and then the cells are cultured in media for enrichment of the cells. In a typical MSCs culturing from bone marrow, MNCs contained in the interphase layer are collected in a tube and centrifuged. The separated MNCs are resuspended in a fresh culture medium in well plate and the cells are incubated in a 5% CO_2 environment at 37 °C for a specific period of time, with the addition of fresh medium at a certain time interval after repeated washing of the adherent cells with PBS solution. Once the culture reaches to confluence about 80–90%, the adherent cells are trypsinized by adding trypsin-EDTA solution with stirring for their detachment from the well plate and the resulting mixture is then centrifuged. After discarding the supernatant, the cells in the pellet are resuspended in a fresh culture medium for further expansion. This one cycle of cell culturing constitutes the passage. Similar methods can be used for obtaining MSCs from different cell sources with a slight variation in the procedure of cell sample preparation (Ferrin et al. 2017). An advanced DMEM/F12 media supplemented with HEPES (N-2-hydroxyethylpiperazine-N'-2-ethanesulfonic acid), penicillin-streptomycin, and glutamax was used for the cultivation of adult stem cells. The medium was additionally introduced with Primocin, N_2, gastrin, B27, and N-acetylcysteine and also supplemented with growth factors for 3 days following each clonal step with antibody, Wnt3a-conditioned medium, Noggin, and solution for the recovery of stem cell cloning. An advanced DMEM/F12 media supplemented with HEPES, penicillin-streptomycin, and glutamax was used to cultivate intestinal stem cell lines. Primocin, recombinant human noggin, and recombinant human Epidermal growth factor (EGF) were added to this media, along with Wnt3a and R-Spondin-conditioned media, B27, N-acetylcysteine, and Nicotinamide. Antibody was added to the intestinal organoid medium for the first 3 days following each clonal stage (Kuijk et al. 2020).

STEM CELL DIFFERENTIATION

Differentiation is a process by which unspecialized stem cells are transformed into specialized cells with specific functions and morphology. Two types of signalling cues that aid in this type of transformation include: intrinsic (within the cell) and extrinsic (outside the cell) (Dua et al. 2003; Lo and Parham 2009). PSC has the potency to form another stem cell or a differentiated cell. The mature cells in a stage just before the terminally differentiated stage are called progenitor cells (e.g. osteoblast) (Lin, Niparko, and Ferrucci 2014b). The intermediate cells between the pluripotent cell stage and the progenitor cell stage are referred to as precursor cells. Whereas, the undifferentiated population of cells between the stem cell stage and the differentiated

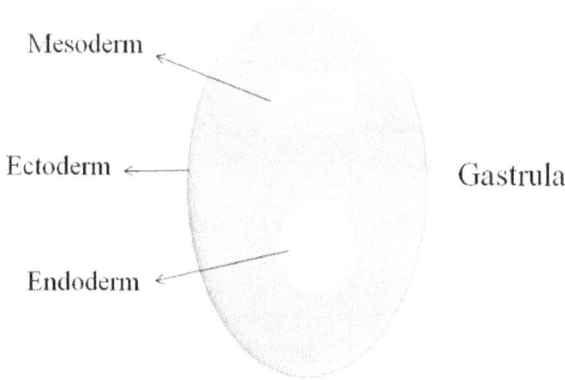

FIGURE 6.4   Three germ layers of embryos.

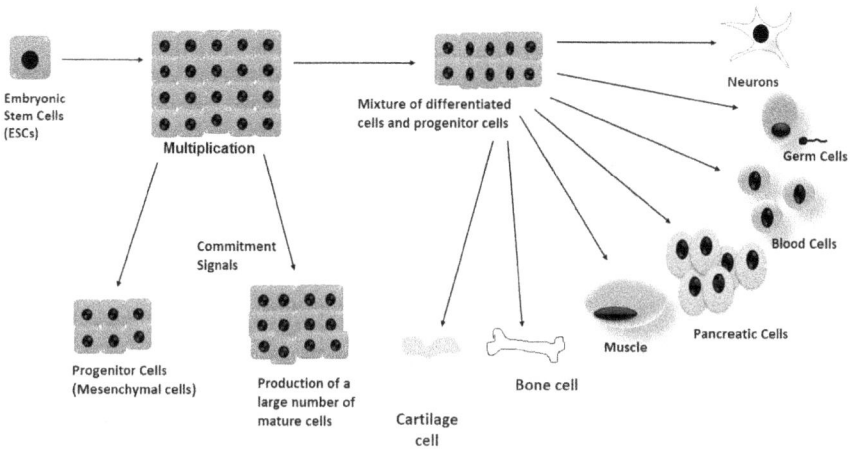

FIGURE 6.5   Various stages of the differentiation of embryonic stem cells into different ineages of mammalian cells.

cell stage are known as transit-amplifying cells. These cells possess high mitotic activity (Rezza et al. 2016).

DIFFERENTIATION OF ESCs

ESCs have unlimited self-regenerating ability and continue to be in an undifferentiated state when grown in an appropriate environment. But when these cells are aggregated together, they form embryoid bodies, which differentiate spontaneously to develop embryonic germ layers of the progeny, *viz.,* mesoderm, endoderm, and ectoderm (Figure 6.4). These germ layers accelerate the differentiation into any type of somatic cells, thereby paving the way towards new mammalian development models and regenerative science. Differentiation of ESCs must be occurred to avoid tumor formation. Spontaneous differentiation of hESCs reults in the formation of a mixture of differentiated cells and progenitor cells. When ESCs exposes to specific commitment signals (growthfactors and culture environment), it converts to a specific progenitor cells. This progenitor cells as well as ESCs have the ability to differentiate into specific mature cells (Figure 6.5) (Zakrzewski et al. 2019; Murry and Keller 2008; Dang et al. 2004).

In brief, the different modes of ESCs differentiation are: (i) aggregation of ESCs to form a 3D colony called embryoid bodies, (ii) direct culturing of ESCs over the stromal cells, and (iii) formation of monolayer of ESCs on extracellular matrix proteins. By altering the chemical composition and surface characteristics of the culture medium and by introducing growth factors and specific genes into the ESCs, the ESCs are promoted to differentiate into various lineages of mammalian cells, for example, blood cells, neuron cells, muscle cells, and pancreatic cell (Keller 1995; Keller 2005).

The differentiation of ESCs has various challenges, which include (i) difficulty in establishing the appropriate cues for differentiation and maintaining the same, (ii) risk of tumour formation, (iii) whether the differentiated cells would be functional or not, (iv) chance of immune rejection and genome instability, (v) difficulty in clinical translation from animal models, and (vi) ethical controversy concerning human application (Fujita et al. 2008).

ADULT STEM CELL DIFFERENTIATION

ASCs are found in various tissues with similar differentiating pathways like ESCs. However, this kind of cells can transform only into certain specified cell types of that particular tissue in which they are found (Cho et al. 2010). Some examples of differentiation of ASCs are described below and shown in Figure 6.6. Haematopoietic stem cell, a multipotent cell, can differentiate into lymphoid and myeloid progenitor cells. Lymphoid cell produces lymphoblast and myeloid progenitor cell giving rise to myeloblast, erythrocytes, and platelets. Lymphoblast can differentiate into B-lymphocyte, T- lymphocyte, and natural killer cell. Myeloblast can differentiate into basophils, eosinophils, neutrophils, monocyte, and macrophages (Figure 6.6).

Haematopoietic stem cells can mature into all types of blood cells like RBC, macrophages, B lymphocytes, neutrophils, T lymphocytes, eosinophils, basophils, natural killer cells, and monocytes (Dzierzak and Speck 2008). Mesenchymal stem cells present in bone marrow mature into many different cell and corresponding tissue types (such as bone cells like osteoblasts and bone tissue like osteocytes, cartilage cells like chondrogenic cells and cartilage tissue like chondrocytes, fat cells like adipogenic cells and adipocytes as fat tissue, and fibrous connective tissue (Ding, Shyu, and Lin 2011).

Neural stem cells extracted from the brain can mature into a variety of cell types, for example, neurons as nerve cells and non-neuronal cells like astrocytes and

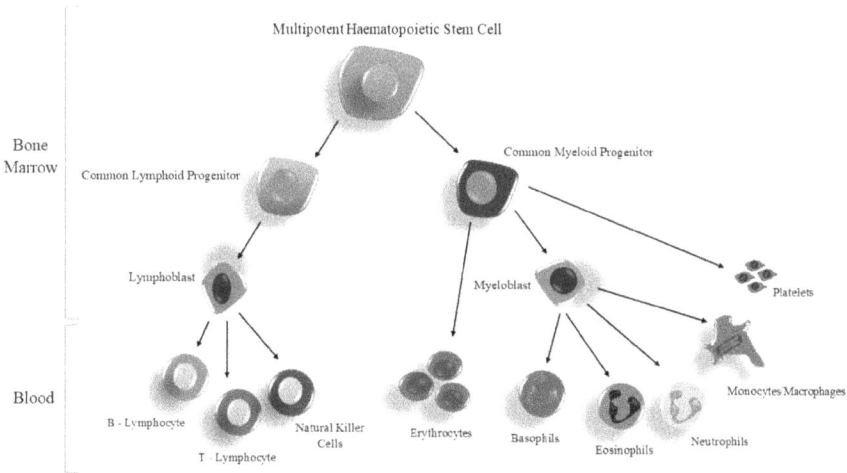

FIGURE 6.6   Various stages of differentiation of haematopoietic stem cells.

oligodendrocytes (Kubis and Catala 2015). Epithelial stem cells extracted from the digestive tract can mature into different cell types including goblet cells, paneth cells, [and] enteroendocrine cells (Schoch et al. 2004). Skin stem cells harvested from the basal layer of the epidermis can mature into keratinocytes. Whereas, stem cells isolated from the base of hair follicles can be transformed into the hair follicle and epidermis (Fuchs 2008).

Even though ASCs differentiate into certain specialized cell types of a particular tissue, there are certain ASC types that are capable of differentiating into cell types of another lineage, for example, stem cells derived from the brain tissue can differentiate into blood cells. This unusual phenomenon is called trans-differentiation (Hombach-Klonisch et al. 2008).

iPSCs DIFFERENTIATION

iPSCs are genetically reprogrammed adult somatic cells that acquire pluripotency and act as ESCs (Ye, Swingen, and Zhang 2013). iPSCs can be generated from any type of somatic cells (e.g. fibroblast) by introducing the necessary factors, for example, Oct3/4, Sox2, c-Myc, and Klf4, through a factor delivery mechanism (retroviral) followed by screening for genetic and protein expression (Fbx15) to validate their pluripotency (Maherali and Hochedlinger 2008). Even though iPSCs have tremendous capability, they have a lower intrinsic differentiation capacity in comparison to ESCs (Robinton and Daley 2012). Researchers were successful in developing iPSCs and promoted them to differentiate into oligodendrocytes, photoreceptor cells, neural cells, odontogenic mesenchymal cells, and cardiomyocytes (Cao et al. 2012; Czepiel et al. 2011).

STEM CELL SIGNALLING MOLECULES

Cell signalling is a process through which cells can communicate or interact with other cells within or outside (external environment) the body. Signalling molecules have the potency to give specific signals to cells through the occurrence of several complex sequencing events, those involving phosphorylation of cytoskeleton protein, metabolic changes, ion fluxes, gene expression, and protein synthesis, resulting in an integrated biological response. They also exhibit diffusion through the extracellular matrix and can act locally due to their slow diffusion. Nonetheless, these signalling molecules can transform different signals that depend on the intracellular signalling pathways, which may differ from one cell type to another (Friedman 2012). Human mesenchymal stem cells (hMSCs) of bone marrow origin have excellent potentiality to differentiate into many tissue-specific lineages following different signalling pathways. The diversification of hMSCs differentiation pathways is due to the activities of various signalling molecules, such as growth factors and genes, among which Cbfa1/Runx2, osterix, lipoprotein-related receptor 5, and Wnt genes are well-known signalling molecules controlling the differentiation of hMSCs into osteoblastic cells. TGF-β family, bone morphogenic proteins, nodal, and activins play an important role in developing and maintaining the many organs that are derived from stem cells. These signalling molecules are also involved in the protection of ESCs identity. At the early stage of differentiation, the levels of expressions of these growth factors are low; however, high level of expressions are observed in the undifferentiated human ESCs. There is often a variation observed between the self-renewal and the early differentiation of ESCs. The fibroblast growth factor (FGF)/Erk signalling pathway needs to attain the differentiation threshold value that defends against this fluctuating state and therefore promote ESCs differentiation. The protein retinoic acid has the ability to stimulate retinoic acid receptor beta and vascular endothelial growth factor (VEGF) gene expression in amnion cells and thereby {promoting} the growth of vascular endothelial cells in ESCs (Cheung et al. 2019). Fibroblast growth factor-2 (FGF-2) and bone morphogenetic protein 2 (BMP-2) promote cardiomyogenic differentiation of ESCs proactively. The nerve growth factor in combination with other growth factors controls the proliferation and terminal differentiation of neural epithelial stem cells (Cattaneo and McKay 1990), whereas growth factor-BB obtained from platelet promotes ESCs to differentiate into smooth muscle cell (Xie et al. 2011). The VEGF promotes multipotent adult progenitor cells to differentiate into endothelial cells via MAPK/ERK1/2 (Mitogen activated protein kinase/Extracellular signal-regulated kinase1/2) signalling pathway (Xu et al. 2008).

There are two types of signalling molecules which can regulate osteogenic differentiation of MSCs, *viz.*, systemic hormones and growth factors. The systemic hormones such as parathyroid hormone, glucocorticoids, and oestrogens have a major role in controlling the osteogenic differentiation. BMP, TGF-β 1/2, insulin-like growth factor (IGF), FGF-2 (VEGF, cytokine modulators (prostaglandins), and Wnt/β-catenin are the local growth factors aiding in osteogenic differentiation. All these signalling molecules regulate the expression of specific transcription factors. Runx2, a frequently occuring transcription factor, plays a remarkable role in osteoblast commitment and osteogenic differentiation of MSCs (Carbonare, Innamorati, and Valenti 2012). There are numerous cytokines and growth factors that have been involved in chondrogenesis and these signalling molecules also have functional overlap with osteogenesis. It is because the differentiation pathway of chondrogenesis has close resemblance with osteogenesis pathway (Heng, Cao, and Lee 2004).

MATRIX MICROENVIRONMENT INFLUENCING STEM CELLS DIFFERENTIATION

As stem cells possess excellent self-renewal and differentiation ability, thereby making them potential cell sources for repairing the bone, cartilage, and other tissues, they also play important role in tissue regeneration (Saroia et al. 2018; Ding and Schultz 2004). The overall stem cell fate including the cell adhesion, proliferation, and differentiation is dependent on diverse microenvironmental factors. Generally, the control of stem cell differentiation is ascribed to molecular and genetic mediators. Several studies have demonstrated that the substrate surface environment, such as mechanical properties, pore, porosity, surface stiffness, surface topography, 3D structures, and mechanical stimulation, has a great influence on the stem cell pro-liferation and differentiation (Xing et al. 2019; Chen et al. 2018). Recent studies have demonstrated that the elasticity of the ECM can affect stem cell fate as can be seen in human MSCs whose substrate elasticity is found to influence the lineage commitment of the cells. When grown on scaffold materials having elasticity similar to that of the desired tissue type, it is seen that stem cells transformed more efficiently into lineages present in that tissue type. For example, freshly isolated muscle stem cells, when placed in a muscle microenvironment, are able to initiate skeletal muscle regeneration upon transplantation in *in vivo* animal models, but the same cells, when introduced to conventional tissue culture plates, differentiated to progenitor cells with reduced regenerative potential. Substrate elasticity is also known to affect cell morph-ology, phenotype, and focal adhesions, particularly in 2D culture. Cells grown on soft materials with a low stiffness were found to express morphologies similar to that of neurons and express neural markers such as P-NFH and β-III tubulin, while cells grown on stiffer materials express myogenic markers and mimic muscle-guided hMSCs. Similarly, the human foetal osteoblastic cell line, when cultured over a scaffold with a high stiffness, expressed the osteogenic marker Runx2 with 1.5 times higher expression intensity than that obtained with hMSCs. Focal adhesion and elong-ation are promoted by stiff substrates. hMSCs are influenced by their microenvir-onment as focal adhesions of stem cells via actin-myosin contractions to its matrix determine the force transmission pathways of the cells (Higuchi et al. 2013). Thus, stiff culture substrates give rise to highly tensed cells. To deform a stiffer matrix, cells alter the expression of the non-muscle myosin such that it generates greater levels of force on the actin cytoskeleton. Stem cell differentiation is hypothesized to be influenced by these forces generated on the actin cytoskeleton (Ghasemi-Mobarakeh 2015). Numerous studies have demonstrated that scaffolds with 370–400 μm pore sizes are more favourable for chondrogenic differentiation of adult stem cells (Oh et al. 2010). The biomimetic 3D porous matrix with interconnected micropores plays a vital role in bone tissue regeneration (Al. 2018; Yoshikawa et al. 2009). Similarly, the surface topography such as roughness and texture of the scaffold structure also has an important role in bone tissue regeneration and in regulating cell behaviours both *in vitro* and *in vivo* (Zhou et al. 2018). Topography may also have an adverse effect on the chondrogenic and osteogenic differentiation of stem cells (Ji et al. 2015; Cooper, Leung, and Zhang 2012). The culture system also has an influence on the cell differentiation. In comparison to 2D culture, 3D culture shows better performance in simulating the microenvironment of cells *in vivo* and can promote proliferation and differentiation, and cellular function. In several studies, 3D cultures of stem cells were found to promote osteogenic, chodrogenic, and osteochondral tissue regeneration by differentiating stem cells (Baharvand et al. 2006; Lin et al. 2014; Zhang, Sun et al. 2019; Cox et al. 2015).

CHALLENGES IN STEM CELL THERAPY

While stem cells provide an ideal solution to cure many diseases, even the chronic ones, still several concerns need to be addressed before their use especially on a large scale. Ethical concerns are the first and foremost among other challenges. ESCs are the most common but widely used PSCs, nonetheless, therapies involving their usage still face ethical conflicts, which were started from the beginning of their discovery in 1998 when scientists found potential for extracting ESCs from the human embryo and stem cell therapy was believed to be the best method for treating all types of diseases including chronic incurable diseases. However, the problem arose when ESCs were isolated from the embryo, which having potential to become a human was sacrificed. Therefore, scientists began to make efforts to isolate the ESCs while avoiding the death of the embryo. To date hESCs are considered a controversial source of stem cells while still bearing tremendous potential as a therapeutic agent for regenerating tissues. The other challenges associated with the use of ESCs are (i) lack of understanding regarding their signalling and complex control systems as well as tumour risk; these must be assessed before their widespread use, (ii) the second issue is the immunological acceptance of the stem cells by the patient's body. In this context, extracting stem cells from the patient's body and transforming them into the state of pluripotency is considered to be the best strategy (Ota 2008). The isolated cells should be able to replace any damaged, malfunctioning, or lost cells in the patient's body, and (iii) the concern of obtaining stem cells without causing any pain or morbidity to the patient or the donor needs to be ensured. The assessment of the uncontrolled cell proliferation and differentiation before their application for tissue regeneration in the patient's body is important (Harris et al. 2004). Tumourigenicity is another concern that limits the use of induced PSCs as there is a chance that oncogenes may be upregulated during the reprogramming of the cells. To avoid this situation, a technique that is able to extract the oncogenes when the cell reaches to the state of pluripotency was established in 2008. However, this is an inefficient and time-consuming method. Enhancing the re-programmability of cells may be achieved by deleting the *p53* gene. However, this gene also functions as an important cancer suppressor, making its removal impossible in order to avoid the presence of increased mutations in the reprogrammed cell. This process also suffers from low efficiency, but is improving each year. Another issue is the use of transcription factors, which risks genomic insertion and further mutations of the genome of the target cell. The injection of hESCs into mouse embryos to evaluate pluripotency is considered as the only ethically acceptable procedure (Mascetti and Pedersen 2016). The International Society for Stem Cell Research (ISSCR) designated the "14-day rule" which prohibits any kind of research involving stem cells after two weeks of fertilization, which coincides with the growth of the primitive streak. ISSCR has formulated some rules like all steps of stem cell research and gene editing should be transparent as the recent advancements in gene editing have given rise to several opportunities for ethical cross-questioning. Lately, there have been reports claiming that the first gene-edited babies were born in China; however, the authentication of this claim is still pending (De Wert and Mummery 2003).

Understanding the mechanisms of the functioning of stem cells requires animal models, which is of prime importance to help in removing the fear of newer technologies involved in stem cell generation and their applications in the public's mind. There is a need for the development of reliable and trustworthy techniques to improve the efficiency of stem cell differentiation. The procedures associated with stem cell therapy starts from their isolation to differentiation need to be scaled up. Future stem cell technology may face many hurdles as it may involve the creation of fully functional organs for transplantation into the patient, thus requiring millions of works on biological accuracy and cooperating cells. Introducing such complex procedures into the field of medicine will involve extensive interdisciplinary and international collaborations. Another major hurdle is the specification and extraction of stem cells from the donor's tissues. Immunogenicity is another pivotal issue that needs to be addressed as transplant rejection may occur in certain procedures or in response to specific kind of stem cells. Further advancements in the field of stem cells will eventually lead to the curtailing of treatment costs for the currently expensive and chronic diseases. For example, in the case of organ failure, the patient can opt for stem cell therapy to heal the organ rather than depend on the prolonged usage of expensive drugs which have side effects. This way the patient will avoid chronic pharmacological treatment while also experiencing prompt relief from the problem. In spite of these concerns associated with stem cell therapy, great progress is being made in the field day by day, with several therapies being already approved for the cure of many diseases. Thus, the impact of stem cells on future medicine is of great significance (Yamanaka 2012; Ota 2008).

EXERCISE

1. What are stem cells? What are their important characteristics?
2. What are the different sources of stem cells?
3. Classify stem cells on the basis of their potency and origin.
4. Explain the method of expansion of embryonic stem cells *in vitro*.
5. What are the important applications of stem cells as therapeutic agents?
6. What are induced pluripotent stem cells?
7. Explain the different methods used in stem cell isolation.

8. Compare embryonic stem cells and adult stem cells.
9. Differentiate between totipotent stem cells and unipotent stem cells.
10. Give two examples of each of the multipotent stem cells, oligopotent stem cells, and unipotent stem cells.
11. Discuss the various challenges involved in stem cell therapy.
12. Explain the influences of scaffold properties on the differentiation of stem cells.
13. Give a brief account of the role of signalling molecules in stem cells differentiation.
14. Write the importance of induced pluripotent stem cells.
15. Give a brief account of adult stem cell culture in the laboratory.
16. Explain the importance of stem cell in tissue engineering and regenerative medicine.
17. What progenitor stem cells? Define stem cell differentiation. Show the various stages of transformation of stem cells to differentiated stem cells with a flow diagram.
18. What is feeder layer? Write the importance of feeder layer. Mention any two feeder layers that are alternative to conventional feeder layer.
19. Explain the different methods of transfer of ICM from the blastocyst.
20. What are the techniques of isolating adult stem cells from different sources? Explain any two methods.
21. Explain the importance of stem cells in disease modeling.
22. What is FACS? Explain its principle with a neat diagram.
23. Discuss the major barrier in stem cell therapy and the future strategy to overcome the obstacle.
24. What are the different methods used for producing iPSCS?
25. Give some examples of signalling molecules which are important for differentiating stem cells to bone tissue.

REFERENCES

Akopian, V., P. W. Andrews, S. Beil, N. Benvenisty, J. Brehm, M. Christie, A. Ford, et al. 2010. "Comparison of defined culture systems for feeder cell free propagation of human embryonic stem cells." *In Vitro Cellular and Developmental Biology – Animal* 46 (3–4): 247–258. https://doi.org/10.1007/s11626-010-9297-z

Al., Taiyang Zhang et al. 2018. "D M Pt." *Journal of Physics D: Applied Physics* Ii: https://doi.org/10.1088/1361-6463/aad7de

Armstrong, L., K. Tilgner, G. Saretzki, S. P. Atkinson, M. Stojkovic, R. Moreno, S. Przyborski, and M. Lako. 2010. "Human induced pluripotent stem cell lines show stress defense mechanisms and mitochondrial regulation similar to those of human embryonic stem cells." *Stem Cells* 28 (4): 661–673. https://doi.org/10.1002/stem.307

Baharvand, H., S. M. Hashemi, S. K. Ashtiani, and A. Farrokhi. 2006. "Differentiation of human embryonic stem cells into hepatocytes in 2D and 3D culture systems in vitro." *International Journal of Developmental Biology* 50 (7): 645–652. https://doi.org/10.1387/ijdb.052072hb

Baker, C. L., and M. F. Pera. 2018. "Capturing totipotent stem cells." *Cell Stem Cell* 22 (1): 25–34. https://doi.org/10.1016/j.stem.2017.12.011

Basu, S., H. M. Campbell, B. N. Dittel, and A. Ray. 2010. "Purification of specific cell population by fluorescence activated cell sorting (FACS)." *Journal of Visualized Experiments* 41: 5–8. https://doi.org/10.3791/1546

Bigdeli, N., M Andersson, R. Strehl, K. Emanuelsson, E. Kilmare, J. Hyllner and A. Lindahl. 2008. "Adaptation of human embryonic stem cells to feeder-free and matrix-free culture conditions directly on plastic surfaces." *Journal of Biotechnology* 133 (1): 146–153. https://doi.org/10.1016/j.jbiotec.2007.08.045

Bissels, U., D. Eckardt and A. Bosio. 2013. "Characterization and classification of stem cells." *Regenerative Medicine*, 155–176. https://doi.org/10.1007/978-94-007-5690-8_6

Cao, N., Z. Liu, Z. Chen, J. Wang, T. Chen, X. Zhao, Y. Ma, et al. 2012. "Ascorbic acid enhances the cardiac differentiation of induced pluripotent stem cells through promoting the proliferation of cardiac progenitor cells." *Cell Research* 22 (1): 219–236. https://doi.org/10.1038/cr.2011.195

Cattaneo, E., & McKay, R. 1990. "Proliferation and differentiation of neuronal stem cells regulated by nerve growth factor." *Nature* 347 (6295): 762–765.

Chen, G., Z. Hou, D. R. Gulbranson, and J. A. Thomson. 2010. "Actin-Myosin contractility is responsible for the reduced viability of dissociated human embryonic stem cells." *Cell Stem Cell* 7 (2): 240–248. https://doi.org/10.1016/j.stem.2010.06.017

Chen, X., H. Fan, X. Deng, L. Wu, T. Yi, L. Gu, C. Zhou, Y. Fan, and X. Zhang. 2018. "Scaffold structural microenvironmental cues to guide tissue regeneration in bone tissue applications." *Nanomaterials* 8 (11): 1–15. https://doi.org/10.3390/nano8110960

Cheung, C. Y., Anderson, D. F., Rouzaire, M., Blanchon, L., Sapin, V., & Brace, R. A. 2019. "Retinoic acid pathway regulation of vascular endothelial growth factor in ovine amnion." *Reproductive Sciences* 26 (10): 1351–1359.

Cho, M., I. Titushkin, S. Sun and J. Shin. 2010. "Physicochemical control of adult stem cell differentiation: Shedding light on potential molecular mechanisms." *Journal of Biomedicine and Biotechnology* 2010: 1–14. https://doi.org/10.1155/2010/743476

Chung, T. L., J. P. Turner, N. Y. Thaker, G. Kolle, J. J. Cooper-White, S. M. Grimmond, M. F. Pera, and E. J. Wolvetang. 2010. "Ascorbate promotes epigenetic activation of CD30 in human embryonic stem cells." *Stem Cells* 28 (10): 1782–1793. https://doi.org/10.1002/stem.500

Clevers, H.. 2015. "What is an adult stem cell?" *Science* 350 (6266): 1319–1320. https://doi.org/10.1126/science.aad7016

Cooper, A., M. Leung, and M. Zhang. 2012. "Polymeric fibrous matrices for substrate-mediated human embryonic stem cell lineage differentiation." *Macromolecular Bioscience* 12 (7): 882–892. https://doi.org/10.1002/mabi.201100269

Cox, S. C., J. A. Thornby, G. J. Gibbons, M. A. Williams, and K. K. Mallick. 2015. "3D printing of porous hydroxyapatite scaffolds intended for use in bone tissue engineering applications." *Materials Science and Engineering C* 47: 237–247. https://doi.org/10.1016/j.msec.2014.11.024

Czepiel, M., V. Balasubramaniyan, W. Schaafsma, M. Stancic, H. Mikkers, C. Huisman, E. Boddeke, and S. Copray. 2011. "Differentiation of induced pluripotent stem cells into functional oligodendrocytes." *Glia* 59 (6): 882–892. https://doi.org/10.1002/glia.21159

Dang, S. M., S. Gerecht-Nir, J. Chen, J. Itskovitz-Eldor, and P. W. Zandstra. 2004. "Controlled, scalable embryonic stem cell differentiation culture." *Stem Cells* 22 (3): 275–282. https://doi.org/10.1634/stemcells.22-3-275

Daniel H., L. D. Buttery, K. M. Shakesheff, and S. J. Roberts. 2008. "Tissue engineering: Strategies, stem cells and scaffolds." *Journal of Anatomy* 213 (1) (July): 66–72. DOI: 10.1111/j.1469-7580.2008.00878.x

Dejosez, M., and T. P. Zwaka. 2012. "Pluripotency and nuclear reprogramming." *Annual Review of Biochemistry* 81: 737–765. https://doi.org/10.1146/annurev-biochem-052 709-104948

Dellatore, S. M., A. Sofia Garcia, and W. M. Miller. 2008. "Mimicking stem cell niches to increase stem cell expansion." *Current Opinion in Biotechnology* 19 (5): 534–540. https://doi.org/10.1016/j.copbio.2008.07.010

Ding, D. C., W. C. Shyu, and S. Z. Lin. 2011. "Mesenchymal stem cells." *Cell Transplantation* 20 (1): 5–14. https://doi.org/10.3727/096368910X

Ding, S., and P. G. Schultz. 2004. "A role for chemistry in stem cell biology." *Nature Biotechnology* 22 (7): 833–840. https://doi.org/10.1038/nbt987

Dottori, M., M. Familari, S. Hansson, and K. Hasegawa. 2012. "Stem cells as in vitro models of disease." *Stem Cells International*, 0–3. https://doi.org/10.1155/2012/565083

Draper, J. S., H. D. Moore, L. N. Ruban, P. J. Gokhale, and P. W. Andrews. 2004. "Culture and characterization of human embryonic stem cells." *Stem Cells and Development* 13 (4): 325–336. https://doi.org/10.1089/1547328041797525

Dua, H. S., A. Joseph, V. A. Shanmuganathan, and R. E. Jones. 2003. "Stem cell differentiation and the effects of deficiency." *Eye* 17 (8): 877–885. https://doi.org/10.1038/sj.eye.6700573

Dzierzak, E., and N. A. Speck. 2008. "Of lineage and legacy: The development of mammalian hematopoietic stem cells." *Nature Immunology* 9 (2): 129–136. https://doi.org/10.1038/ni1560

Egashira, T., Yuasa, S., & Fukuda, K. 2011. "Induced pluripotent stem cells in cardiovascular medicine." *Stem Cells International* 2011: 1–7.

Eslaminejad, M. B.. 2014. "Mesenchymal stem cells as a potent cell source for articular cartilage regeneration." *World Journal of Stem Cells* 6 (3): 344. https://doi.org/10.4252/wjsc.v6.i3.344

Ferrin, I., I. Beloqui, L. Zabaleta, J. M. Salcedo, C. Trigueros, and A. G. Martin. 2017. "Isolation, culture, and expansion of mesenchymal stem cells." *Methods in Molecular Biology* 1590: 177–190. https://doi.org/10.1007/978-1-4939-6921-0_13

Friedenstein, A. J., I. I. Piatetzky-Shapiro, and K. V. Petrakova. 1966. "Osteogenesis in transplants of bone marrow cells." *Journal of Embryology and Experimental Morphology* 16 (3): 381–390. https://doi.org/10.1242/dev.16.3.381

Friedman, W.. 2012. *Growth Factors. Basic Neurochemistry*. Eighth Edition. Elsevier Inc. https://doi.org/10.1016/B978-0-12-374947-5.00029-8

Fuchs, E.. 2008. "Skin stem cells: Rising to the surface." *Journal of Cell Biology* 180 (2): 273–284. https://doi.org/10.1083/jcb.200708185

Fujita, J., A. M. Crane, M. K. Souza, M. Dejosez, M. Kyba, R. A. Flavell, J. A. Thomson, and T. P. Zwaka. 2008. "Caspase activity mediates the differentiation of embryonic stem cells." *Cell Stem Cell* 2 (6): 595–601. https://doi.org/10.1016/j.stem.2008.04.001

Gerrard, L., Debiao Zhao, A. J. C., and W. Cui. 2005. "Stably Transfected human embryonic stem cell clones express OCT4-specific green fluorescent protein and maintain self-renewal and pluripotency." *Stem Cells* 23 (1): 124–133. https://doi.org/10.1634/stemce lls.2004-0102

Ghasemi-Mobarakeh, L.. 2015. "Structural properties of scaffolds: Crucial parameters towards stem cells differentiation." *World Journal of Stem Cells* 7 (4): 728. https://doi.org/10.4252/wjsc.v7.i4.728

Giachino, C., Basak, O., & Taylor, V. 2009. "Isolation and manipulation of mammalian neural stem cells in vitro." *Stem Cells in Regenerative Medicine* 143–158.

Goodell, M. A. 2005. "Stem cell identification and sorting using the hoechst 33342 side population (SP) staining and analysis of stem cell side population in murine bone marrow." *Journal of Experimental Medicine* 183 (4): 1797–1806.

Goodell, M. A., K. Brose, G. Paradis, A. Stewart Conner, and R. C. Mulligan. 1996. "Isolation and functional properties of murine hematopoietic stem cells that are replicating in vivo." *Journal of Experimental Medicine* 183 (4): 1797–1806. https://doi.org/10.1084/jem.183.4.1797

Guo, G., F. Von Meyenn, F. Santos, Y. Chen, W. Reik, P. Bertone, A. Smith, and J. Nichols. 2016. "Naive pluripotent stem cells derived directly from isolated cells of the human inner cell mass." *Stem Cell Reports* 6 (4): 437–446. https://doi.org/10.1016/j.stemcr.2016.02.005

Harris, M. T., D. L. Butler, G. P. Boivin, J. B. Florer, E. J. Schantz, and R. J. Wenstrup. 2004. "Mesenchymal stem cells used for rabbit tendon repair can form ectopic bone and express alkaline phosphatase activity in constructs." *Journal of Orthopaedic Research* 22 (5): 998–1003. https://doi.org/10.1016/j.orthres.2004.02.012

Haynesworth, S. E., J. Goshima, V. M. Goldberg, and A. I. Caplan. 1992. "Characterization of cells with osteogenic potential from human marrow." *Bone* 13 (1): 81–88. https://doi.org/10.1016/8756-3282(92)90364-3

Heng, B. C., Cao, T., & Lee, E. H. 2004. "Directing stem cell differentiation into the chondrogenic lineage in vitro." *Stem Cells* 22 (7): 1152–1167.

Higuchi, A., Q. D. Ling, Y. Chang, S. T. Hsu, and A. Umezawa. 2013. "Physical cues of biomaterials guide stem cell differentiation fate." *Chemical Reviews* 113 (5): 3297–3328. https://doi.org/10.1021/cr300426x

Hombach-Klonisch, S., S. Panigrahi, I. Rashedi, A. Seifert, E. Alberti, P. Pocar, M. Kurpisz, K. Schulze-Osthoff, A. MacKiewicz, and M. Los. 2008. "Adult stem cells and their trans-differentiation potential – perspectives and therapeutic applications." *Journal of Molecular Medicine* 86 (12): 1301–1314. https://doi.org/10.1007/s00109-008-0383-6

Hong, J., H. He, P. Bui, B. Ryba-White, M. A.K. Rumi, M. J. Soares, D. Dutta, et al. 2013. "A focused microarray for screening rat embryonic stem cell lines." *Stem Cells and Development* 22 (3): 431–443. https://doi.org/10.1089/scd.2012.0279

Inoue, H., and S. Yamanaka. 2011. "The use of induced pluripotent stem cells in drug development." *Clinical Pharmacology and Therapeutics* 89 (5): 655–661. https://doi.org/10.1038/clpt.2011.38

Ireland, R. G., M. Kibschull, J. Audet, M. Ezzo, B. Hinz, S. J. Lye, and C. A. Simmons. 2020. "Combinatorial extracellular matrix microarray identifies novel bioengineered substrates for xeno-free culture of human pluripotent stem cells." *Biomaterials* 248 (August 2019): 120017. https://doi.org/10.1016/j.biomaterials.2020.120017

Jaatinen, T., and J. Laine. 2007. "Isolation of mononuclear cells from human cord blood by ficoll-paque density gradient." *Current Protocols in Stem Cell Biology* 2 (June): 1–4. https://doi.org/10.1002/9780470151808.sc02a01s1

Javazon, E. H., K. J. Beggs, and A. W. Flake. 2004. "Mesenchymal stem cells: paradoxes of passaging." *Experimental Hematology* 32 (5): 414–425.

Ji, J., X. Tong, X. Huang, T. Wang, Z. Lin, Y. Cao, J. Zhang, L. Dong, H. Qin, and Q. Hu. 2015. "Sphere-shaped nano-hydroxyapatite/chitosan/gelatin 3D porous scaffolds increase proliferation and osteogenic differentiation of human induced pluripotent stem cells from gingival fibroblasts." *Biomedical Materials (Bristol)* 10 (4): 45005. https://doi.org/10.1088/1748-6041/10/4/045005

Johnson, K.W., M. Dooner, and P. J. Quesenberry. 2007. "Fluorescence activated cell sorting: A window on the stem cell." *Current Pharmaceutical Biotechnology* 8 (3): 133–139. https://doi.org/10.2174/138920107780906487

Juopperi, T. A., W. Schuler, X. Yuan, M. I. Collector, C. V. Dang, and S. J. Sharkis. 2007. "Isolation of bone marrow-derived stem cells Using density-gradient separation." *Experimental Hematology* 35 (2): 335–341. https://doi.org/10.1016/j.exphem.2006.09.014

Keller, G.. 2005. "Embryonic stem cell differentiation: Emergence of a new era in biology and medicine." *Genes and Development* 19 (10): 1129–1155. https://doi.org/10.1101/gad.1303605

Keller, G. M. 1995. "Es cell diff." *Current Opinion in Cell Biology* 7: 862–869. https://ac.els-cdn.com/0955067495800719/1-s2.0-0955067495800719-main.pdf?_tid=a1b0348e-cabb-4b98-be11-3729e8511cc5&acdnat=1538845545_2d71bf1e78c8116c222061bbe9ac646c

Kobold, S., A. Guhr, A. Kurtz, and P. Löser. 2015. "Human embryonic and induced pluripotent stem cell research trends: Complementation and diversification of the field." *Stem Cell Reports* 4 (5): 914–925. https://doi.org/10.1016/j.stemcr.2015.03.002

Kubis, N., and M. Catala. 2015. "Neural stem cells." *Stem Cell Biology and Regenerative Medicine*, 477–497. https://doi.org/10.1161/01.res.0000065580.02404.f4

Kuijk, E., M. Jager, B. van der Roest, M. D. Locati, A. Van Hoeck, J. Korzelius, R. Janssen, et al. 2020. "The mutational impact of culturing human pluripotent and adult stem cells." *Nature Communications* 11 (1): 2493. https://doi.org/10.1038/s41467-020-16323-4

Lee, O. K., T. K. Kuo, W. M. Chen, K. D. Lee, S. L. Hsieh, and T. H. Chen. 2004. "Isolation of multipotent mesenchymal stem cells from umbilical cord blood." *Blood* 103 (5): 1669–1675. https://doi.org/10.1182/blood-2003-05-1670

Li, D., J. Zhou, F. Chowdhury, J. Cheng, N. Wang, and F. Wang. 2011. "Role of mechanical factors in fate decisions of stem cells." *Regenerative Medicine* 6 (2): 229–240. https://doi.org/10.2217/rme.11.2

Lin, C. Y., C. H. Huang, Y. K. Wu, N. C. Cheng, and J. Yu. 2014. "Maintenance of human adipose derived stem cell (HASC) differentiation capabilities using a 3D culture." *Biotechnology Letters* 36 (7): 1529–1537. https://doi.org/10.1007/s10529-014-1500-y

Lin, F. R., J. K. Niparko, and L. Ferrucci. 2014a. "基因的改变NIH Public access." *Bone* 23 (1): 1–7. https://doi.org/10.1038/ni1560.Of

Lo, B., and L. Parham. 2009. "Ethical issues in stem cell research." *Endocrine Reviews* 30 (3): 204–213. https://doi.org/10.1210/er.2008-0031

Ma, S., N. Xie, W. Li, B. Yuan, Y. Shi, and Y. Wang. 2014. "Immunobiology of mesenchymal stem cells." *Cell Death and Differentiation* 21 (2): 216–225. https://doi.org/10.1038/cdd.2013.158

MacIntyre, D. A., D. Melguizo Sanchís, B. Jiménez, R. Moreno, M. Stojkovic, and A. Pineda-Lucena. 2011. "Characterisation of human embryonic stem cells conditioning media by 1H-Nuclear magnetic resonance spectroscopy." *PLoS ONE* 6 (2). https://doi.org/10.1371/journal.pone.0016732.

Maherali, N., and K. Hochedlinger. 2008. "Guidelines and techniques for the generation of induced pluripotent stem cells." *Cell Stem Cell* 3 (6): 595–605. https://doi.org/10.1016/j.stem.2008.11.008

Martin, I., H. Baldomero, C. Bocelli-Tyndall, M. Y. Emmert, S. P. Hoerstrup, H. Ireland, J. Passweg, and A. Tyndall. 2014. "The survey on cellular and engineered tissue therapies in europe in 2011." *Tissue Engineering – Part A* 20 (3–4): 842–853. https://doi.org/10.1089/ten.tea.2013.0372

Mascetti, V. L., and R. A. Pedersen. 2016. "Human-mouse chimerism validates human stem cell pluripotency." *Cell Stem Cell* 18 (1): 67–72. https://doi.org/10.1016/j.stem.2015.11.017

Matahine, T., I. Supriatna, D. Sajuthi, A. Boediono, J. Produksi Ternak, P. Peternakan, U. Nusa Cendana, et al. 2008. "Produksi embryonic stem cells dari inner cell mass blastosis yang diisolasi dengan metode enzimatik dan immunosurgery." *Jurnal Veteriner* 9 (1): 13–19..

Maury, Y., M. Gauthier, M. Peschanski, and C. Martinat. 2012. "Human pluripotent stem cells for disease modelling and drug screening." *BioEssays* 34 (1): 61–71. https://doi.org/10.1002/bies.201100071

McEwen, K. R., H. G. Leitch, R. Amouroux, and P. Hajkova. 2013. "The impact of culture on epigenetic properties of pluripotent stem cells and pre-implantation embryos." *Biochemical Society Transactions* 41 (3): 711–719. https://doi.org/10.1042/BST2 0130049

Mimeault, M., and S. K. Batra. 2009. "Characterization of nonmalignant and malignant prostatic stem/progenitor cells by hoechst side population method." *Methods in Molecular Biology (Clifton, N.J.)* 568: 139–149. https://doi.org/10.1007/978-1-59745-280-9_8

Miura, M., S. Gronthos, M. Zhao, B. Lu, L. W. Fisher, P. G. Robey, and S Shi. 2003. "SHED: Stem cells from human exfoliated deciduous teeth." *Proceedings of the National Academy of Sciences of the United States of America* 100 (10): 5807–5812. https://doi.org/10.1073/pnas.0937635100

Mori, H., and M. Hara. 2013. "Cultured stem cells as tools for toxicological assays." *Journal of Bioscience and Bioengineering* 116 (6): 647–652. https://doi.org/10.1016/j.jbiosc.2013.05.028

Murry, C. E., and G. Keller. 2008. "Differentiation of embryonic stem cells to clinically relevant populations: Lessons from embryonic development." *Cell* 132 (4): 661–680. https://doi.org/10.1016/j.cell.2008.02.008

Ogawa, M. 1993. "Differentiation and proliferation of hematopoietic stem cells." *Blood* 81 (11): 2844–2853. https://doi.org/10.1182/blood.v81.11.2844.2844

Oh, S. H., T. H. Kim, G. I. Im, and J. H. Lee. 2010. "Investigation of pore size effect on chondrogenic differentiation of adipose stem cells using a pore size gradient scaffold." *Biomacromolecules* 11 (8): 1948–1955. https://doi.org/10.1021/bm100199m

Ota, K. I.. 2008. "Fuel cells: Past, present and future." *IEEJ Transactions on Fundamentals and Materials* 128 (5): 329–332. https://doi.org/10.1541/ieejfms.128.329

Pereira, T., G. Ivanova, A. R. Caseiro, P. Barbosa, P. J. Bártolo, J. D. Santos, A. L. Luís, and A. C. Maurício. 2014. "MSCs conditioned media and umbilical cord blood plasma metabolomics and composition." *PLoS ONE* 9 (11): 1–31. https://doi.org/10.1371/journal.pone.0113769

Pierre Amarenco, J. B., A. Callahan 3rd, L. B. Goldstein, M. Hennerici, A. E. Rudolph, H. Sillesen, L. Simunovic, M. Szarek, K. M. A. Welch, and J. A. Zivin. 2011. "Stroke prevention by aggressive reduction in cholesterol levels (SPARCL) investigators.. "需要引用的霍奇金第二肿瘤New England Journal." *New England Journal of Medicine* 365: 687–696.

Preston, S. L., M. R. Alison, S. J. Forbes, N. C. Direkze, R. Poulsom, and N. A. Wright. 2003. "The new stem cell biology: Something for everyone," 86–96.

Rebelatto, C. K., A. M. Aguiar, M. P. Moretão, A. C. Senegaglia, P. Hansen, F. Barchiki, J. Oliveira, et al. 2008. "Dissimilar differentiation of mesenchymal stem cells from bone marrow, umbilical cord blood, and adipose tissue." *Experimental Biology and Medicine* 233 (7): 901–913. https://doi.org/10.3181/0712-RM-356

Rezza, A., Z. Wang, R. Sennett, W. Qiao, D. Wang, N. Heitman, K. W. Mok, et al. 2016. "Signaling networks among stem cell precursors, transit-amplifying progenitors, and their niche in developing hair follicles." *Cell Reports* 14 (12): 3001–3018. https://doi.org/10.1016/j.celrep.2016.02.078

Robinton, D. A., and G. Q. Daley. 2012. "The promise of induced pluripotent stem cells in research and therapy." *Nature* 481 (7381): 295–305. https://doi.org/10.1038/nature10761

Rowntree, R. K., and J. D. McNeish. 2010. "Induced pluripotent stem cells: Opportunities as research and development tools in 21st century drug discovery." *Regenerative Medicine* 5 (4): 557–568. https://doi.org/10.2217/rme.10.36

Sánchez Alvarado, A., and S. Yamanaka. 2014. "Rethinking differentiation: Stem cells, regeneration, and plasticity." *Cell* 157 (1): 110–19. https://doi.org/10.1016/j.cell.2014.02.041

Saroia, J., W. Yanen, Q. Wei, K. Zhang, T. Lu, and B. Zhang. 2018. "A review on biocompatibility nature of hydrogels with 3D printing techniques, tissue engineering application and its future prospective." *Bio-Design and Manufacturing* 1 (4): 265–279. https://doi.org/10.1007/s42242-018-0029-7

Sarugaser, R., D. Lickorish, Dolores Baksh, M. Morris Hosseini, and John E. Davies. 2005. "Human umbilical cord perivascular (HUCPV) cells: A source of mesenchymal progenitors." *Stem Cells* 23 (2): 220–229. https://doi.org/10.1634/stemcells.2004-0166

Schmitz, B., A. Radbruch, T. Kummel, H. Korb, C. Wickenhauser, J. Thiele, M. L. Hansmann, and R. Fischer. 1994. "Magnetic activated cell sorting (MACS) – a new imrnunomagnetic method for megakarvocvtic cell isolation." *European Journal of Heamatology* 52 (5): 267–275.

Schoch, K. G., A. Lori, K. A. Burns, T. Eldred, J. C. Olsen, and S. H. Randell. 2004. "A subset of mouse tracheal epithelial basal cells generates large colonies in vitro." *American Journal of Physiology – Lung Cellular and Molecular Physiology* 286 (4): 631–642. https://doi.org/10.1152/ajplung.00112.2003

Scott, C. W., M. F. Peters, and Y. P. Dragan. 2013. "Human induced pluripotent stem cells and their use in drug discovery for toxicity testing." *Toxicology Letters* 219 (1): 49–58. https://doi.org/10.1016/j.toxlet.2013.02.020

Seita, J., and I. L. Weissman. 2010. "Published in final edited form as: Hematopoietic stem cell: Self-Renewal versus differentiation." *Wiley Interdisciplinary Reviews: Systems Biology and Medicine* 2 (5): 1–20. https://doi.org/10.1002/wsbm.86.Hematopoietic

Shirasawa, S., I. Sekiya, Y. Sakaguchi, K. Yagishita, S. Ichinose, and T. Muneta. 2006. "In vitro chondrogenesis of human synovium-derived mesenchymal stem cells: Optimal condition and comparison with bone marrow-derived cells." *Journal of Cellular Biochemistry* 97 (1): 84–97. https://doi.org/10.1002/jcb.20546

Sobhani, A., N. Khanlarkhani, M. Baazm, F. Mohammadzadeh, A. Najafi, S. Mehdinejadiani, and F. S. Aval. 2017. "Multipotent stem cell and current application." *Acta Medica Iranica* 55 (1): 6–23.

Sousa, B. R., R. C. Parreira, E A. Fonseca, M J. Amaya, F. M. P. Tonelli, S. M. S. N. Lacerda, P. Lalwani, et al. 2014. "Human adult stem cells from diverse origins: An overview from multiparametric immunophenotyping to clinical applications." *Cytometry Part A* 85 (1): 43–77. https://doi.org/10.1002/cyto.a.22402

Stacey, G. N. 2009. "Consensus guidance for banking and supply of human embryonic stem cell lines for research purposes: The international stem cell banking initiative." *Stem Cell Reviews and Reports* 5 (4): 301–314. https://doi.org/10.1007/s12015-009-9085-x

Sukoyan, M. A., S. Y. Vatolin, A. N. Golubitsa, A. I. Zhelezova, L. A. Semenova, and O. L. Serov. 1993. "Embryonic stem cells derived from morulae, inner cell mass, and blastocysts of mink: Comparisons of their pluripotencies." *Molecular Reproduction and Development* 36 (2): 148–158. https://doi.org/10.1002/mrd.1080360205

Tang, F., C. Barbacioru, S. Bao, C. Lee, E. Nordman, X. Wang, K. Lao, and M. A. Surani. 2010. "Tracing the derivation of embryonic stem cells from the inner cell mass by single-cell RNA-Seq analysis." *Cell Stem Cell* 6 (5): 468–478. https://doi.org/10.1016/j.stem.2010.03.015

Trounson, A., and N. D. DeWitt. 2016. "Pluripotent stem cells progressing to the clinic." *Nature Reviews Molecular Cell Biology* 17 (3): 194–200. https://doi.org/10.1038/nrm.2016.10

Wen, D., N. Saiz, Z. Rosenwaks, A. K. Hadjantonakis, and S. Rafii. 2014. "Completely ES cell-derived mice produced by tetraploid complementation using inner cell mass (ICM) deficient blastocysts." *PLoS ONE* 9 (4). https://doi.org/10.1371/journal.pone.0094730

Wert, G. D., and C. Mummery. 2003. "Human embryonic stem cells: Research, ethics and policy." *Human Reproduction* 18 (4): 672–682. https://doi.org/10.1093/humrep/deg143

Wray, J., and C. Hartmann. 2012. "WNTing embryonic stem cells." *Trends in Cell Biology* 22 (3): 159–168. https://doi.org/10.1016/j.tcb.2011.11.004

Xiao, L., X. Yuan, and S. J. Sharkis. 2006. "Activin a maintains self-renewal and regulates fibroblast growth factor, wnt, and bone morphogenic protein pathways in human embryonic stem cells." *Stem Cells* 24 (6): 1476–1486. https://doi.org/10.1634/stemcells.2005-0299

Xie, C., Ritchie, R. P., Huang, H., Zhang, J., & Chen, Y. E. 2011. "Smooth muscle cell differentiation in vitro: models and underlying molecular mechanisms." *Arteriosclerosis, Thrombosis, and Vascular Biology* 31 (7): 1485–1494.

Xing, F., L. Li, C. Zhou, C. Long, L. Wu, H. Lei, Q. Kong, Y. Fan, Z. Xiang, and X. Zhang. 2019. "Regulation and directing stem cell fate by tissue engineering functional microenvironments: Scaffold physical and chemical cues." *Stem Cells International* 2019 Article ID 2180925: 1–16. https://doi.org/10.1155/2019/2180925

Yamanaka, S. 2012. "Induced pluripotent stem cells: Past, present, and future." *Cell Stem Cell* 10 (6): 678–684. https://doi.org/10.1016/j.stem.2012.05.005

Ye, L., C. Swingen, and J. Zhang. 2013. "Send orders of reprints at Bspsaif@emirates.Net. Ae induced pluripotent stem cells and their potential for basic and clinical sciences." *Current Cardiology Reviews* 9 (1): 63–72.

Yoshikawa, H., N. Tamai, T. Murase, and A. Myoui. 2009. "Interconnected porous hydroxyapatite ceramics for bone tissue engineering." *Journal of the Royal Society Interface* 6 (Suppl.3): S341–348. https://doi.org/10.1098/rsif.2008.0425.focus

Zakrzewski, W., Dobrzyński, M., Szymonowicz, M., & Rybak, Z. 2019. "Stem cells: past, present, and future." *Stem Cell Research & Therapy*, 10 (1): 1–22.

Zhang, B., H. Sun, L. Wu, L. Ma, F. Xing, Q. Kong, Y. Fan, C. Zhou, and X. Zhang. 2019. "3D printing of calcium phosphate bioceramic with tailored biodegradation rate for skull bone tissue reconstruction." *Bio-Design and Manufacturing* 2 (3): 161–171. https://doi.org/10.1007/s42242-019-00046-7

Zhang, S., T. Chen, N. Chen, D. Gao, B. Shi, S. Kong, R. C. West, et al. 2019. "Implantation initiation of self-assembled embryo-like structures generated using three types of mouse blastocyst-derived stem cells." *Nature Communications* 10 (1). https://doi.org/10.1038/s41467-019-08378-9

Zhou, C., Y. Jiang, Z. Sun, Y. Li, B. Guo, and Y. Hong. 2018. "Biological effects of apatite nanoparticle-constructed ceramic surfaces in regulating behaviours of mesenchymal stem cells." *Journal of Materials Chemistry B* 6 (35): 5621–5632. https://doi.org/10.1039/c8tb01638k

Zuba-Surma, E. K., W. Wojakowski, Z. Madeja, and M. Z. Ratajczak. 2012. "Stem cells as a novel tool for drug screening and treatment of degenerative diseases." *Current Pharmaceutical Design* 18 (18): 2644–2656. https://doi.org/10.2174/138161212800492859

Zuk, P. A., M. Zhu, H. Mizuno, J. Huang, J. W. Futrell, A. J. Katz, P. Benhaim, H. P. Lorenz, and M. H. Hedrick. 2001. "Multilineage cells from human adipose tissue: Implications for cell-based therapies." *Tissue Engineering* 7 (2): 211–228. https://doi.org/10.1089/107632701300062859

7 Bioreactor and Tissue Graft Generation

INTRODUCTION

In tissue engineering, the culture environment has a great influence not only on the cell expansion but also on the formation and properties of tissue constructs; this can be achieved by providing necessary biochemical, physiochemical, and biomechanical cues (Zurina et al. 2020; Han et al. 2019; Ahmed et al. 2019). For example, delivery of oxygen and nutrients and mechanical stimulation encourage cell proliferation and differentiation, and results in an uniform cell distribution in the culture system. Bioreactor has the ability to provide necessary biochemical and physical regulatory signals to the cells for their proliferation and growth, and also inspire cells to undergo differentiation during the process of construct or tissue graft generation *in vitro*. Besides, an ideal bioreactor can facilitate continuous nutrient transfer and gas exchange, waste product removal, maintain a sterile environment, to implement other stimuli like electrical signals, mechanical and magnetic stimulation, etc., the engineered tissue. Moreover, bioreactors have the ability to improve the applicability of tissue engineering processes, thereby helping to translate basic tissue engineering research knowledge into alternative strategies to classical donor organs and animal testing.

The use of bioreactor for bone and cartilage tissue regeneration involving 3D culture offers a novel approach and hence has been under active research in recent years. This has evolved a number of bioreactor systems with different designs like spinner flask, perfusion flow, rotating vessel, hollow fiber, microfluidic devices, and others to achieve adequate interaction among the scaffolds, cells, and signalling molecules, thereby promoting rapid and homogeneous production of engineered bone and cartilage ECMs with desired functional properties. This chapter presents the various types of bioreactors that are suitable for stem cell expansion and production of cell-scaffold construct or tissue graft along with their advantages and disadvantages. The various steps involved in the neo tissue formation including the techniques for seeding of cells onto the scaffold, cell–scaffold interaction such as cell adhesion, cell migration and cell aggregation, along with their assessment have been described. The various examples of bioreactors that have been designed and used by several researchers worldwide for the regeneration of bone and cartilage tissue, and more complex joint tissue have also been highlighted in this chapter

 DOI: 10.1201/9781003245353-7

BIOREACTOR CONFIGURATIONS

The commonly applied 2D culture systems are usually static culture vessels such as culture or petri dishes, well plates, and T-flasks. In the last decade, there was a paradigm change from 2D to 3D cell culture systems that was driven by the massive development in the tissue engineering field. However, the major disadvantage of conventional 2D cell culture system is that the results obtained in these monolayer environments do not reflect in the *in vivo* microenvironment. Due to the paradigm change in cell culture, various types of bioreactors have been evolved in tissue engineering that include spinner flask, rotating vessel, hollow fiberre, perfusion flow, microfluidic devices, magnetic bioreactors, ultrasonic bioreactors, and others, which are described in the following sections.

Spinner Flask Bioreactor

Spinner flask, a cylindrical glass vessel, is the simplest configuration of bioreactor used in tissue engineering. In this culture system, scaffolds are suspended through a wire or string in the culture medium. Typically, the volume of spinner flasks is about 120 mL, although flasks of 20 litres or even higher volume have been designed. The culture vessel is agitated by a magnetic bar placed at the bottom of the vessel and rotating at a typical rotation of 50 r/min to maintain a homogeneous culture medium. Figure 7.1 shows a typical spinner flask bioreactor system. It consists of two ports that are used for gas exchange and addition of nutrients. In this 3D culture, the bioreactor can produce convective flow and hydrodynamic force that enhance the mass transport within the construct as well as efficiency of seeding of the cells onto the scaffold

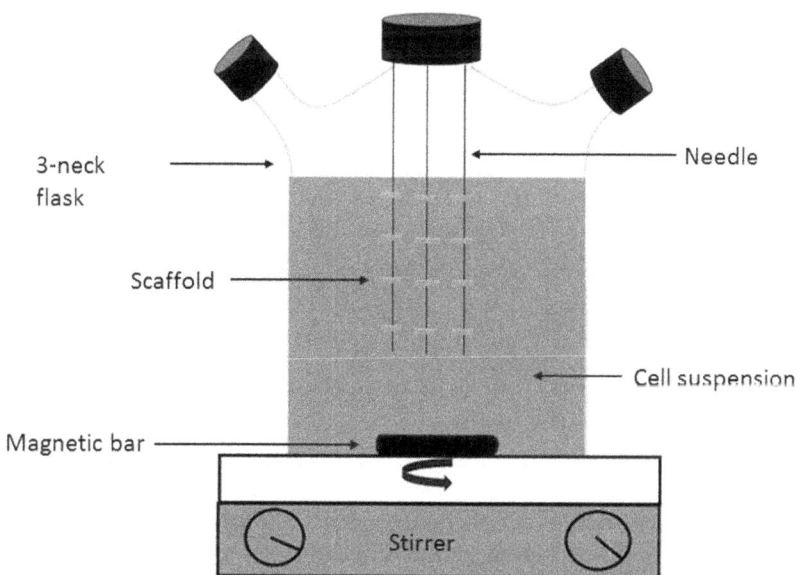

FIGURE 7.1 Spinner flask dynamic bioreactor system.

(Ahmed et al. 2019; Gaspar, Gomide, and Monteiro 2012). The advantages of spinner flask include its simple design, ease of operation, cost effective and and scaling up maintenance of uniform cell distribution throughout the tissue construct. However, it has limitations in nutrient diffusion, requirement of significant labor for cleaning, sterilizing, and reassembling, and shear stress generation.

Spinner flask bioreactors can be designed and operated in both batch and continuous culture modes. The batch type consists of a closed culture system that normally does not allow the addition of fresh medium to the culture vessel and also cannot remove the waste from it, thus providing limited product yield, but with low risk of contamination. This culture method, therefore has the drawbacks of accumulation of harmful waste metabolic by-products produced during culturing. On the contrary, the continuous culture can overcome many limitations of the spinner flask bioreactor systems including the waste removal, and offers prolonged period of culturing, thereby providing higher tissue production, automation and consequently less labor requirement. However, this method requires high capital investment and exposes the culture to a high risk of contamination.

ROTATING WALL VESSEL

Rotating wall vessel was developed by Schwarz and colleagues at Johnson Space Center of the National Aeronautics and Space Administration (NASA) with the aim of creating a model microgravity environment associated with the space, and later it was used to create more precise features of human tissue *in vivo*. This bioreactor is comprised of a rotating cylinder that is filled with culture media in which the scaffolds are suspended. These bioreactors are designed based on two basic design principles: one uses solid body rotation and the other one uses a silicon rubber membrane for oxygenation (Altman et al. 2002). In the former design, a cylinder rotates along a horizontal axis and is filled with culture medium, in which the cell aggregates depending on their natural cellular affinities are suspended under microgravity. The gravitational vectors may induce cell signalling and facilitate cell differentiation. In these bioreactors, cells are grown under low fluid–shear condition that facilitates oxygen and nutrient transport, thereby enabling cells to form complex 3D tissue-like aggregates (Mabvuure, Hindocha and Khan 2012; Rauh et al. 2011; Skardal et al. 2010). The configuration of a typical rotating wall vessel bioreactor is shown in Figure 7.2.

HOLLOW-FIBRE BIOREACTOR (HFB)

This bioreactor offers a 3D culture system and a novel approach for tissue regeneration. Two types of HFB configurations have been designed for tissue engineering applications: cylindrical and rectangular. In cylindrical HFB, a bundle of hollow fibers of semipermeable capillary membranes is encased in a cylindrical polycarbonate shell forming a bioreactor cartridge, which is fitted with ports that allow the flow of media surrounding the fibers. It comprises two-compartment modules having intracapillary and extracapillary spaces that ensure uniform axial distribution of nutrients. The cells are seeded into the bioreactor space and are expanded. The culture medium is pumped through the intracapillary space and the nutrients and oxygen are delivered to the cells through the hollow fiber membrane perfusion. When the cells expand, the produced metabolic waste products as well as CO_2 perfuse the membranes and are diffused away by the flow of medium via its intracapillary space. The accumulation of waste products due to increased cell mass can increase the medium flow rate, thereby resisting the inhibition of cell growth caused by the produced toxic waste (Marlovits et al. 2003). In a rectangular HFBs, the hollow fibre membrane is embedded in the scaffold with a rectangular shape. The cell culture medium flows through the internal lumen of the hollow fibres and cell sheets are cultured on the top of the polymeric HF membrane scaffold as shown in Figure 7.3 (Eghbali et al. 2016). HFB with its highest surface

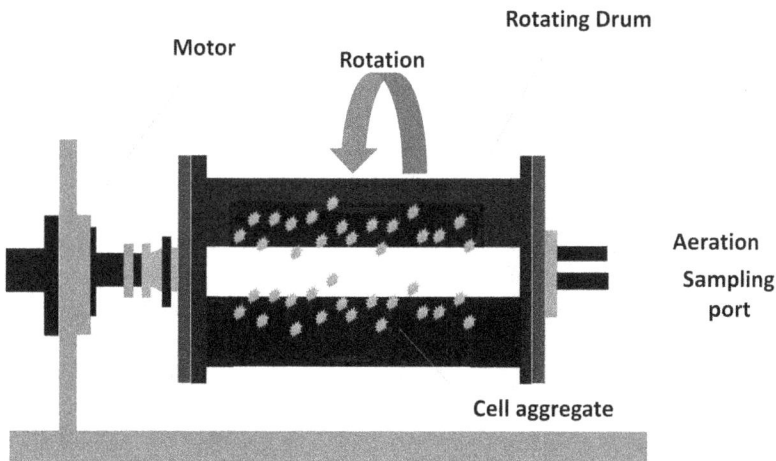

FIGURE 7.2   Rotating wall vessel bioreactor.

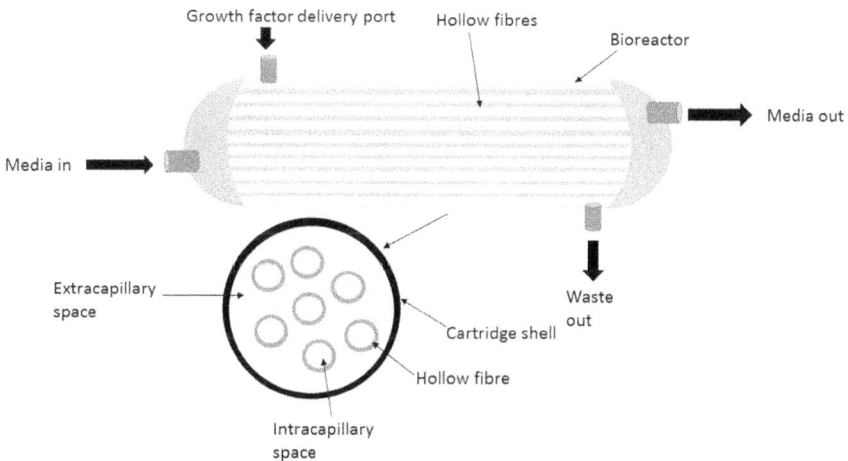

FIGURE 7.3   Hollow fibre bioreactor.

area to volume ratio among all the bioreactor configurations has many advantages like excellent nutrient transport, which often becomes a hurdle to engineer sizable constructs *in vitro*. In *in vivo*-like culture microenvironment, it can produce a high quantity of desired cellular products with less population variation, and at reasonable operating costs.

PERFUSION BIOREACTORS

Perfusion bioreactors are equipped with a pumping system, a culture media reservoir, and a perfusion cartridge for holding scaffolds. These bioreactors make 3D culture system and culture cells in a continuous mode by supplying fresh media containing cells and remove spent media continuously while maintaining the cells in the culture vessel. The cells can be maintained in the bioreactor by different means such as (i) using capillary fibers or membranes to which the cells are attached, (ii) using a filtration system that allows the removal of media while keeping the cells intact, and (iii) using a centrifuge that separates the cells and recycles them to the bioreactor. The flow perfusion bioreactor delivers cells to the scaffolds that are cascaded in a cartridge by a controlled flow of media using a suitable pumping system like peristaltic pump, where the flow of media reverses back and forth within the cell-seeded scaffold, the so-called construct. Thus, the culture medium forced through the internal porous network of the 3D matrix can overcome the limitation of the internal diffusion, thereby enhancing the transport of oxygen and nutrients to the cell culture media through the pores of the scaffolds (Salehi-Nik et al. 2013) as well as the removal of metabolic waste from the culture. Besides improving mass transfer and maintaining homogeneous cell suspension, the bioreactor can also provide high cell seeding efficiency. However, the mechanical stress produced may lead to the denaturation of the cultured cells. Therefore, the flow rate should be optimized in this bioreactor systems, to avoid cells from damage due to high flow rates, or insufficient nutrient and oxygen supply at low flow rate (Grayson et al. 2008). Figure 7.4 shows a typical perfusion bioreactor system.

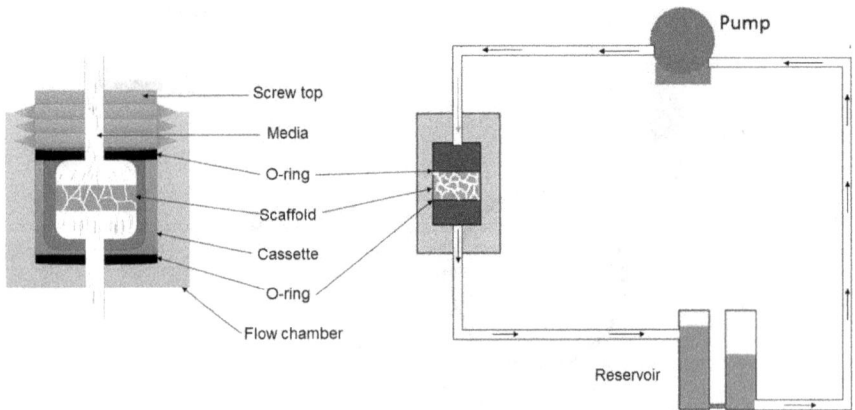

FIGURE 7.4 Flow perfusion bioreactor.

The perfusion bioreactor consists of four to six chambers which are usually made of polycarbonate. Transparent fluorinated ethylene propylene (FEP) membranes (copolymer of hexafluoropropylene and tetrafluoroethylene) are attached to both ends of each chamber using stainless steel bolts. These FEP membranes prevent the attachment of cells to the wall during long-time cultivation (Kleinhans et al. 2015). Furthermore, O-rings are used between perfusion chamber body and FEP membranes to prevent contamination. The perfusion chamber is linked to the media reservoir and the peristaltic pump through a silicon hose.

Quasi Vivos are the commercially available perfusion bioreactor systems that have been designed with different configurations. These bioreactors have several advantages, such as their simplicity, ease of operation, and design flexibility that provides a single flow of fresh medium, or recirculation of media, thereby protecting the cells from damage due to shock during media feeding; furthermore maintain laminar flow rate and chamber pressure making them suitable for different tissue types, promotse cellular activity and provide the ease of retrieving scaffolds from the culture. The bioreactors can be connected to multiple chambers and thus enabling culturing of multiple or the same cell types, thereby promoting better cell-cell or tissue–tissue interactions which are important phenomena for ECM synthesis or specific organ interactions (Sikavitsas et al. 2003). Moreover, the shear force generated from fluid-flow perfusion has shown enhanced expression of the osteoblast phenotype. In a study, when MSCs derived from bone marrow were cultured under static and perfusion conditions, the similar proliferation rate and alkaline phosphatase activity patterns were observed in both the cuture conditions, however, a significant increase in calcium deposition was achieved when the cell-seeded scaffolds (constructs) was cultured under perfused conditions (Gomes et al. 2003).

WAVE BIOREACTOR

This bioreactor is also known as cell bags bioreactor. These bioreactors consist of disposable plastic bags, in which cells and medium are housed and have ports for air circulation. The bags containing cells are kept in a electric rocking platform that provides efficient mixing of cells and medium by shaking the plastic bag alternating similar to wave motion under controlled rock frequency, thereby resulting in a homogeneous cell suspension and effective mass transfer while avoiding bubble formation and decreasing shear stress damage that often occurs in a conventional stir tank bioreactor. This bioreactor was first commercialized by GE Healthcare Life Sciences with Wave Bioreactor as a brand name (Singh 1999).

The use of disposable bags in these bioreactors Healthcare Life Sciences has the advantage of greatly reducing the risk of cross-contamination, thereby improving process safety and also offering easy scalability and oxygen transport efficiency. These bioreactors are suitable for the production of functional tissues following tissue engineering approach and also the expansion of human cells as therapeutic agents and other applications like production of virus for gene therapies and therapeutic proteins (Eibl and Eibl 2009). A typical wave bioreactor is shown in Figure 7.5. The German company Sartorius has developed a similar bioreactor under the trade name "BIOSTAT RM". Large-scale production of neutrophils from

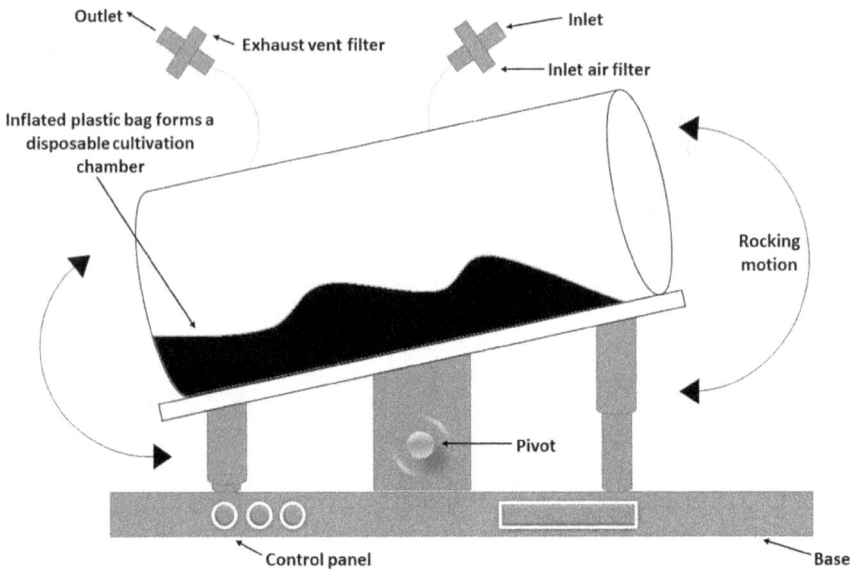

FIGURE 7.5 Wave bioreactor.

HSC's T cells in a 10 L wave bioreactor achieved higher than ten fold production in comparison to that obtained by using traditional 2D culture method. However, a disposable wave bioreactor systems may be expensive.

ROLLER BOTTLE CULTURES

Roller bottles (RBs) are disposable and cylindrical plastic container used for cell culturing. RBs with surface area of about 500–1700 cm² are kept in a rack rolling inside an incubator and rotated slowly at a range from 5 to 240 rph to bathe the cells. RBs are suitable for cell culture volumes of 0.1–0.3 L and higher volumes like 1–1.5 L. A typical roller bottle culture system is depicted in Figure 7.6. In these types of bioreactors, cells having adhering or anchorage-dependent characteristics are attached to the interior surface of the bottles and the attached cells are alternately exposed to gases in the bottle headspace and nutrients from culture medium through the rotating motion. These systems are manually controlled, which makes it difficult to monitor culturing parameters like pH and DO, as well as their scale up even by increasing the bottle size. Apart from adherent culture, these are also used for laboratory-scale suspension culture.

Corning roller bottles (CRBs) are popular for cell culturing and CRBs rotating between 5 and 60 rph are most commonly used for initial scale-up of the attached cells. The cells are attached to the inner surface of the bottles. It can provide a large surface area for the cells to be attached and for their growth. Therefore, a large quantity of anchorage-dependent cells can be cultured economically without much labor requirement in comparison to the conventional cell culture flask. This type of cell culturing system offers the advantages like its mild agitation does not damage the cells and also prevents the formation of gradients within the medium that may affect

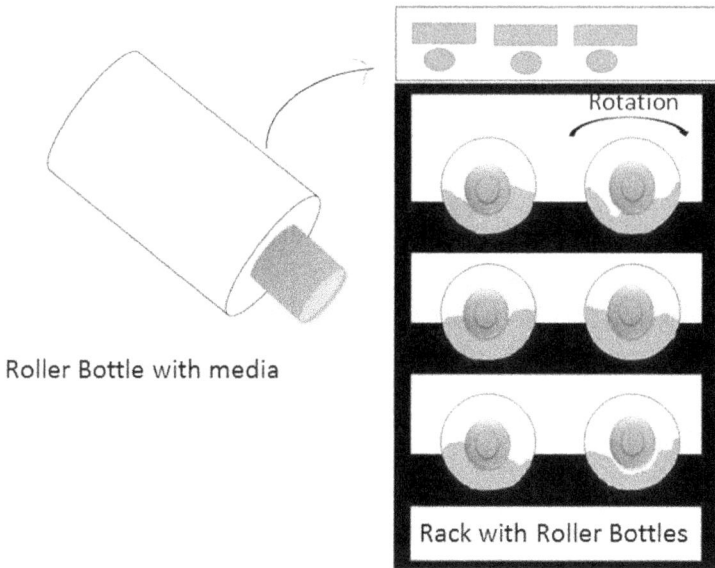

Roller Bottle with media

Rotation

Rack with Roller Bottles

FIGURE 7.6 Roller bottle culture system.

cellular growth and superior gas exchange because cells are mostly covered by a thin layer of medium.

MICROCARRIER-BASED BIOREACTOR

The microcarrier culture system was first reported by Van Wezel in 1967 (Van Wezel 1967). Microcarriers have the advantage of providing a large surface area to volume ratio favourable for the attachment of a large number of cells under controlled and homogeneous culture conditions and overcoming the limitation of traditional flask culture system that often leads to inadequate cell density because of having low surface area to volume ratio. Figure 7.7 represents a microcarrier-based bioreactor system. One of the major categories of the commercially available microcarriers is the solid, either spherical or disk-shaped, particles that are made from polymers such as dextran, cellulose and polystyrene. The porous microcarrier is another category that is made of biopolymers like gelatin, collagen, and fibrin and the porous structures can facilitate cell growth within their internal pores. The microcarriers prepared from collagen-coated dextran and matrigel-coated cellulose showed their ability to promote the proliferation of hESCs in stirred bioreactors with higher cell yields.

Bioreactors when combined with micro-carriers enhance the rate of cell proliferation, reduce production cost, and considerably improves relative repeatability. Micro-carriers are able to promote cell adhesion and maintain cell suspension in the culture system, thereby increasing the number of cultured cells (Jorgenson et al. 2018; Chen et al. 2006; Lam et al. 2017). Bioreactor in combination with microcarriers were employed for the expansion of hMSCs with superior process control and

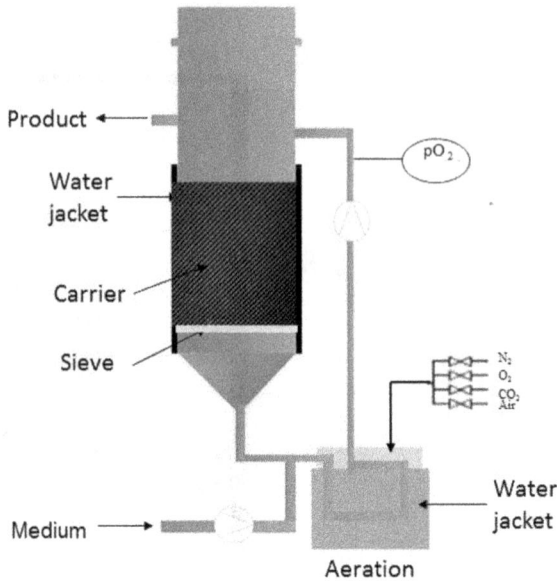

FIGURE 7.7   Micro-carriers based bioreactor.

monitoring and thereby maintaining a higher consistency and efficiency, resulting in hMSC based products that were more accessible and affordable (Couto et al. 2020). In another study, matrigel-coated microcarriers also supported the culture and differentiation of hESCs into the endoderm. However, the applications of microcarrier based bioreactor systems suffer from the difficulty in recovering the cells from the microcarriers (Skardal et al. 2010).

In an *in vitro* cell culture experiment, the cocultured bovine chondrocytes and cytodex-3 microcarriers in a rotating -wall vessel bioreactor indicated that the 3D environment of the coculture system have a role in the cell growth, differentiation, and cartilage ECM formation. The coculture systems reduce the cost and also enhance oxygen exchange, maintain extracellular environment, and regulate oxygen partial pressure and pH of the cell culture media, thereby effectively regulating the tissue-engineered cells (Fu et al. 2021). In a study, bioreactors combined with biodegradable poly (epsilon-caprolactone) microcarriers remarkably enhanced the expansion of hMSCs and various cell secretion factors (Lam et al. 2017). The microcarrier-based bioreactor system is reported to be an attractive and efficient method for culturing cells and augmenting the phenotype expression. Microcarriers has also played a role in delivering both undifferentiated and differentiated cells to the defect tissue region, rendering them suitable for tissue engineering applications, especially in repairing of damaged cartilage and bone (Malda and Frondoza 2006). Microcarrier-based spinner flask culture system has been successfully used to propagate chondrocytes and osteoblasts, for the analysis of cell response and various tissue engineering applications.

Microencapsulation-Based Bioreactors

Microencapsulation based bioreactor is a type of bioreactor that uses microcapsule. Cell microencapsulation is an attractive technique that protects the cells from hydrodynamic shear damage, prevents the cells from excessive agglomeration, and facilitates the effective transport of nutrients, gases, and cell signalling molecules like growth factors to the cell culture media through the microcapsule matrix (Zimmermann et al. 2007). hESCs encapsulated in sodium alginate beads were able to maintain their pluripotency for a prolonged period of time, of about 9 months, with higher cell survival rate than that shown in the conventional 2D static flask culturing method and without excessive cell aggregation. However, this method suffers from difficulty in separation and recovery of cells from the encapsulated matrix or hydrogels and hence poses a great challenge. In this context, direct transplantation of cell-encapsulated microcapsules may be an attractive approach.

Microfluidic Bioreactor

Microfluidic bioreactors having length scale at micro level similar to the dimensions of most cells can create *in vivo*-like microenvironment, thus enabling the study of cell behaviour as well as their internal organization in an innate microenvironment. These bioreactors have numerous advantages over the conventionally used macroscale bioreactor systems such as enhanced biological function, quality cell-based information, requirement of smaller sample volume, portability, less power consumption and space requirement, and lower cost (Pasirayi et al. 2011). The microfabrication methods that are usually employed to fabricate microfluidic devices and have been described elsewhere (Becker and Gärtner 2008; Chinn 2010; Rashid et al. 2010). Microfluidic devices often consider organ-on-chips in which a special type of cells can be cultured and continuously perfused inside the chambers with micrometer size dimension, which has the ability to model the physiological functions of the tissue or organ (Bhatia and Ingber 2014). However, the major limitations of these devices are associated with the non-standard culture protocols that often involve complex operational control and chip design. Besides, the changes in scaling may be a constraint in adapting biological procedures to fit experiments based on the microsystem, like media and cell concentration. (Velve-Casquillas et al. 2010). Microfluidic systems using soft lithographic techniques were first introduced by Whitesides, 2001. The most common polymer used for lithography is polydimethylsiloxane (PDMS), which is biocompatible, transparent, elastomeric, and permeable. These systems can be designed with extreme precision and nutrient and gas transfer is also easy at the micron level. Microfluidic chips are now being used to study viability and proliferation in different cell culture conditions, time lapse studies, high throughput screening, and mechanotransduction.

The different bioreactor configurations and applications, and their advantages and disadvantages are presented in Tables 7.1 and 7.2.

TABLE 7.1
Different types of bioreactors and their applications

Type of Bioreactor	Cell Type and Cell Organization	Specific Application	Performance of Cell Culture	Reference
Stirred tank bioreactors	Multipotent embryonic stem cells (mESCs) aggregates	Expansion of mESCs	31-fold expansion in 5 days	(Liu et al. 2014)
	Human pluripotent stem cells (hPSCs) aggregates	Expansion of hPSCs	6–8-fold expansion in 7 days	(Kropp et al. 2016)
	Pluripotent stem cell-derived EBs	Differentiation of cardiomyocyte, haematopoietic progenitors	6–7-fold expansion in 10 days, 30% contracting EBs	(Liu et al. 2014)
	iPSCs aggregates	Derivation, expansion, and differentiation of human iPSCs	58-fold expansion in 4 days	(Ackermann et al. 2022)
	Neural stem cells (NSCs) aggregates	Expansion and transplantation of NSCs	9-fold expansion in 7 days	(Liu et al. 2014)
	Mesenchymal stem cells (MSCs) aggregates	Expansion and differentiation of MSCs	<5% proliferating cells; increased osteogenic differentiation	(King and Miller 2007)
	CSCs aggregates	Expansion of CSCs	20-fold expansion per batch	(Liu et al. 2014)
	Hematopoietic stem cells (HSCs)	Expansion of HSCs	22-fold expansion of colony forming cell (CFC) in 4 weeks	(Andrade-Zaldívar, Santos, and De León Rodríguez 2008)
Rotary cell culture system (RCCS)	PSC-derived EBs	Differentiation of PSCs into cardiomyocytes, neural progenitors; hemotopoietic progenitors	1.5–2-fold more EB forming efficiency; promoted lineage-specific differentiation	(Liu et al. 2014)
	MSCs and HSCs	Expansion of MSCs and HSCs simultaneously	9-fold expansion Stro-1$^+$ CD44$^+$ MSCs in 8 days	(Chen, Xu et al. 2006)

Bioreactor	Cell type	Application	Results	Reference
Wave bioreactors	HSCs	Expansion of haematopoietic cell	10-fold expansion and higher than observed with traditional methods	(Liu et al. 2014)
Microcarrier-based bioreactors	mESCs	Expansion of mESCs	2.5–3.9-fold expansion	(Alfred et al. 2011)
	hPSCs	Expansion of hPSCs	5–7-fold expansion in 5 days	(Badenes et al. 2016)
		Differentiation of hPSCs to cardiomyocyte, endoderm, and neural progenitors	Cardiomyocyte: 2×10^5 cells/mL; Endoderm cells: 1.2×10^6 cells/mL; Neural progenitors: 1.0×10^7 cells/mL	
Scaffold bioreactors	MSCs	Expansion of MSCs	20-fold expansion in 8–10 days	(Lembong et al. 2020)
	PSC-derived EBs	Differentiation of PSCs into vascular and bone cells over alginate polymer scaffolds	2-fold higher differentiation than using static cultures	(Liu et al. 2014)
	MSCs	Osteogenic differentiation	2–3-fold more differentiation	(Zhang, Eyisoylu et al. 2021)
	mESCs	Neuronal differentiation	71% neuronal cells	(Grossemy, Chan, and Doran 2021)
Fibrous bed bioreactors	hESCs	Expansion of hESCs	60-fold expansion in 55 days; 60–70% neural cells	(Oh et al. 2009)
	Amniotic fluid-derived stem cells (AFSCs)	Differentiation into neural cells		(Liu et al. 2014)
		Expansion of amniotic fluid-derived stem cells	Maintain osteogenic and adipogenic differentiation	(Liu, Li, and Yang 2014)
Microencapsulation-based bioreactors	PSCs	For PSC self-renewal	Self-renewal capability shown for 260 days	(Fridley, Kinney, and McDevitt 2012)
	ESCs	Differentiation into cardiomyocytes and osteoblasts	9-fold higher in 15 days	(Pandolfi et al. 2017)
	MSCs	Differentiation into adipocytes in fixed-bed bioreactor	Adipocytes differentiation was similar to stirred tank bioreactor	(Liu et al. 2014)
Hollow-fibre bioreactors	PSCs	Expansion of hPSC	Low harvested cell density	(Liu et al. 2014)
	MSCs	Differentiation into adipocytes	Enhanced adipocyte differentiation	(Nold et al. 2013)

TABLE 7.2
Advantages and Disadvantages of Different Bioreactors

Type of Bioreactor	Purpose	Advantages	Disadvantages	References
Perfusion bioreactor	Growth and differentiation study of bone marrow stromal cells	Convective media flow improved nutrient delivery through the scaffold; Maintenance of cell viability and differentiation; Scalable tissue growth		(Gandhi et al. 2019)
Stirred tank bioreactor	Growth and differentiation of suspended cells	Offers aggregate culture; homogeneous culture environment; scalability	High shear stress	(Mizukami et al. 2016)
Microencapsulation-based bioreactor stirred tank, rotary cell culture systems (RCCS)	Immobilized cells are cultured onto the scaffolds	Protects from shear stress and provides 3D microenvironment	The cells are to be released from the hydrogels	(Liu et al. 2014)
Perfusion-chambered bioreactor	Production of clinically important tissue-engineered product using goat bone marrow stromal cells	Increase in product quantity and reduction in required steps and storage space	Mechanical force-generated fluid flow causes cells shearing	(Janssen et al. 2006)
Autoclavable and modular perfusion bioreactor	Study of large-scale cell culture of tissue-engineered bone	Uniform nutrient transfer in bigger scaffolds, thereby reducing the scaffold core's necrosis		(Bhaskar et al. 2018)
Fixed bed, fluidized bed, and fibrous bed bioreactors	Immobilization of cells in to 3D scaffolds	Can maintain 3D microenvironment; allows spatial organization of cell; regulates proliferation, differentiation, and ECM formation	Difficult to harvest cells	(Liu et al. 2014)

Ultrasonic-assisted microfluidic perfusion bioreactor	Engineering of 3D scaffold-free neocartilage grafts of human articular chondrocytes	Low shear rate; enhanced mass transfer rate	Chances of robust chondrogenesis	(Li et al. 2014)
Wave bioreactor	Culture of cell-seeded scaffolds continuously under motion	Haematopoietic stem cells; low shear stress; scalability	Sophisticated and expensive	(Rousseau, Giarratana, and Douay 2014)
Spinner Flask bioreactor	Cultivation of cartilage and cardiac constructs	Decreases stationary cell layer near the construct surface and provides the cells with a suitable mixed environment	Cartilaginous tissue produced forms an exterior fibrous capsule due to turbulent flow; high shear stress.	(Chen, Lee et al. 2006)
	For growth of suspension cultures in liquid media; Mostly used in bone tissue engineering	Higher proliferation, differentiation, and distribution of cells in scaffolds than static culture; Better oxygen and nutrients transport than rotating wall vessels	Not all the cells are exposed to the same shear loads due to significant variation in the magnitude of shear stresses between various sites	(Zhang et al. 2010)
Recirculation column bioreactor	Development of osteochondral composite constructs	Establishment of direct contact between tissue-engineered cartilage and bone resulting in substantial enhancement in cartilage quality		(Mahmoudifar and Doran 2005)

(continued)

TABLE 7.2 (Continued)
Advantages and Disadvantages of Different Bioreactors

Type of Bioreactor	Purpose	Advantages	Disadvantages	References
Concentric cylinder bioreactor	Cartilage tissue engineering indicating increased construct production (about 16 constructs can be cultivated in the reactor)	Decreased shear stress and massive growth surface area	Non-availability of oxygen probes due to complex instrumentation	(Williams, Saini, and Wick 2002)
Rotating-wall vessel bioreactor	Bone, cartilage, liver, neuronal, adipose epithelial and cardiac tissues engineering	Proper cell morphology, viability, and strong capability to develop bone tissue	---	(Zhang et al. 2009)
Double-chambered bioreactor	Designed for coculturing of chondrocytes and osteoblasts	Efficient cell culturing on biphasic scaffold	Limited culture medium diffusion in the scaffold	(Chang et al. 2004)
Double-chambered stirring bioreactor	Potency study of a tissue-engineered osteochondral graft	Adequate mechanical stimulation	---	(Pei et al. 2014)
Rotating-shaft bioreactor	Dual-phase cultivation of tissue-engineered cartilage	Effective medium and surface-aeration based oxygen transfer	---	(Chen, Lee et al. 2006)

Bioreactor	Application	Advantages	Limitations	Reference
Rotating wall vessel (RWV) bioreactor	Generation of sizeable and fast-growing organoids	Low shear and turbulence environment; High mass transfer with increased level of metabolic function; Controlled oxygen transfer with creation of microgravity environment	Decreased cell viability and disruption of cell agglomeration and differentiation due to bubble formation	(Phelan et al. 2019)
Rotating wall bioreactor vessel	Chondrogenesis study using aged human articular chondrocytes	Low shear, efficient mass transfer, enhanced cell–cell interaction, and less chance of cell damage		(Marlovits et al. 2003)
Hollow fiber membrane bioreactor	Study of scaffold pore morphology (bone tissue engineering)	Proper separation of cell culture media from waste substances; Enhanced nutrient transport	Choice of the solutes depends on the pore size and permeability of the membrane; Potential membrane damage	(Wang et al. 2021)
Hollow fibre membrane bioreactor	Large-scale engineering of 3D bone tissue	Promotes high-density cell growth; Attainment of high flow rates without damaging the cells; Cell growth and proliferation are facilitated by hollow fibres in the gel matrix within the additional capillary gaps; Channels or the lumen region provide an appropriate microenvironment	Sample collection is challenging during tissue formation in the bioreactor	(Mohebbi-Kalhori et al. 2012)
Hollow fibre membrane bioreactor	3D bone tissue growth	Suitable for bulk 3D bone tissue growth	Difficult bioreactor design; higher mass transfer limitation	(Abdullah et al. 2006)

CELL–SCAFFOLD INTERACTION AND TISSUE REGENERATION

Scaffolds that are the analogs of extracellular matrices act as regulators of cellular activities that influence the viability, division, growth, function, and mobility of the seeded cells. This is known as cell– scaffold interaction. The proper interaction between the cells and the scaffold is the most crucial aspect in in vitro production of engineered tissue construct. The different types of cell–biomaterial interactions that occur during the tissue construct/graft production are cell seeding, cell adhesion, cell migration, and cell aggregation, which are described in the next section.

CELL SEEDING

The seeding or loading of cell so called "cell seeding" is the first step in the inter-action between the cells and the scaffold which is one of the vital events for tissue regeneration process. The seeding of the cells involving the initial cell attachment into the scaffold is a significant step to achieve the desired functional properties of the engineered tissues. The seeding process involves cell distribution throughout the scaffold in the culture vessel to obtain adequate cell density and homogeneous cell distribution. The efficiency of the seeding process and cell distribution has a great influence on the biological performance of the scaffold and ultimate tissue regen-eration (Wendt et al. 2006). Therefore, cell seeding is one of the challenging steps for the construction of construct or tissue graft through tissue engineering approach and becomes more critical when cells are seeded onto a 3D highly porous complex scaffold structure. A number of techniques have been developed for the seeding of cells with the progress in tissue engineering field over the past few decades; and some of the important methods are described in the following section.

CELL SEEDING METHODS

The cells can be seeded into the scaffold by diverse methods which can be broadly classified into two categories: static seeding or gravitational seeding and dynamic seeding.

Static or Gravitational Seeding

It is the most common and the simplest seeding process that consists of injecting cell suspension on the surface of the scaffold, allowing the cells to settle or infiltrate into the scaffold by gravitational force, and finally attach and/or adhere to the sur-face over time (Tan, Ren, and Kuijer 2012). A typical static cell seeding method is shown in Figure 7.8. Although it is a simple process, the method suffers from many disadvantages such as poor seeding efficiency, lack of penetration into the scaffold structure and reproducibility, longer seeding time causing contamination, and non-uniform cell distribution within scaffold (Villalona et al. 2010; Bueno, Laevsky, and Barabino 2007; Thevenot et al. 2008) that ultimately result in poor cell attachment. Moreover, cell attachment is restricted mainly to outer surface compared to the interior of the scaffold, which may be due to the rapid flow of cell suspension through

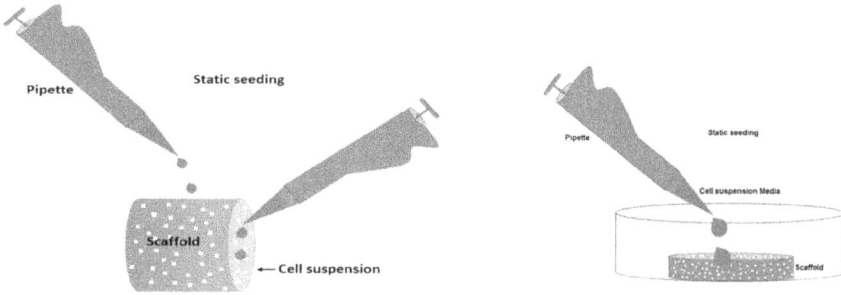

FIGURE 7.8 Static cell seeding method.

the scaffold to the bottom of the culture plate (Kim et al. 1998) and partly due to weak gravitational force limiting the infiltration.

Modified Static Seeding Techniques

To overcome the limitations of the static method, various modified static cell seeding methods have been developed. These methods include centrifugal cell seeding, low-pressure cell seeding, and magnetic cell seeding, which are described next.

Centrifugal Cell Seeding

This method of cell seeding applies centrifugal force that assists the penetration of cells onto the scaffold. The method offers better cell insertion and a more homogeneous cell distribution in the scaffold. The method has the major disadvantage of difficulty in controlling the orientation of scaffold during the seeding process, and the centrifugal forces may affect the function of the cell.

Low-Pressure or Vacuum Cell Seeding

In this method, the desired cell population and the scaffolds are kept into a sterile vacuum desiccator and vacuum is applied to create low pressure in the desiccator for the removal of air from the scaffold that results in enhancement of cell entry into the scaffold as shown in Figure 7.9. This method has the advantage of easy operation and application to a wide variety of porous scaffolds. However, the low-pressure atmosphere may have the adverse impact of altering the cell function and cell characteristics because of genetic mutation (Villalona et al. 2010).

Magnetic Cell Seeding

In this seeding method, magnetic force is applied to attract the nanoparticles to be attached to the cells to be seeded in to the scaffold. In this method, magnetic particles are attached to the desired cell population to enhance their penetration into the porous scaffold and the cells are pulled into the scaffold pores by applying a magnetic force across the scaffold. The process involves the use of a supermagnetic iron with micro-or nano-beads that are capable of separating the desired cell population from a cell suspension through specific binding to the desired cells or proteins (Villalona et al. 2010)

Vacuum Seeding

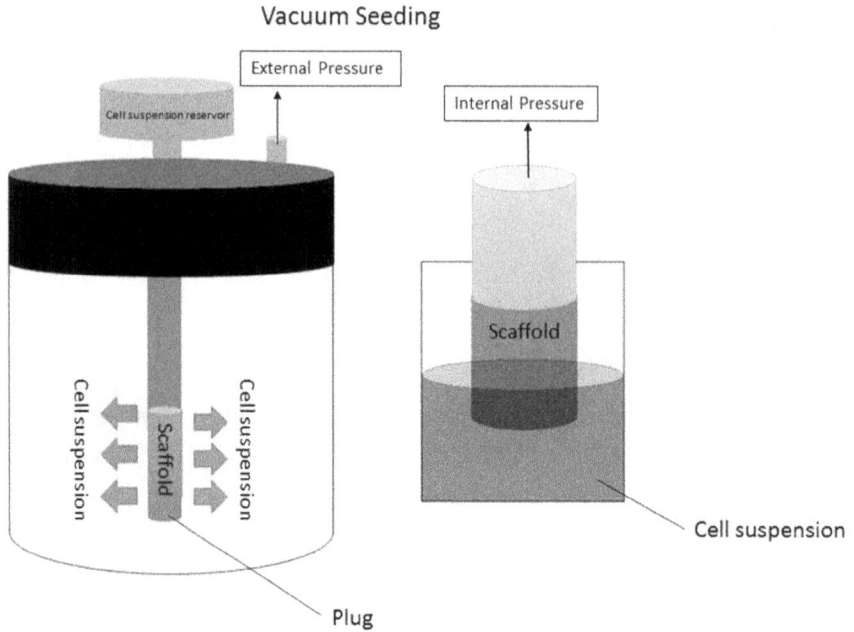

FIGURE 7.9 Vacuum or low-pressure cell seeding technique.

and the magnetically separated cells are characterized by specific surface receptors followed by conjugating the separated cells with the magnetic nanoparticles as shown in Figure 7.10 and then the cells are seeded onto the scaffold. The nanoparticle-conjugated cells are pulled toward the magnet, which is placed below the scaffold and align themselves in the scaffold surface accordingly (Dai et al. 2009).

The advantage of this method includes the enhanced cell seeding efficiency and the selectivity of the desired cell type using antibodies that enable magnetic particles to be attached to the cells (Dar et al. 2002). This method can manipulate cells without direct physical contact and at a distance, and also localize the cells in a specific area and pattern. However, this method may cause nonspecific binding of the magnetic particles with the undesired cells. Moreover, the application of the magnetic particles and subsequently the magnetic force may alter the gene expression levels in the target cells (Sasaki et al. 2008).

Dynamic Cell Seeding

Although diverse static cell seeding methods have been developed, they have several limitations and no method is perfectly efficient for promoting the cell seeding of cells on the scaffold or can improve the function of long-term engineered graft. Therefore, an efficient, fast, and able method to provide a uniform cell seeding and thereby improve the clinical potential of engineered tissue grafts is of great importance. One way to achieve these cell seeding requirements is the design and use of bioreactor.

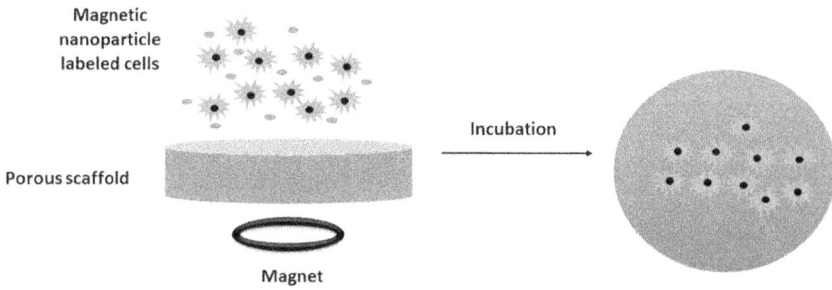

FIGURE 7.10   Magnet-assisted cell seeding technique.

This method is referred to as the dynamic cell seeding technique. Various bioreactors were discussed in the previous section, some of which are also used for seeding cell onto the scaffold efficiently. Dynamic seeding has the advantages of providing higher efficiency of cell seeding, more uniform cell distribution, and penetration of cells onto the scaffold in comparison to static methods (Villalona et al. 2010). Among the bioreactors, spinner flask bioreactor and perfusing bioreactors have widely been used for the seeding of cells in the scaffold matrix.

CELL ADHESION

Cell adhesion is a process or mechanism by which cells interact within themselves and bind to other cells at their surfaces through cell adhesion molecules containing specialized protein molecules, which is represented as cell–cell adhesion or interaction with and binding to an ECM component. In tissue engineering, the adherent or anchorage-dependent cultured cells need to be attached to an insoluble solid surface for their growth, proliferation, and viability. 3D scaffolds provide a more realistic *in vitro* and *in vivo* culture environment for bone and cartilage tissue regeneration. Cell adhesion is usually regulated by cell adhesion molecules present in the scaffold that eventually recognize the different ligands at the cell junctions and in the engineered matrices. Cell adhesion is important for the necessary cell communication and regulation, development and maintenance of tissues, survival and growth of seeded cells, and neotissue formation (Sytnyk, Leshchyns'ka, and Schachner 2017; Benson et al. 2000).

Cell adhesion to a surface matrix is a critical factor because it is greatly influenced by other important factors such as cell morphology and cell spreading, cell migration, and also function of differentiated cells as shown in Figure 7.11. 3D scaffolds are used to achieve a more realistic *in vitro* culture environment and hence sucessful tissue regeneration. Cell adhesion involves three different phenomena including the cell attachment and morphology, cell proliferation and cell spreading, and focal adhesion.

At stage of cell attachment, cells are adhered and/or attached to the surface of the ECM and form monolayer coverage on the scaffold. In cell spreading, the surface attached cells are divided through the process of mitosis and proliferated, thereby covering the surface of the scaffold. The cells are also penetrated within

Extracellular space

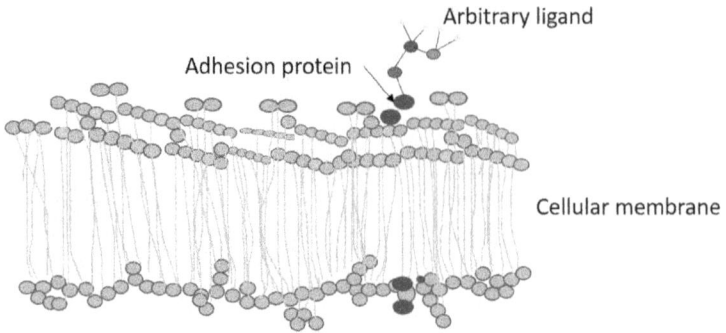

FIGURE 7.11   Cell adhesion.

the interconnected pores of the 3D matrices. Focal adhesions also called cell-matrix adhesion are multi-protein structures which establish mechanical linkages between the ECM matrix and the interacting cells over it. In focal adhesions, the cellular proteins which are cell adhesion molecules link actin filaments within cells to fibronectins. The adapter proteins such as talins, vinculins, and α-actinins form large, dynamic multi-protein complexes. The cytoskeleton proteins such as integrin, actin, and myosin present outside the cytoplasm connects to the ECM or scaffold through these formed dynamic protein complexes. Among these, integrins, the trans-membrane proteins, are mostly bound to ligands present in the ECM, whereas the other end of integrin connects to sub-membrane plaque that subsequently connects to the cytoskeleton (e.g. actin filaments) of the cells. The phenomena of focal adhesion are depicted in Figure 7.12.

ASSESSMENT OF CELL ADHESION

The extent of cell adhesion is determined by various techniques that include (i) sedimentation-detachment assay, (ii) centrifugation assay, and (iii) fluid-flow chamber technique. These techniques are described in the following section.

Sedimentation-Detachment Assay

In this method, cell suspensions are subjected to sedimentation onto a polymer or protein-coated surface of the culture vessel. The sedimented cells are then incubated in culture media for a desired time period. After incubation, the loosely adhered cells are detached by removing the culture medium followed by thorough washing. The extent of cellular adhesion can be quantified either by counting the number of cells that remain attached to the coated surface or by determining the number of cells that

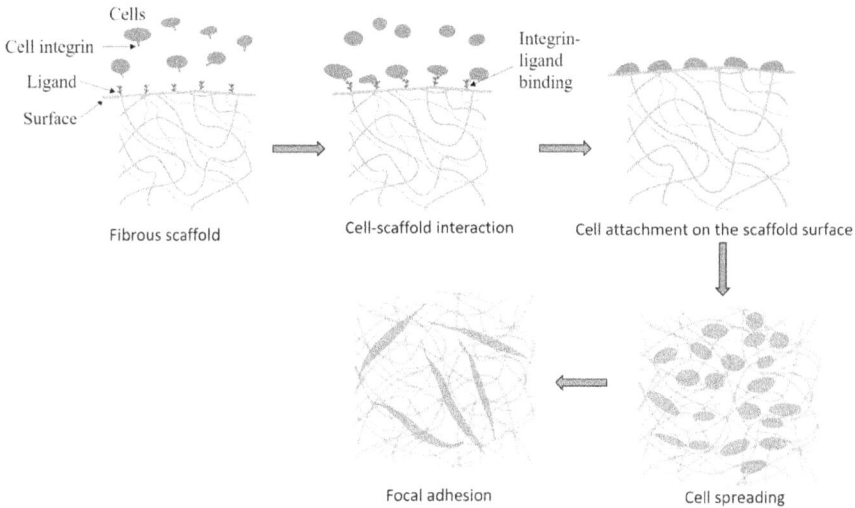

FIGURE 7.12   Focal adhesion.

are separated from the washes. A typical schematic diagram of the sedimentation-detachment assay is presented in Figure 7.13.

Centrifugation Assay

In this assessment method, cells are seeded on the scaffold surface in a coated culture vessel and are incubated in a culture medium for a specific time period. After incubation, the culture plate is inverted and the cells are detached by applying a controlled centrifugal force. Like sedimentation-detachment method, the cell adhesion is quantified by determining the number of cells remaining adhered to the coated surface. The centrifugation method is shown in Figure 7.14.

Fluid-Flow Chambers

In this technique, cells detachment is done by applying the fluid mechanical forces in a well-regulated and quantifiable manner. Cell suspension flows into a rectangular chamber, the bottom surface of which is coated with a polymer or a protein, and the cells are then allowed to settle down and attached onto the coated surface. After incubation, the fluid is forced between two parallel plates and the non-adherent cells are washed away with the flow of fluid, whereas the adhered or attached cells remaining on the surface are quantified. A fluid-flow chamber for the evaluation of cell adhesion is shown in Figure 7.15.

CELL MIGRATION

Cell migration refers to the movement of cells from one location to the other. Cell migration becomes crucial within a tissue for the formation of the appropriate tissue architecture. In any tissue engineering technique, the ability of the movement of the

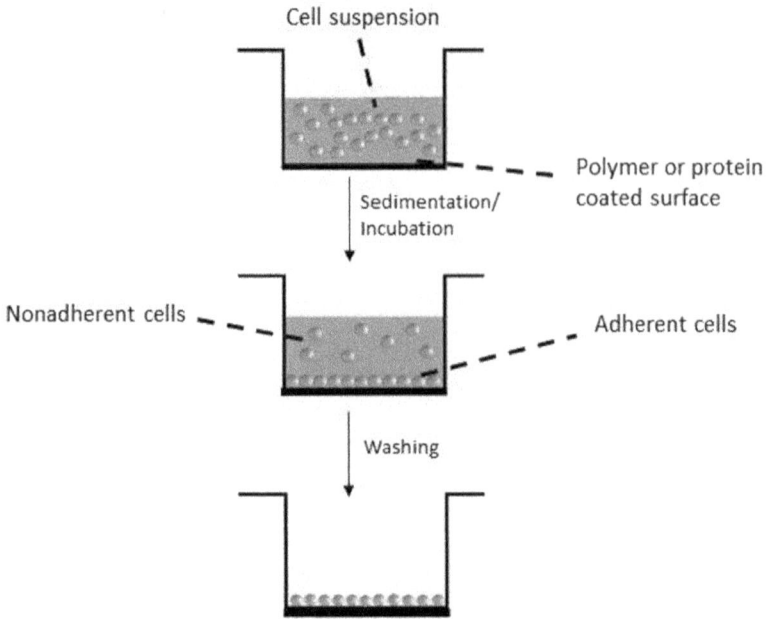

FIGURE 7.13 Sedimentation-detachment assay for cell adhesion.

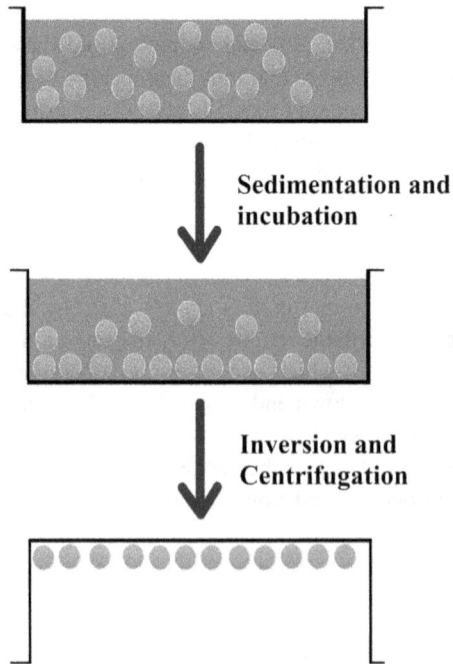

FIGURE 7.14 A schematic diagram showing the centrifugation assay for cell adhesion.

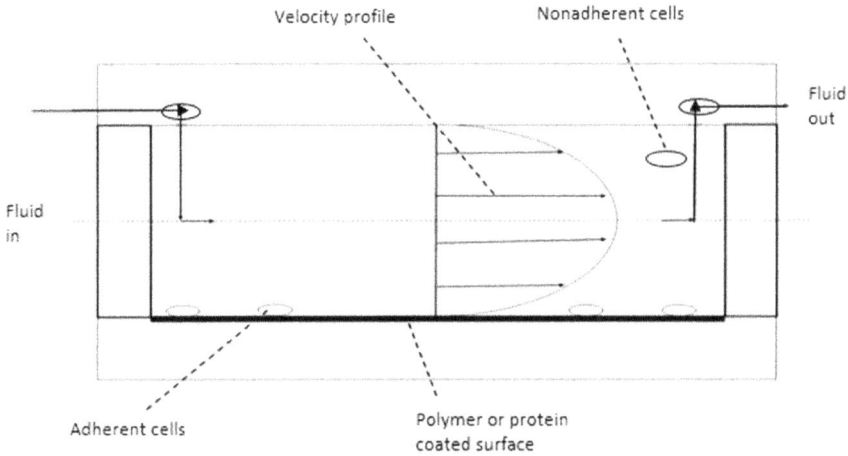

FIGURE 7.15 Fluid-flow chambers for cell adhesion assessment.

cells, in association with the scaffold surface or through the other cells, is a vital event for the neotissue regeneration. The efficiency and the mode of cell migration depends on various factors that are related to cell and ECM properties (Qu, Guilak, and Mauck 2019). The migration or locomotion of cells within a 3D complex scaffold structure is more difficult compared to 2D matrix and it depends on the composition, stiffness, and structure of ECM (Lo et al. 2000; Cukierman et al. 2001; Baker and Chen 2012). Cells are also sensitive to mechanical and biochemical factors influencing their motility (Lo et al. 2000; Stoker and Gherardi 1991). Cell migration is a critical phenomenon for bone and more complex joint tissue regeneration for defects with critical size specifically (Yang et al. 2017). The cell migration in the ECM is assessed by a number of methods, such as Under agarose test, filter assay, and direct visualization. In the Under agarose test, the cell suspension is placed in a well containing semisolid agarose, where the motile cells crawl on the solid substrate underneath the agarose as shown in Figure 7.16.

In the filter assay, the cell suspension is placed on a filter paper having smaller size of pores. The motile cells crawl through these pores to the other side, where they are detected and quantified. Figure 7.17 presents a schematic of this method. In the direct visualization assay, the paths of movement of the individual cells are directly observed by a microscope for cells migrating onto the surfaces and within the solid gels.

CELL AGGREGATION

In tissue engineering, cell aggregation involving the clustering of cells together is an important stage in neotissue development. It is useful for rapid and controlled formation of the targeted ECM structure that mimics the architectural and functional characteristics of the native tissue by correlating and re-establishing the cell–cell interaction, thereby enhancing tissue formation (Mahoney and Saltzman 2001). The

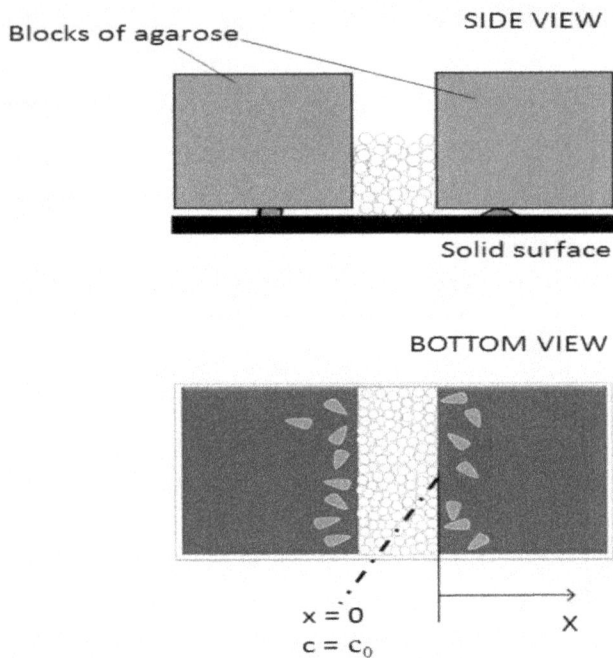

FIGURE 7.16   Under agarose test for cell migration assessment.

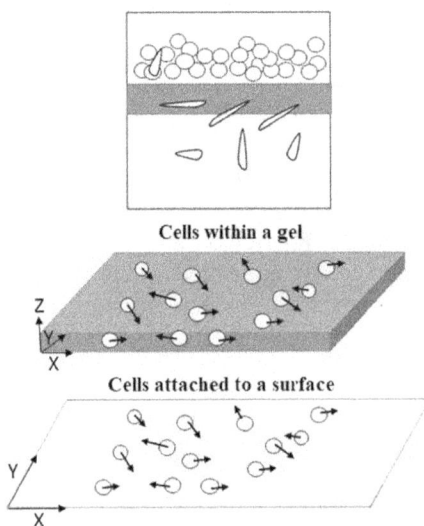

FIGURE 7.17   Filter assay method for cell migration assessment.

morphology of the cell aggregation improves the cell function and cell survival rate in aggregate culture. The cell aggregates are usually formed by incubating cells in suspension with mild rotational agitation. The addition of serum or serum proteins can promote cell aggregation. PEG conjugated with Arginine-Glycine-Aspartic acid (RGD) (fibronectin) and Phenylalanine-Isoleucine-Glycine-Serine-Arginine (YIGSR) (fibronectin) cell-binding peptides promoted cell aggregation in a suspension culture (Boateng et al. 2005).

Cell aggregation is assessed by different techniques, including the direct visualization, electronic particle counter, and aggregometers. This is a widely used method, in which the size of cell aggregate is monitored to determine the extent of aggregation. Electronic particle counter which was invented by Moscona (1961) determines the kinetics of cell aggregation by measuring cell aggregate size distribution over time. This method observes the disappearance of single cells with time by computer-based image analysis. Aggregometers are used to measure the small-angle light scattering through rotating sample cuvettes, thereby making continuous record of the growth of cell aggregate.

BONE, CARTILAGE, AND JOINT TISSUE REGENERATION IN BIOREACTOR

Bioreactors are used in tissue engineering to overcome the drawbacks of the static culturing conditions and to obtain uniform distribution of cells within the scaffolds, and provide sufficient levels of oxygen, nutrients, cytokines, and growth factors, and to expose the cultured cells to mechanical stimuli. Dynamic condition of cell culture has also been shown to influence stem cells differentiation. Spinner flask, the simplest dynamic culture system, provides efficient mass transport and mechanical stimulation, which are beneficial for generating cartilage construct. The phenotype of chondrocytes was observed to be maintained when cultured in spinner flask. However, these studies were limited to the inherent capability of autologous chondrocytes towards forming cell aggregate, thereby generating a 3D structure or getting encapsulated into the gel beads that have limitations associated with aggregate size and rupture on implantation (Agrawal et al. 2018). Therefore, there is a need for systematic research for construct generation in spinner flask bioreactor using the combination of appropriate cells and scaffold, and validating their performance over the widely used static culture technique. Spinner flasks have also been used for bone tissue regeneration because they can mimic native bone environment. However, these bioreactors offer certain limitations such as they restrict the ECM production to the scaffolds surface only and create turbulent shear at the surfaces mixing the media, which affect cell growth and tissue formation (Gaspar, Gomide, and Monteiro 2012). This bioreactor promoted osteogenesis of mesenchymal stem cells that were isolated from rat over 3D scaffolds with respect to alkaline phosphatase (ALP) activity and secretion of osteocalcin. Moreover, the constructs upon culturing showed a higher rate of cell proliferation and calcium content than those obtained with conventional flask system (Sikavitsas, Bancroft, and Mikos 2002). The influence of the flow field was investigated in a spinner flask dynamic culture system that was operated under optimal conditions for cartilage formation (Sucosky et al. 2004).

Cells usually respond to mechanical stimulation; bioreactors can therefore be used to provide required mechanical stimulation to cells, thereby inspiring cells to synthesize ECM in a shorter period of time and in a more homogeneous manner than that achieved using the traditional static culture (Villalona et al. 2010). Besides mechanical stimulation, bioreactors can facilitate interaction among the scaffolds, cells, and signaling molecules, thereby promoting rapid and homogeneous ECM production, triggering stem cells toward a particular direction for their differentiation into the targeted tissue, and enhancing spatial distribution of cells. For example, bone being a dynamic tissue can sense and adapt to mechanical stimulation through the modulation of its mass, geometry, and structure.

In a study, the efficiency of static and dynamic culture systems on the proliferation and osteogenic differentiation of bone marrow stromal cells (BMSCs) derived from rat seeded on scaffolds was investigated and that resulted in higher osteogenic differentiation under dynamic condition using flow perfusion bioreactor than the static culture condition (Gomes et al. 2003). Similarly, in another study, an increased ALP activity, level of bone-specific protein transcript, and mineralized matrix production representing an enhanced osteogenic differentiation of human BMSCs resulted in a dynamic bioreactor system with applied mechanical stimulation. It is further reported that the influence of mechanical stimulation towards the differentiation of stem cells is yet to be studied in detail (Mauney et al. 2004). In a study conducted by Marlovits et al., differentiated chondrocytes cultured in a rotating wall vessel under microgravity were able to form cartilage-like neotissue, encapsulated by fibrous tissue that closely resembled the perichondrium, without using any scaffold (Marlovits et al. 2003). In another set of studies, umbilical cord blood-derived hMSCs seeded in polymeric composite matrices and culturing under dynamic spinner flask bioreactor system promoted hMSCs attachment, proliferation, and subsequently chondrogenic differentiation, thereby producing cartilage-specific ECM matrices (Agrawal and Pramanik 2019; Agrawal, et al. 2018).

A perfusion bioreactor system was sucessfully used to regenerate joint hyaline cartilage on the over the calcium carbonate surface. (Krelau et al.1999). An osteochondral construct comprising chondrocytes-seeded (PGA) and periosteal cells-seeded matrices (PLA/PGA/PEG) was cultures in an orbital shaker to construct osteochondral tissue (Schaefer D et al 2000). A dual chamber novel bioreactor by modifying spinner flask and perfusion bioreactors was developed for osteochondral tissue regeneration by co-culturjng chondrocytes and osteoblasts, or, to induce simultaneous differentiation of chondrocytes and osteoblasts (Chih-Hung et al.)

There are a number of commercially available bioreactor systems for bone tissue engineering application aiming to produce mineralized cell–scaffold constructs. The Bell-Flow spinner flask made of autoclavable borosilicate glass and manufactured by Bellco Biotechnology is available in capacity ranging from 100 mL to 3 L and more, whereas autoclavable spinner flasks and disposable systems made of plastic are manufactured by Lifesciences Corning. MINUCELLS and MINUTISSUE GmbH offer a wide variety of perfusion chambers that are referred to as indirect perfusion method for the generation of cartilage constructs and others. The compact design of autoclavable OsteoGen Bioreactor based on direct perfusion developed by Tissue Growth Technologies, which is commercially available. The chambers of these bioreactors are designed to fit for cylindrical scaffolds. Zellwerk GmbH offers the Good manufacturing Practice (GMP)-conforming RBB tissue culturing bio-reactor system with an inbuilt GMP breeder, and a control unit, under the trade name BIOSTAT Bplus RBS (www.zellwerk.biz/). The other rotating cell culture micro-gravity bioreactors with autoclavable and disposable features which are originally designed and developed by NASA are available from Synthecon, Inc. (www.synthe con.com). This company also offers perfusion bioreactor with online monitoring system for measuring important process parameters, such as pH and oxygen levels. Another design of dynamic bioreactor system with an RBB meeting GMP standards is offered by B. Braun Biotech International GmbH. Dynamic bioreactor systems pro-viding tension, compression, and shear stress are available from Flexcell International Corporation; for example, Flexcell FX-5000 tension System and Flexcell FX-5000 Compression Systems provide cell culturing on flexible-bottomed culture plates and allow to observe signalling responses under strain stimulation in real time at a micro-scopic level.

EXERCISE

1. Write the various phenomena occurring during cell =scaffold interaction.
2. Write the advantages of dynamic culture in comparison to static culture during cell–biomaterial interaction.
3. What are the different configurations of bioreactors that are used in producing tissue grafts?
4. What is cell adhesion and how is it important in tissue regeneration?
5. What are cell adhesion molecules and what are their function?
6. Explain how you measure the extent of focal adhesion during tissue graft generation.
7. What do you mean by cell aggregation and cell migration? Explain their importance in neotissue regeneration.
8. What are the different methods used for seeding cells on the scaffold? In which type of cell seeding is the bioreactor used? With a neat diagram, describe the most effective bioreactor to achieve cell seeding with the highest efficiency.
9. Write short notes on the following:
   I. Perfusion bioreactor
   II. Micro-carrier based bioreactor
10. Explain how cell seeding is important in tissue engineering. What are the forces you have come across for seeding of cells onto the scaffold? Name the different modified techniques developed for improving cell seeding efficiency.
11. Explain the dynamic cell seeding technique.
12. Write the various steps involved in tissue regeneration process. What are the factors that influence tissue regeneration in bioreactor?
13. What do you mean by cell adhesion? Explain the methods of assessing cell attachment and cell morphology.
14. Give a brief account of bone and related joint tissue regeneration in bioreactor.

15. In your opinion which type of bioreactor is the most suitable for bone regeneration and why? Give few bioreactor systems which are commercially available for regenerating bone and cartilage.

REFERENCES

Abdullah, N. S., D. B. Das, H. Ye, and Z. F. Cui. 2006. "3D bone tissue growth in hollow fibre membrane bioreactor: Implications of various process parameters on tissue nutrition." *The International Journal of Artificial Organs* 29 (9): 841–851.

Ackermann, M., A. R. Hashtchin, F. Manstein, M. C. Oliveira, H. Kempf, R. Zweigerdt, and N. Lachmann. 2022. "Continuous human iPSC-macrophage mass production by suspension culture in stirred tank bioreactors." *Nature Protocols* 17 (2): 513–539.

Agrawal, P., K. Pramanik, V. Vishwanath, A. Biswas, A. Bissoyi, and P. K. Patra. 2018. "Enhanced chondrogenesis of mesenchymal stem cells over silk fibroin/chitosan-chondroitin sulfate three dimensional scaffold in dynamic culture condition." *Journal of Biomedical Materials Research Part B: Applied Biomaterials* 106 (7): 2576–2587. DOI: 10.1002/jbm.b.34074

Agrawal, P., and K. Pramanik. 2019. "Enhanced chondrogenic differentiation of human mesenchymal stem cells in silk fibroin/chitosan/glycosaminoglycan scaffolds under dynamic culture condition." *Differentiation* 110: 36–48.

Agrawal, P., K. Pramanik, A. Biswas, and R. K. Patra. 2018. "In vitro cartilage construct generation from silk fibroin-chitosan porous scaffold and umbilical cord blood derived human mesenchymal stem cells in dynamic culture condition." *Journal of Biomedical Materials Research Part A* 106 (2): 397–407.

Ahmed, S., V. M. Chauhan, A. M. Ghaemmaghami, and J. W. Aylott. 2019. "New generation of bioreactors that advance extracellular matrix modelling and tissue engineering." *Biotechnology Letters* 41 (1): 1–25.

Alfred, R., J. Radford, J. Fan, K. Boon, R. Krawetz, D. Rancourt, and M. S. Kallos. 2011. "Efficient suspension bioreactor expansion of murine embryonic stem cells on microcarriers in serum-free medium." *Biotechnology Progress* 27 (3): 811–823.

Altman, G. H., R. L. Horan, I. Martin, J. Farhadi, P. R. H. Stark, V. Volloch, J. C. Richmond, G. Vunjak-Novakovic, and D. L. Kaplan. 2002. "Cell differentiation by mechanical stress." *The FASEB Journal* 16 (2): 1–13.

Andrade-Zaldívar, H., L. Santos, and A. De León Rodríguez. 2008. "Expansion of human hematopoietic stem cells for transplantation: Trends and perspectives." *Cytotechnology* 56 (3): 151–160.

Badenes, S. M., T. G. Fernandes, C. A. V. Rodrigues, M. M. Diogo, and J. M. S. Cabral. 2016. "Microcarrier-based platforms for in vitro expansion and differentiation of human pluripotent stem cells in bioreactor culture systems." *Journal of Biotechnology* 234: 71–82.

Baker, B. M., and C. S. Chen. 2012. "Deconstructing the third dimension-how 3D culture microenvironments alter cellular cues." *Journal of Cell Science* 125 (13): 3015–3024.

Becker, H., and C. Gärtner. 2008. "Polymer microfabrication technologies for microfluidic systems." *Analytical and Bioanalytical Chemistry* 390 (1): 89–111.

Benson, D. L., L. M. Schnapp, L. Shapiro, and G. W. Huntley. 2000. "Making memories stick: Cell-adhesion molecules in synaptic plasticity." *Trends in Cell Biology* 10 (11): 473–482.

Bhaskar, B., R. Owen, H. Bahmaee, P. S. Rao, and G. C. Reilly. 2018. "Design and assessment of a dynamic perfusion bioreactor for large bone tissue engineering scaffolds." *Applied Biochemistry and Biotechnology* 185 (2): 555–563.

Bhatia, S. N., and D. E. Ingber. 2014. "Microfluidic organs-on-chips." *Nature Biotechnology* 32 (8): 760–772.

Boateng, S. Y., Lateef, S. S., Mosley, W., Hartman, T. J., Hanley, L., & Russell, B. (2005). "RGD and YIGSR synthetic peptides facilitate cellular adhesion identical to that of laminin and fibronectin but alter the physiology of neonatal cardiac myocytes." *American Journal of Physiology-Cell Physiology* 288 (1): C30-C38.

Bueno, E. M., G. Laevsky, and G. A. Barabino. 2007. "Enhancing cell seeding of scaffolds in tissue engineering through manipulation of hydrodynamic parameters." *Journal of Biotechnology* 129 (3): 516–531.

Chang, C.-H., F.-H. Lin, C-C. Lin, C.-H. Chou, and H.-C. Liu. 2004. "Cartilage tissue engineering on the surface of a novel gelatin–calcium-phosphate biphasic scaffold in a double-chamber bioreactor." *Journal of Biomedical Materials Research Part B: Applied Biomaterials: An Official Journal of the Society for Biomaterials, the Japanese Society for Biomaterials, and the Australian Society for Biomaterials and the Korean Society for Biomaterials* 71 (2): 313–321.

Chen, H. C., H. P. Lee, Y. C. Ho, M. L. Sung, and Y. C. Hu. 2006. "Combination of baculovirus-mediated gene transfer and rotating-shaft bioreactor for cartilage tissue engineering." *Biomaterials* 27 (16): 3154–3162. DOI: 10.1016/j.biomaterials.2006.01.018

Chen, R., S. J. Curran, J. M. Curran, and J. A. Hunt. 2006. "The use of poly (l-lactide) and RGD modified microspheres as cell carriers in a flow intermittency bioreactor for tissue engineering cartilage." *Biomaterials* 27 (25): 4453–4460.

Chen, X., H. Xu, C. Wan, and G. Li. 2006. "Expansion of mesenchymal stem cells in 3-D bioreactor system." *Orthopaedic Proceedings* 88: 402.

Chih-Hung Chang, Chien-Cheng Lin, Chen-Hung Chou, Feng-Huel Lin, Hwa-Chang Liu. 2005. "Novel Bioreactors for Osteochondral Tissue Engineering." *Biomed Eng Appl Basis Comm* 17: 38–43.

Chinn, D.. 2010. "Microfabrication techniques for biologists: A primer on building micromachines." *Microengineering in Biotechnology*: 583: 1–53.

Couto, P. S., M. C. Rotondi, A. Bersenev, C. J. Hewitt, A. W. Nienow, F. Verter, and Q. A. Rafiq. 2020. "Expansion of human mesenchymal stem/stromal cells (hMSCs) in bioreactors using microcarriers: Lessons learnt and what the future holds." *Biotechnology Advances* 45: 107636.

Cukierman, E., R. Pankov, D. R. Stevens, and K. M. Yamada. 2001. "Taking cell-matrix adhesions to the third dimension." *Science* 294 (5547): 1708–1712.

Dai, W., J. Dong, G. Chen, and T. Uemura. 2009. "Application of low-pressure cell seeding system in tissue engineering." *Bioscience Trends* 3 (6): 216–219.

Dar, A., M. Shachar, J. Leor, and S. Cohen. 2002. "Optimization of cardiac cell seeding and distribution in 3D porous alginate scaffolds." *Biotechnology and Bioengineering* 80 (3): 305–312.

Eghbali, H., M. M. Nava, D. Mohebbi-Kalhori, and M. T. Raimondi. 2016. "Hollow fiber bioreactor technology for tissue engineering applications." *The International Journal of Artificial Organs* 39 (1): 1–15.

Eibl, R., and D. Eibl. 2009. "Application of disposable bag bioreactors in tissue engineering and for the production of therapeutic agents." *Bioreactor Systems for Tissue Engineering* 112: 183–207.

Fridley, K. M., M. A. Kinney, and T. C. McDevitt. 2012. "Hydrodynamic modulation of pluripotent stem cells." *Stem Cell Research & Therapy* 3 (6): 1–9.

Fu, L., P. Li, H. Li, C. Gao, Z. Yang, T. Zhao, W. Chen, Z. Liao, Y. Peng, and F. Cao. 2021. "The application of bioreactors for cartilage tissue engineering: Advances, limitations, and future perspectives." *Stem Cells International* 2021: 1–13.

Gandhi, J. K., S.-W. Kao, B. M. Roux, R. A. Rodriguez, S.-J. Tang, J. P. Fisher, M.-H. Cheng, and E. M. Brey. 2019. "Perfusion bioreactor culture of bone marrow stromal cells enhances cranial defect regeneration." *Plastic and Reconstructive Surgery* 143 (5): 993e–1002e.

Gaspar, D. A., V. Gomide, and F. Jorge Monteiro. 2012. "The role of perfusion bioreactors in bone tissue engineering." *Biomatter* 2 (4): 167–175.

Gomes, M. E., V. I. Sikavitsas, E. Behravesh, R. L. Reis, and A. G. Mikos. 2003. "Effect of flow perfusion on the osteogenic differentiation of bone marrow stromal cells cultured on starch-based three-dimensional scaffolds." *Journal of Biomedical Materials Research Part A: An Official Journal of the Society for Biomaterials, the Japanese Society for Biomaterials, and the Australian Society for Biomaterials and the Korean Society for Biomaterials* 67 (1): 87–95.

Grayson, W. L., S. Bhumiratana, C. Cannizzaro, P.-H. Grace Chao, D. P. Lennon, A. I. Caplan, and G. Vunjak-Novakovic. 2008. "Effects of initial seeding density and fluid perfusion rate on formation of tissue-engineered bone." *Tissue Engineering Part A* 14 (11): 1809–1820.

Grossemy, S., P. P. Y. Chan, and P. M. Doran. 2021. "Enhanced neural differentiation using simultaneous application of 3D scaffold culture, fluid flow, and electrical stimulation in bioreactors." *Advanced Biology* 5 (4): 2000136.

Han, Y., X. Li, Y. Zhang, Y. Han, F. Chang, and J. Ding. 2019. "Mesenchymal stem cells for regenerative medicine." *Cells* 8 (8): 886.

Janssen, F. W., J. Oostra, A. van Oorschot, and C. A. van Blitterswijk. 2006. "A perfusion bioreactor system capable of producing clinically relevant volumes of tissue-engineered bone: in vivo bone formation showing proof of concept." *Biomaterials* 27 (3): 315–323.

Jorgenson, K. D., D. A. Hart, R. Krawetz, and A. Sen. 2018. "Production of adult human synovial fluid-derived mesenchymal stem cells in stirred-suspension culture." *Stem Cells International* 2018: 1–16.

Kim, B.-S., A. J. Putnam, T. J. Kulik, and D. J. Mooney. 1998. "Optimizing seeding and culture methods to engineer smooth muscle tissue on biodegradable polymer matrices." *Biotechnology and Bioengineering* 57 (1): 46–54.

King, J. A., and W. M. Miller. 2007. "Bioreactor development for stem cell expansion and controlled differentiation." *Current Opinion in Chemical Biology* 11 (4): 394–398.

Kleinhans, C., R. R. Mohan, G. Vacun, T. Schwarz, B. Haller, Y. Sun, A. Kahlig, P. Kluger, A. Finne-Wistrand, and H. Walles. 2015. "A perfusion bioreactor system efficiently generates cell-loaded bone substitute materials for addressing critical size bone defects." *Biotechnology Journal* 10 (11): 1727–1738.

Kreklau B, Sittinger M, Mensing MB, et. al. 1999. "Tissue engineering of biphasic joint cartilage transplants." *Biomaterials* 20: 1743–1749.

Kropp, C., H. Kempf, C. Halloin, D. Robles-Diaz, A. Franke, T. Scheper, K. Kinast, T. Knorpp, T. O. Joos, and A. Haverich. 2016. "Impact of feeding strategies on the scalable expansion of human pluripotent stem cells in single-use stirred tank bioreactors." *Stem Cells Translational Medicine* 5 (10): 1289–1301.

Lam, A. T.-L., J. Li, J. Pei-Wen Toh, E. Jia-Hui Sim, A. Kuan-Liang Chen, J. Kok-Yen Chan, M. Choolani, S. Reuveny, W. R. Birch, and S. Kah-Weng Oh. 2017. "Biodegradable poly-ε-caprolactone microcarriers for efficient production of human mesenchymal stromal cells and secreted cytokines in batch and fed-batch bioreactors." *Cytotherapy* 19 (3): 419–432.

Lembong, J., R. Kirian, J. D. Takacs, T. R. Olsen, L. T. Lock, J. A. Rowley, and T. Ahsan. 2020. "Bioreactor parameters for microcarrier-based human MSC expansion under xeno-free conditions in a vertical-wheel system." *Bioengineering* 7 (3): 73.

Li, S., P. Glynne-Jones, O. G. Andriotis, K. Y. Ching, U. S. Jonnalagadda, R. OC Oreffo, M. Hill, and R. S. Tare. 2014. "Application of an acoustofluidic perfusion bioreactor for cartilage tissue engineering." *Lab on a Chip* 14 (23): 4475–4485.

Liu, M., Yan Li, and S.-T. Yang. 2014. "Expansion of human amniotic fluid stem cells in 3-dimensional fibrous scaffolds in a stirred bioreactor." *Biochemical Engineering Journal* 82: 71–80.

Liu, N., R. Zang, S.-T. Yang, and Y. Li. 2014. "Stem cell engineering in bioreactors for large-scale bioprocessing." *Engineering in Life Sciences* 14 (1): 4–15.

Lo, C.-M., H.-B. Wang, M. Dembo, and Y.-L. Wang. 2000. "Cell movement is guided by the rigidity of the substrate." *Biophysical Journal* 79 (1): 144–152.

Mabvuure, N., S. Hindocha, and W. S. Khan. 2012. "The role of bioreactors in cartilage tissue engineering." *Current Stem Cell Research & Therapy* 7 (4): 287–292.

Mahmoudifar, N., and P. M. Doran. 2005. "Tissue engineering of human cartilage and osteochondral composites using recirculation bioreactors." *Biomaterials* 26 (34): 7012–7024.

Mahoney, M. J., and W. Mark Saltzman. 2001. "Transplantation of brain cells assembled around a programmable synthetic microenvironment." *Nature Biotechnology* 19 (10): 934–939.

Malda, J., and C. G. Frondoza. 2006. "Microcarriers in the engineering of cartilage and bone." *Trends in Biotechnology* 24 (7): 299–304.

Marlovits, S., B. Tichy, M. Truppe, D. Gruber, and V. Vécsei. 2003. "Chondrogenesis of aged human articular cartilage in a scaffold-free bioreactor." *Tissue Engineering* 9 (6): 1215–1226.

Mauney, J. R., S. Sjostorm, J. Blumberg, R. Horan, J. P. O'Leary, G. Vunjak-Novakovic, V. Volloch, and D. L. Kaplan. 2004. "Mechanical stimulation promotes osteogenic differentiation of human bone marrow stromal cells on 3-D partially demineralized bone scaffolds in vitro." *Calcified Tissue International* 74 (5): 458–468. DOI: 10.1007/s00223-003-0104-7

Mizukami, A., A. Fernandes-Platzgummer, J. G. Carmelo, K. Swiech, D. T. Covas, J. M. S. Cabral, and C. L. da Silva. 2016. "Stirred tank bioreactor culture combined with serum-/xenogeneic-free culture medium enables an efficient expansion of umbilical cord-derived mesenchymal stem/stromal cells." *Biotechnology Journal* 11 (8): 1048–1059.

Mohebbi-Kalhori, D., A. Behzadmehr, C. J. Doillon, and A. Hadjizadeh. 2012. "Computational modeling of adherent cell growth in a hollow-fiber membrane bioreactor for large-scale 3-D bone tissue engineering." *Journal of Artificial Organs* 15 (3): 250–265.

Nold, P., C. Brendel, A. Neubauer, G. Bein, and H. Hackstein. 2013. "Good manufacturing practice-compliant animal-free expansion of human bone marrow derived mesenchymal stroma cells in a closed hollow-fiber-based bioreactor." *Biochemical and Biophysical Research Communications* 430 (1): 325–330.

Oh, S. K. W., A. K. Chen, Y. Mok, Xiaoli Chen, U-M. L., A. Chin, A. B. H. Choo, and S. Reuveny. 2009. "Long-term microcarrier suspension cultures of human embryonic stem cells." *Stem Cell Research* 2 (3): 219–230.

Pandolfi, V., U. Pereira, M Dufresne, and C. Legallais. 2017. "Alginate-based cell microencapsulation for tissue engineering and regenerative medicine." *Current Pharmaceutical Design* 23 (26): 3833–3844.

Pasirayi, G., V. Auger, S. M. Scott, Pattanathu K. S. M. Rahman, M. Islam, L. O'Hare, and Z. Ali. 2011. "Microfluidic bioreactors for cell culturing: A review." *Micro and Nanosystems* 3 (2): 137–160.

Pei, Y., J.-J. Fan, X.-Q. Zhang, Z.-Y. Zhang, and M. Yu. 2014. "Repairing the osteochondral defect in goat with the tissue-engineered osteochondral graft preconstructed in a double-chamber stirring bioreactor." *BioMed Research International* 2014: 1–11.

Phelan, M. A., A. L. Gianforcaro, J. A. Gerstenhaber, and P. I. Lelkes. 2019. "An air bubble-isolating rotating wall vessel bioreactor for improved spheroid/organoid formation." *Tissue Engineering Part C: Methods* 25 (8): 479–488.

Qu, F., F. Guilak, and R. L. Mauck. 2019. "Cell migration: Implications for repair and regeneration in joint disease." *Nature Reviews Rheumatology* 15 (3): 167–179.

Rashid, M., Y.-H. Dou, V. Auger, and Z. Ali. 2010. "Recent developments in polymer microfluidic devices with capillary electrophoresis and electrochemical detection." *Micro and Nanosystems* 2 (2): 108–136.

Rauh, J., F. Milan, K.-P. Günther, and M. Stiehler. 2011. "Bioreactor systems for bone tissue engineering." *Tissue Engineering Part B: Reviews* 17 (4): 263–280.

Rousseau, G. F., M.-C. Giarratana, and L. Douay. 2014. "Large-scale production of red blood cells from stem cells: What are the technical challenges ahead?" *Biotechnology Journal* 9 (1): 28–38.

Salehi-Nik, N., G. Amoabediny, B. Pouran, H. Tabesh, M. Ali Shokrgozar, N. Haghighipour, N. Khatibi, F. Anisi, K. Mottaghy, and B. Zandieh-Doulabi. 2013. "Engineering parameters in bioreactor's design: A critical aspect in tissue engineering." *BioMed Research International* 2013: 1–15.

Sasaki, T., N. Iwasaki, K. Kohno, M. Kishimoto, T. Majima, S.-I. Nishimura, and A. Minami. 2008. "Magnetic nanoparticles for improving cell invasion in tissue engineering." *Journal of Biomedical Materials Research Part A: An Official Journal of the Society for Biomaterials, the Japanese Society for Biomaterials, and the Australian Society for Biomaterials and the Korean Society for Biomaterials* 86 (4): 969–978.

Schaefer D, Martin I, Shastri P, et. al. 2000. "In vitro generation of osteochondral composites." *Biomaterials* 21: 2599-2606.

Sikavitsas, V. I., G. N. Bancroft, and A. G. Mikos. 2002. "Formation of three-dimensional cell/polymer constructs for bone tissue engineering in a spinner flask and a rotating wall vessel bioreactor." *Journal of Biomedical Materials Research* 62 (1): 136–148. DOI: 10.1002/jbm.10150

Sikavitsas, V. I., G. N. Bancroft, H. L. Holtorf, J. A. Jansen, and A. G. Mikos. 2003. "Mineralized matrix deposition by marrow stromal osteoblasts in 3D perfusion culture increases with increasing fluid shear forces." *Proceedings of the National Academy of Sciences* 100 (25): 14683–14688.

Singh, V.. 1999. "Disposable bioreactor for cell culture using wave-induced agitation." *Cytotechnology* 30 (1): 149–158.

Skardal, A., S. F. Sarker, A. Crabbé, C. A. Nickerson, and G. D. Prestwich. 2010. "The generation of 3-D tissue models based on hyaluronan hydrogel-coated microcarriers within a rotating wall vessel bioreactor." *Biomaterials* 31 (32): 8426–8435.

Stoker, M., and E. Gherardi. 1991. "Regulation of cell movement: The motogenic cytokines." *Biochimica et Biophysica Acta (BBA)-Reviews on Cancer* 1072 (1): 81–102.

Sucosky, P., D. F. Osorio, J. B. Brown, and G. P. Neitzel. 2004. "Fluid mechanics of a spinner-flask bioreactor." *Biotechnology and Bioengineering* 85 (1): 34–46.

Sytnyk, V., I. Leshchyns'ka, and M. Schachner. 2017. "Neural cell adhesion molecules of the immunoglobulin superfamily regulate synapse formation, maintenance, and function." *Trends Neurosci* 40 (5): 295–308. DOI: 10.1016/j.tins.2017.03.003

Tan, L., Y. Ren, and R. Kuijer. 2012. "A 1-min method for homogenous cell seeding in porous scaffolds." *Journal of Biomaterials Applications* 26 (7): 877–889.

Thevenot, P., A. Nair, J. Dey, J. Yang, and L. Tang. 2008. "Method to analyze three-dimensional cell distribution and infiltration in degradable scaffolds." *Tissue Engineering Part C: Methods* 14 (4): 319–331.

Van Wezel, A. L. 1967. "Growth of cell-strains and primary cells on micro-carriers in homogeneous culture." *Nature* 216 (5110): 64–65.

Velve-Casquillas, G., M. L. Berre, M. Piel, and P. T. Tran. 2010. "Microfluidic tools for cell biological research." *Nano Today* 5 (1): 28–47.

Villalona, G. A., B. Udelsman, D. R. Duncan, E. McGillicuddy, R. F. Sawh-Martinez, N. Hibino, C. Painter, T. Mirensky, B. Erickson, and T. Shinoka. 2010. "Cell-seeding techniques in vascular tissue engineering." *Tissue Engineering Part B: Reviews* 16 (3): 341–350.

Wang, S., H. Suhaimi, M. Mabrouk, S. Georgiadou, J. P. Ward, and D. B. Das. 2021. "Effects of scaffold pore morphologies on glucose transport limitations in hollow fibre membrane bioreactor for bone tissue engineering: experiments and numerical modelling." *Membranes* 11 (4): 257.

Wendt, D., S. Stroebel, M. Jakob, G. T. John, and I. Martin. 2006. "Uniform tissues engineered by seeding and culturing cells in 3D scaffolds under perfusion at defined oxygen tensions." *Biorheology* 43 (3–4): 481–488.

Williams, K. A., S. Saini, and T. M. Wick. 2002. "Computational fluid dynamics modeling of steady-state momentum and mass transport in a bioreactor for cartilage tissue engineering." *Biotechnology Progress* 18 (5): 951–963.

Yang, D., Z. Zhao, F. Bai, S. Wang, A. P. Tomsia, and H. Bai. 2017. "Promoting cell migration in tissue engineering scaffolds with graded channels." *Advanced Healthcare Materials* 6 (18): 1700472.

Zhang, J., H. Eyisoylu, X.-H. Qin, M. Rubert, and R. Müller. 2021. "3D bioprinting of graphene oxide-incorporated cell-laden bone mimicking scaffolds for promoting scaffold fidelity, osteogenic differentiation and mineralization." *Acta Biomaterialia* 121: 637–652.

Zhang, Z.-Y., S. H. Teoh, W.-S. Chong, T.-T. Foo, Y.-C. Chng, M. Choolani, and J. Chan. 2009. "A biaxial rotating bioreactor for the culture of fetal mesenchymal stem cells for bone tissue engineering." *Biomaterials* 30 (14): 2694–2704.

Zhang, Z.-Y., S. Hin Teoh, E. Yiling Teo, M. Seow Khoon Chong, C. Woon Shin, F. Toon Tien, M. A. Choolani, and J. K.Y. Chan. 2010. "A comparison of bioreactors for culture of fetal mesenchymal stem cells for bone tissue engineering." *Biomaterials* 31 (33): 8684–8695.

Zimmermann, H., F. Wählisch, C. Baier, M. Westhoff, R. Reuss, D. Zimmermann, M. Behringer, F. Ehrhart, A. Katsen-Globa, and C. Giese. 2007. "Physical and biological properties of barium cross-linked alginate membranes." *Biomaterials* 28 (7): 1327–1345.

Zurina, I. M., V. S. Presniakova, D. V. Butnaru, A. A. Svistunov, P. S. Timashev, and Y. A. Rochev. 2020. "Tissue engineering using a combined cell sheet technology and scaffolding approach." *Acta Biomaterialia* 113: 63–83.

8 *In Vitro* Assessment of Engineered Bone and Cartilage Tissue Grafts

INTRODUCTION

In vitro study is a proof of concept testing which is used to assess the compatibility of the any cell or tissue and biologically functionalized implanted devices with the host tissue. (Motamedian 2015). *In vitro* study happens in a controlled environment, which is similar to the body's environment to some extent (Przekora 2019). This study provides prior ideas about suitability of the implant for *in vivo* studies, pre-clinical trials, and clinical trials (Nöth et al. 2002). *In vitro* study is an essential aspect of biological safety as well as cost-effective exercise. In tissue engineering field, *in vitro* studies, prior to pre-clinical and clinical trials of any new devices including the scaffolds, cell-seed scaffold construct, and tissue graft, are performed with these tissue engineered products. Besides cell and tissue compatibility, these studies provide useful information on the compatibility of the regenerative devices implanted in the defect site, thereby ensuring the safety of their use for tissue regeneration as well as shedding light on possible cellular and tissue actions in vivo, using simpler systems than the complicated in vivo milieu. Therefore, a battery of in vitro testing procedures have been standardized which are performed routinely during the tissue construct or tissue graft formation processes in the past few decades. These studies provide an idea about the cell proliferation and cell growth, as well as differentiation of cells towards neotissue formation and hence success of tissue regeneration in vitro. Therefore, *In vitro* cellular models are potential to replace *in vivo* animal tests effectively in initial evaluation of cytotoxicity of the engineered tissue scaffold, growth and adhesion of osteoblasts on the scaffold, bone extracellular matrix (ECM) formation on the scaffold surface, and the risk associated with the post-surgery inflammation (Przekora 2019).

Several *in vitro* studies are performed for the assessment of engineered bone and cartilage tissue products. In bone tissue engineering, some of the important characteristics such as mineralization, calcium content, and osteogenic potential by gene expressions for ALP, osteocalcin, osteoprotegrin, and RUNX2; studies that are specific to bone tissue or bone cell are performed. In addition, some commonly used assays such as cell morphology, live/dead assay of cells, cell proliferation, cell viability, and cell adhesion are also performed (Rodrigues et al. 2003). Although the

DOI: 10.1201/9781003245353-8

bone and cartilage structures and functions are similar, some specific tests like collagen II staining in the case of cartilage tissue scaffold in addition to the common assays as mentioned above are performed (Woodfield et al. 2004). Besides scaffold, the regenerated bone and cartilage constructs are also assessed by these *in vitro* tests (Rhee et al. 2016; Rouwkema, De Boer, and Van Blitterswijk 2006). Through these *in vitro* tests several issues involved in these tissue engineering products can be rectified easily. In this chapter, a review of the various in *vitro* assays that have been performed as the proof-of-concept testings, during the various stages of engineered tissue development pertaining to bone and cartilage as well as their complex derivatives like joint (osteochondral) has been presented.

IN VITRO ASSESSMENT OF BONE CONSTRUCTS

Bone defects, which often occur due to accidents, diseases, etc., are challenging issues for researchers and surgeons for their repairand maintenance of their normal function. Bone construct, a custom-tailored material, is developed from stem cells and biocompatible material and has the potential to accelerate the healing process at the defect site. Stem cells involved in this process are pluripotent and either autologous or allogenic in nature. In this scenario, the stem cells are cultured on the scaffold for proper cell attachment and proliferation. These cell-seeded scaffolds also referred to as constructs are implanted at the defect site of the patient for tissue regeneration, thereby filling up the gap (Logeart-Avramoglou et al. 2005). A number of *in vitro* studies including the microscopic studies for morphological, cell attachment and cell spreading, MTT assay for cell viability, alamar blue and DNA quantification for proliferation, Alizarin Red S staining, ALP assay for diffrentiation, immunocytochemistry study, have been performed to understand the level of interaction of the cells with the materials (Park, Lee, and Kim 2011) and hence overall outcome of the bone tissue regeneration. These assays are described below.

CELL ADHESION, CELL MORPHOLOGY, AND CELL SPREADING/DISTRIBUTION

The interaction between the cell and the artificial ECM plays an important role in cell attachment, morphology, and ultimately neotissue formation. It is, therefore, vital to study cell attachment over the scaffold surface (Khalili and Ahmad 2015). In general, after incubation, the cell-seeded scaffolds (constructs) are removed from the culture vessel and thoroughly cleaned with phosphate buffered saline (PBS) and dehydrated by using gradient ethanol of 35%, 50%, 70%, 90%, and 100 % usually for 5 min each. The cells are then fixed with 2% glutaraldehyde or paraformaldehyde solution. The fixed samples are then coated with gold or platinum by sintering process and are observed under SEM (Scanning Electron Microscope) (Chen et al. 2014). In an *in vitro* study, after 24 hr of cell culture, the distribution of human mesenchymal stem cells (hMSCs) over alginate/O-carboxymethyl chitosan/*Cissus quadrangularis* extract and alginate/O-carboxymethyl chitosan scaffold were investigated under SEM (Soumya et al. 2012). Cell adhesion on scaffold was quantified by the extraction of DNA from the attached cells and quantification of the extracted DNA using Hoechst 33258 DNA assay. Yang et al. (2012) examined the attachment of MSCs over poly l-lactide-co-e-caprolactone (PLCL) and PLCL/chitosan scaffolds. After 16 hr of incubation, SEM micrographs of the constructs revealed that the distribution of MSCs on the PLCL/chitosan scaffold was uniform and the morphology of MSCs noticeably changed from round to spherical, whereas the distribution of cells on the PLCL scaffold was not uniform and the cells were round in shape. In another study, the elongated morphology of the stem cells due to the actin fibre polymerization in the cytoplasm of the MSCs on PLCL/chitosan scaffold was studied (Yang et al. 2012). Bharadwaj et al. (2012) studied the attachment of rat mesenchymal stem cells (rMSCs) on the surface of the silk fibroin/chitosan (SF/CH) scaffold, in which silk fibroin derived from both *Antheraea myliita* (SFAM) and *Bombyx mori* (SFBM) was used. The confocal microscopy study revealed that MSCs cultured on the SF/CH and SFAM scaffolds were well spread, prominent, and round in shape, whereas the attachment of cells was found to be lesser in SFBM scaffold (Bhardwaj and Kundu 2012). Human adipose-derived stem cells (ADSCs) were cultured over PCL/graphene 3D fibrous scaffold and the resulting constructs to delete were assessed for bone regenerating activity. The cellular adhesion was observed under SEM as well as laser confocal microscopy. The SEM micrographs of the cell-seeded scaffold showed the confluent cell growth and several orthogonal bridges made by cells over the scaffold filaments, which signify that an appropriate environment was provided by the scaffold for cell growth and proliferation (Wang et al. 2016). Electrospun scaffolds made up of polylactic acid (PLA)/polyethylene glycol (PEG)/multi wall carbon nanotubes showed osteogenic differentiation on rat bone marrow stromal cells (RBMSCs). These cells were seeded on scaffolds of different compositions of PLA, 0.5C (multi wall carbon nanotubes), 0.5C/1PEG (0.5 multi wall carbon nanotubes/1 PEG) and 0.5 C/10PEG (0.5 multi wall carbon nanotubes/10 PEG. The distribution of differentiated cells on

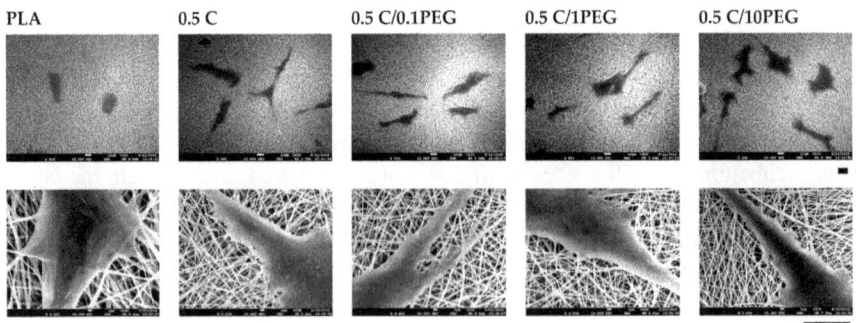

FIGURE 8.1   SEM micrographs showing cell attachment on different nanofibrous scaffolds of polylactic acid (PLA), multi-wall carbon nanotubes (0.5C), 0.5 multi-wall carbon nanotubes/1 polyethylene glycol (0.5C/1PEG), and 0.5 multi-wall carbon nanotubes/10 polyethylene glycol (0.5 C/10PEG).

Source: Polyethylene and Scaffolds (2021).

the scaffolds was seen under SEM and the captured SEM micrographs showed that the cells were profusely distributed in electrospun fibres and deposited calcium in ECM (Figure 8.1) (Polyethylene and Scaffolds 2021).

Similarly, several studies have been performed to observe the attachment of cells over the cartilage and bone constructs as well as the scaffolds to assess their respective tissue regenerating activity (Motamedian 2015). hMSCs were seeded on the developed porous chitosan-hydroxyapatite (CH-HA) scaffolds and cultured followed by differentiation in a dynamic perfusion bioreactor resulting in bone constructs as shown in Figure 8.2 (Rogina et al. 2017).

After 21 days of culture, the cell attachment of the construct was observed under fluorescence microscope, after staining with nuclear stain Hoechst which is cell permeable. It was observed that grafts having 30% and 50% HA showed the highest and lowest cell attachment, respectively, as shown in Figure 8.3. The higher HA content might have negative effects on the bone cell survival (Rogina et al. 2017).

A bone construct was developed by culturing and differentiating MSCs on the PCL nanofibrous scaffold using osteogenic differentiation media in a static culture condition. In this static culture system, MSCs were grown on the PCL fibre in culture media at 37°C and 5% CO_2. The resulting cell-seeded PCL (construct) was shifted to a rotational oxygen-permeable bioreactor system, in which 35ml osteogenic media was added for proper growth and differentiation of MSCs on the scaffold. After 4 weeks of dynamic culture of cells on PCL fibre, the cell-seeded scaffold was probed using SEM to check the distribution and morphology of cells in the construct. The analysis of SEM micrograph of the cell-seeded scaffold revealed that the surface of the scaffold was covered with several layers of cells, and the presence of osteoblast-like cells and globular accretions with collagen bundles was also observed (Shin, Yoshimoto, and Vacanti 2004). Frohlich al. (2010) developed a bone construct by seeding and culturing human adipose-derived stem cells (hASCs) over the decellularized bone scaffold in a perfusion bioreactor. After 2 days of proper growth and attachment of cells over the scaffold surface, cell-seeded scaffolds were differentiated in the perfusion bioreactor with osteogenic media and were cultured in the normal culture media (static culture) separately. The cell distribution on the constructs has been assessed by SEM analysis, for which the constructs were fixed with 2% glutaraldehyde for 2 hr in sodium cacodylate buffer followed by thorough washing in buffer and finally dried overnight. The fixed constructs were seen under SEM after coating with gold or platinum and SEM micrographs revealed that the cells were grown properly and filled the pores within and outer region of the scaffold. In static culture, a thin layer of cells was evident over the surface, whereas in perfusion reactor cells were grown homogeneously in large amount over the surface of the construct (Frohlich 2010).

CELL VIABILITY AND CELL PROLIFERATION

MTT (3-(4,5-dimethylthiazol-2-yl)-2,5-diphenyl-2H-tetrazolium bromide) assay is performed to evaluate the cytotoxicity and viability of the cells cultured on the scaffold. In this assay, the tetrazolium rings on MTT are reduced by the reductase

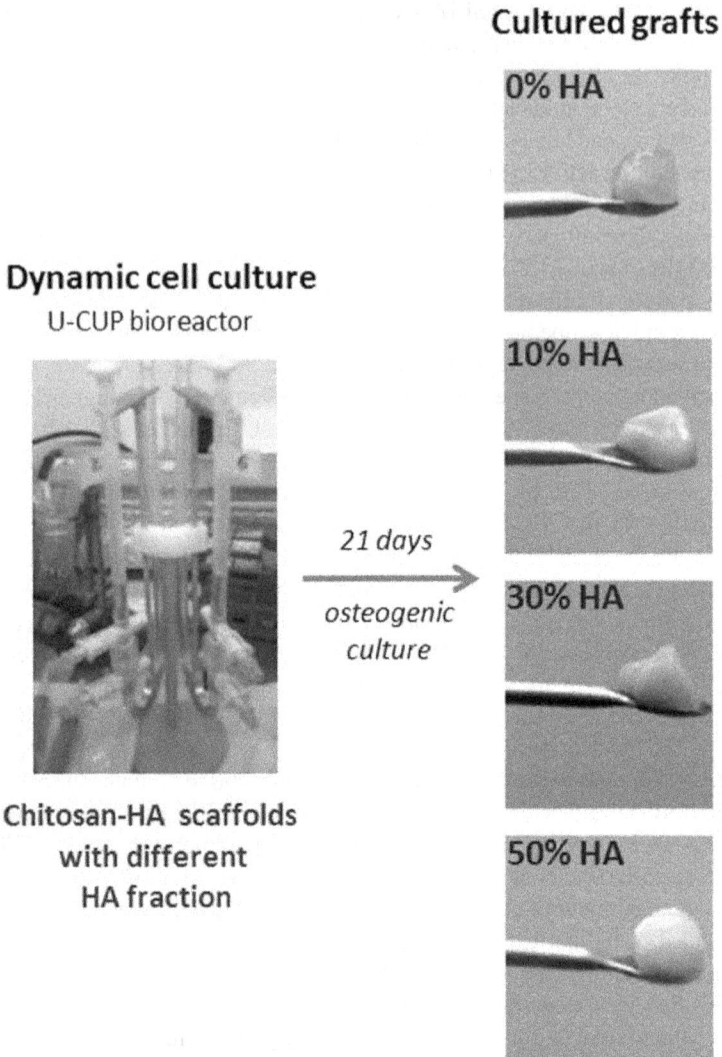

FIGURE 8.2 Dynamic culture of hMSCs over chitosan-hydroxyapatite (CH-HA) scaffolds in a perfusion bioreactor for generating bone construct.

Source: (Rogina et al. 2017).

enzymes present in the mitochondria that change the colour of MTT solution from pale yellow to dark blue. This active mitochondria study measures the cell viability (Thein-Han and Misra 2009). In an *in vitro* study, the cell-seeded scaffold was constructed by culturing cells on the sterilized scaffold in Dulbecco's Modified Eagle's Medium (DMEM) cell culture media supplemented with 10% foetal bovine serum (FBS) and 1% antibiotic antimycotic solution. After 7 days of incubation,

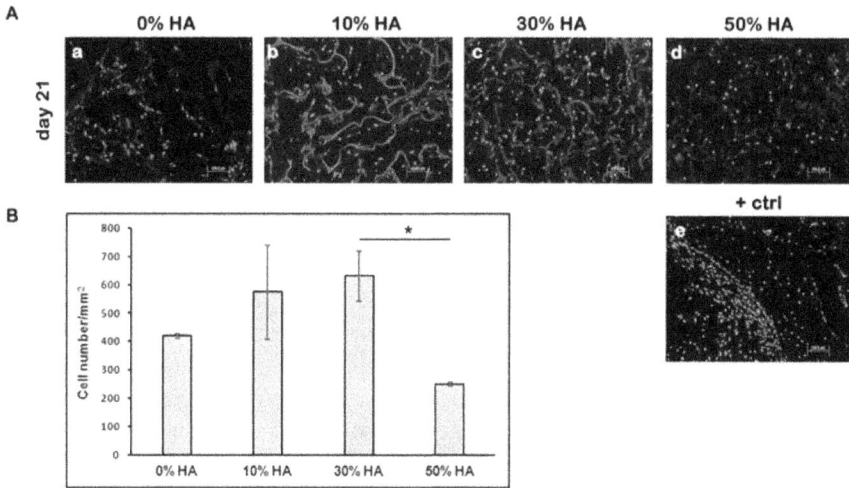

FIGURE 8.3 Cell distribution study on bone tissue grafts generated by culturing and differentiating hMSCs over different compositions of chitosan-hydroxyapatite (CH-HA) in a perfusion bioreactor tissue grafts. (A) Fluorescence microscopic images of Hoechst stained cells on the grafts. (B) Graphical representation of the cell number distribution in each graft observed under the fluorescence microscope.

Source: Rogina et al. (2017).

supernatants were discarded from the culture wells and an amount of 10 µL MTT solution was added to each well followed by the addition of 90 µL culture media and kept for 4 hr. After incubation, the supernatant of each well was removed and the formed formazan was dissolved in DMSO which was added to each plate in appropriate proportion. The sample was incubated for 20–30 min at 37°C in a shaker incubator and the absorbance of the colour sample was measured at 590 nm in ELISA (Enzyme-Linked Immunosorbent Assay) reader (Mostofi et al. 2022). In another study, the cytotoxicity test of a porous hydroxyapatite (HAp) scaffold for bone tissue engineering application was performed on the mouse fibroblast cells and the cell viability was evaluated by MTT assay. RBMSCs isolated from the femora of male rats (Fischer 344/N rats) were cultured in Eagle's minimum essential medium (MEM) with 15% FBS and 1% antibiotic-antimycotic solutions. The cultured cells were seeded on an HAp porous scaffold at different cell densities and incubated for 7 days. The cell viability was assessed by determining the total adenosine triphosphate (ATP) content present in the cell-seeded constructs by a CellTiter-Glo1 luminescent cell viability assay that measures the luminescence of the construct under microplate reader using an opaque-walled multi-well plate. The ATP content was found to be directly proportional to the viable cells (Oliveira et al. 2009). In a study, the viability of MC 3T3-E1 (pre-osteoblasts) cells on 3D porous chitosan–nanohydroxyapatite scaffold for bone tissue engineering was measured by the MTT assay (Thein-Han and Misra 2009). The viability of MG63 cells seeded and cultured on a developed chitosan/poly(caprolactone) nanofibrous scaffold was investigated by alamar blue (rezasurin) assay, which is a non-fluorescent dye. After incubation, 10% alamar blue solution was added to the construct and incubated for 5 hr. The absorbance of each sample was measured in ELISA reader and the cell viability was assessed in triplicate and plotted in terms of percentage of optical density. In this assay, the dye is reduced by mitochondrial enzymes present in active cells and converts into bright red fluorescent resorufin, which ultimately shows the presence of active or viable cells in the construct (Shalumon et al. 2011). The cell viability or cytotoxicity of hMSCs seeded on porous scaffolds, made of tricalcium phosphate (TCP) and marine plankton-derived whitlockite (MP-WH), was evaluated by using calcein acetoxymethyl ester as well as ethidium homodimer-1. The cells were cultured on the scaffold in a culture media and the resulting cell-seeded scaffolds were rinsed properly with PBS and stained with different dyes like calcein acetoxymethyl ester (calcein AM) and ethidium homodimer. The stained samples were observed under fluorescence microscope for cell viability. The fluorescence image Figure 8.4 showed that most of the cells were viable on different scaffolds (stained green by calcein AM) and no dead cells were observed (stained red by ethidium homodimer-1). Simultaneously, more

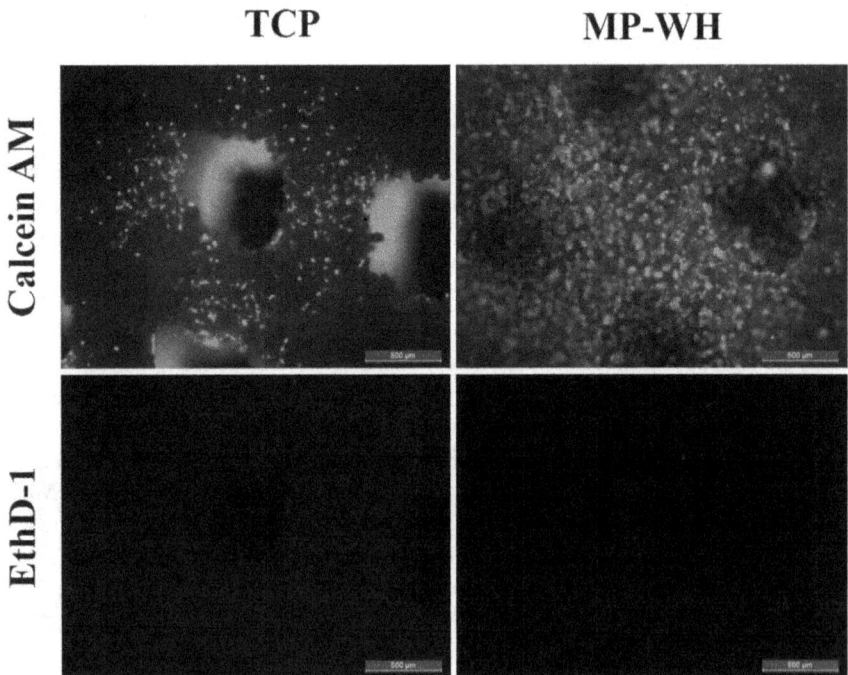

FIGURE 8.4 Cell viability study of tested scaffolds (MP-WH (marine plankton derived whitlockite) and TCP (tricalcium phosphate)) seeded with hMSCs under fluorescence microscope.

Source: Baek et al. (2022).

number of cells adhered to the surface of MP-WH scaffold than the TCP scaffold (Baek et al. 2022).

Live/dead assay was performed for mouse embryonic fibroblast (MEF) cells cultured on the porous PLLA/PEG scaffold by using live/dead assay kit. Different stains were used, such as 4',6-diamidino-2-phenylindole (DAPI), calcein-AM, and EthD-1 to label the nucleus, live cell, and dead cell, respectively, and the stained samples were observed under florescence microscope. Calcein-AM stains live cells and EthD-1 stains dead cells with green and red fluorescence, respectively. DAPI generally stains DNA region rich in adenine–thymine which is analysed by fluorescence microscopy. The fluorescence images showed that the number of viable cells was higher than the nonviable cells and cells were flattened on the surface of the scaffold, which indicates the strong interaction of MEFs over the surface of PLLA/PEG scaffold (Ju et al. 2019). The live/dead assay of hASCs-seeded decellularized bone scaffold was evaluated on osteogenic media and normal cell culture media. The hASC/decellularized bone construct was stained with calcein AM and ethidium homodimer-1 and the stained samples were observed under confocal microscope., that depicted the viable cells demononstrating the hASC proliferative activity both in osteogenic and normal media (Frohlich 2010). The rate of proliferation of hASCs on a decellularized bone scaffold was measured by DNA content of the cultured cells in the regenerated bone graft. For DNA isolation, cell-seeded scaffolds were rinsed repeatedly in PBS solution with digestion buffer and stored for overnight at 56°C. The samples were centrifuged and supernatants were collected for further studies. Picogreen dye, a molecular probe, was added to the sample in 1:1 ratio and the samples were observed under fluorescent plate reader. The constructs grown in osteogenic media displayed higher cell proliferation and differentiation rates than the constructs grown in normal media (Frohlich 2010).

OSTEOGENIC DIFFERENTIATION

Cells like bone marrow-derived mesenchymal stem cells (BMSCs), dental pulp stem cells (DPSCs), and adipose-derived mesenchymal stem cells (ADMSCs), are converted to osteogenic cells for bone tissue growth. In bone tissue engineering, cell-seeded scaffolds are cultured by adding osteogenic differentiation medium that consists of 10% FBS, 2 mM sodium phosphate, 2 mM L-glutamine, dexamethasone (100 nM), 100 units/mL penicillin, 50 mg/mL ascorbic acid, 100 lg/mL streptomycin, and 5 lg/mL amphotericin B. The media is usually changed every 2 days of culture. After incubation, the expression of osteoblast marker genes like alkaline phosphatase (ALP), osteocalcin (OCN), and osteoprotegrin (OPN), are determined (Chuenjitkuntaworn et al. 2016). ALP is an early marker of osteoblast activity and characteristic feature of osteoblast phenotype. The osteogenic differentiation activities of MSCs cultured on PCL/HA scaffold using osteogenic media were assessed by determining gene expressions such as type I collagen (COL 1), Runt-related transcription factor 2 (RUNX-2), and osteocalcin using real-time reverse transcription polymerase chain reaction (RT-PCR) (Chuenjitkuntaworn et al. 2016). Murphy et al. (2010) lysed the MC3T3-E1 cells, a pre-osteoblastic cell line, seeded on a porous collagen/ glycosaminoglycan scaffold by papain enzyme and quantified the extracted DNA using Hoechst 33258 DNA assay. In this assessment, the extracted DNA was fluorescently labelled with Hoechst 33258 and observed under a fluorescence spectrophotometer. The cell attachment on the scaffold was analysed by converting the reading of the fluorescent DNA to cell number through the standard curve (Murphy, Haugh, and O'Brien 2010). Similarly, in an *in vitro* study, the effect of pore size of a 3D-printed silicon-based porous scaffold (SiOC(N) on stem cell differentiation was investigated. The hMSCs were seeded on the scaffolds and cultured in osteogenic medium, resulting in bone tissue grafts. The expressions of differentiating marker genes such as ALP, COL 1, RUNX2, and secreted protein acidic and cysteine rich (SPARC) were examined in different incubation periods of 7, 14, and 21 days by RT-PCR. The expressions of these genes were compared with the expression of a glyceraldehyde-3-phosphate dehydrogenase, a housekeeping gene, and the relative expressions of these marker genes are shown in Figure 8.5. The expression of ALP gene was initially high in small pore size scaffold, while at 21 days the expression level was same in both small and large pore size of [SiOC(N)] scaffolds. At 14 days, the expression of COL 1 was same in both the scaffolds and by increasing the incubation period to 21 days the expression level was dropped almost to zero. The level of RUNX2 was lowered in both the groups, but small pore size SiOC(N) scaffold showed a higher level of expression of this gene in the first week compared with the large pore size SiOC(N). Both groups showed a similar pattern of expression of SPARC (Secreted Protein Acidic and Rich in Cysteine) protein helps in cell proliferation with similar trend during the 3 weeks of culture (Yang et al. 2021). Osteogenic differentiation of hMSCs-laden bi-phasic osteochondral scaffold was evaluated by morphological analysis using Alizarin red and von Kossa staining, by light microscopy and SEM. qPCR was used to measure the transcript levels of ALP, bone gamma-carboxyglutamate, RUNX2, osteopontin (SPP1), and Osteonectin(SPARC) (Csaba Matta et al 2019).

BIOMINERALIZATION ACTIVITY

Biomineralization is an important process by which cells form carbonated apatite layer over the surface of the implanted scaffold at the bone defect site, thereby aiding its attachment with living bone tissue and thus facilitates bone tissue regeneration. Alizarin red Sis a commonly used stain to determine calcium deposits in the differentiated culture of stem cells. It is an important characteristic of bone tissue engineering, as calcium deposition is an essential factor for bone cell growth and proliferation. In this method, after the cell culture on the scaffold, the cells in the construct are fixed by 4% paraformaldehyde and then 2% Alizarin Red is added for staining the calcium deposited by cells on the scaffold. The alizarin red dye is then removed by washing with distilled water and PBS solution. The calcium deposition is assessed by observing the samples under phase-contrast light microscope to (Mostofi et al. 2022). Kim et al. (2012) reported the mineralization on the bone construct derived from PCL/β-TCP scaffold seeded with MG63 cells. MG63 cells were cultured on PCL and different compositions of PCL/β-TCP scaffolds

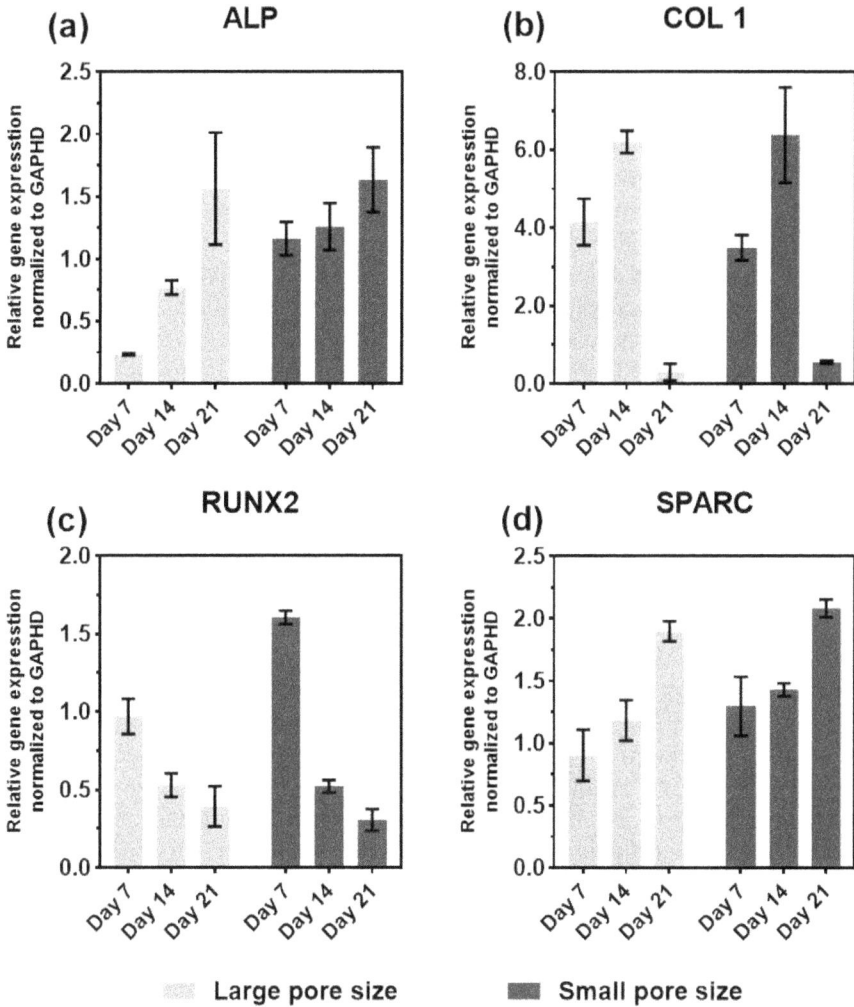

FIGURE 8.5 Relative gene expression of ALP (a), COL 1 (b), RUNX2 (c), and SPARC (d) of hMSCs cultured over SiOC(N) scaffolds with different pore sizes in osteogenic medium for days 7, 14, and 21 days. GAPDH was used as a housekeeping gene for the study.

Source: Yang et al. (2021).

in DMEM medium. After proper growth of cells on the scaffolds, the cell-seeded scaffolds (constructs) were stained with alizarin red S and then all the samples were destained with cetylpyridium chloride. Finally, the absorbance of the samples was recorded at 562 nm using a microplate reader. An increased mineral deposition with increased β-TCP concentration in PCL/β-TCP scaffold was achieved as compared to that obtained with pure PCL scaffold. In this case, β-TCP helped in the growth of MG63 cells, which stimulated mineralization and thereby promoting osteogenic differentiation (Kim and Kim 2012). Chuenjitkuntaworn et al. (2016) performed the Alizarin Red staining assay to assess the calcium deposition due to the culture of different stem cells including the BMSCs (Bone marrow derived stem cell), DPSCs (Dental pulp stem cells), and ADSCs (Adipose tissue-derived stem cells) on the PCL/HA scaffolds in an osteogenic induction media for 21 days. The resulting cell-seeded scaffolds were fixed in cold methanol and washed thoroughly with deionized water. The fixed construct samples were stained with 1% Alizarin Red-S. Then the samples were subjected to destaining with 10% cetylpyridinium chloride monohydrate in 10 Mm sodium phosphate solution for 15 min at 37°C and the absorbance was measured at 570 nm in a microplate reader. The actual value of the deposited calcium was calculated by subtracting the measured absorbance of the control comprising scaffolds without cells from the absorbance value obtained with the cell-scaffold construct. Mineral deposition was found to be more significant in PCL/HAp scaffold seeded with BMSCs and DPSCs than ADSCs (Chuenjitkuntaworn et al. 2016). In an *in vitro* study, a significant deposition of calcium on the surface of butterfly wings, which was acted as scaffold, seeded with MSCs was reported (Mostofi et al. 2022). In this study, alizarin S Red staining was performed to evaluate the biomineralization activity of the MSCs on the matrix. hASCs on the generated construct (hASCs/decellularized bone construct) were fixed by ethanol at 48°C for 1 hr and washed with deionized water followed by staining of the deposited minerals with 2% Alizarin Red. The fixed samples were then seen under phase-contrast microscopy. The stain was removed by cetylpyridinium chloride monohydrate and absorbance of the sample was recorded at 540 nm. The mineralization was significantly higher in construct grown under osteogenic media in perfusion bioreactors than the control construct which was cultured in normal media. So, the media involved in the differentiation of hASCs to osteogenic cell were more pronounced in mineral deposition over matrix. The calcium assay was performed with the cells extracted from the bone construct using 5% trichloroacetic acid solution. The calcium content was measured by adding O-Cresolphthalein complex to the sample and absorbance was recorded at 550 nm. The result showed that calcium content was more in construct grown under osteogenic media than the normal media (Frohlich 2010). Rogina et al. (2017) evaluated the mineralization of hMSCs on Chitosan-Hydroxyapatite grafts having different ratios of HAp: CH by alizarin red S and von Kossa staining methods. Though von Kossa staining is not specific for calcium ions, it can stain calcium carbonate or phosphate derivatives. The observed result showed that scaffold with 10% HAp had bright staining of mineralized tissue, whereas bone nodules stained in dark brown colour with HAp 30% (Figure 8.6). In contrast, 50% HAp scaffold showed less von Kossa and alizarin staining, which indicates its poor extracellular mineralization property (Rogina et al. 2017).

Alkaline Phosphatase Activity

ALP activity is a vital tool that is used to assess the cell differentiation including the osteogenic differentiation of the stem cells over the scaffold. In ALP activity assessment, the organic phosphate esters present in the bone matrix are cleaved by the ALP enzyme which helps in the supply the free phosphate ions to the zones of

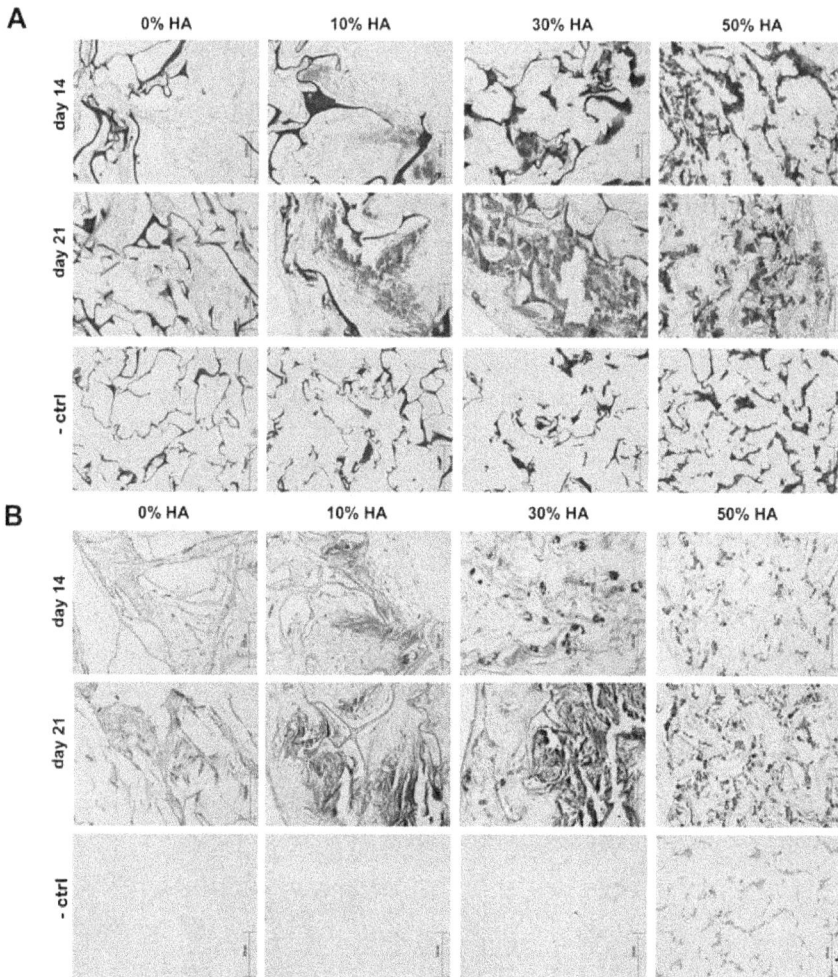

FIGURE 8.6   Illustrating mineralization on Chitosan-Hydroxyapatite grafts after 21 days of hMSCs culture in perfusion bioreactor. Scaffolds without cells were used as control of the study. (A) Calcium deposition in extracellular matrix was stained by alizarin red S at 14 and 21 days and (B) evaluation of mineralization in extracellular matrix by von Kossa staining.

Source: Rogina et al. (2017).

mineral nucleation. It is an early osteogenic marker which denotes the differentiation and mineralization of the osteoblast phenotype (Kang et al. 2008). In an ALP activity assay, cells were subjected to lysis for proper release of solubilized ALP protein by RIPA (Radio-Immunoprecipitation Assay) buffer solution after 7 and 14 days of cell culture on decellularized butterfly wing surface. The ALP activity was determined as per instructions in the manufacturer's kit. Eventually, the absorbance of the extracted sample was measured at 405 nm in an ELISA plate reader and the total protein content was then calculated (Mostofi et al. 2022). Scaffolds of hydroxyapatite/collagen/chitosan (HAp/Col/CH), hydroxyapatite/chitosan (HAp/CH), CH, and TCP were seeded with iPSC-MSCs. After 2 weeks of culture in osteogenic media, ALP activity was evaluated by using alkaline phosphatase colour development kit following the manufacturer's protocol (Xie et al. 2016). The absorbance of each sample was measured in a microplate reader at 405 nm. The ALP activity of the HAp/Col/CH scaffold was more pronounced than the other scaffolds (Xie et al. 2016). Ruckh et al. (2010) examined the ALP activity on PCL nanofibrous scaffold. The method involved the lysis of the cells adhered on the scaffold followed by the quantification of the ALP using ALP colorimetric assay kit. The ALP enzyme converted p-nitrophenolphosphate to p-nitrophenol and phosphate and the absorbance of p-nitrophenol was measured at 405 nm in a microplate reader to evaluate the expression of ALP. The level of ALP expression was significant over PCL nanofibres (Ruckh et al. 2010). In another study, ALP activities of MSCs cultured on the 3D-printed polycaprolactone (PCL) and PCL/tricalcium phosphate (PCL/β-TCP) scaffolds were investigated in growth media and osteogenic media for 7 and 14 days. There was no significant difference found in ALP activity of both the cell-seeded scaffolds in growth media, whereas in osteogenic media cell-seeded PCL/β-TCP scaffold showed significantly higher ALP activity than the PCL activity as shown in Figure 8.7 (López-gonzález et al. 2021).

Frohlich (2010) observed the alkaline phosphatase activity of hASCs/decellularized bone construct following the same protocol for ALP estimation as described above. The construct grown in osteogenic media showed pronounced ALP activity than the undifferentiated cell culture media. The study concluded that media, matrix/

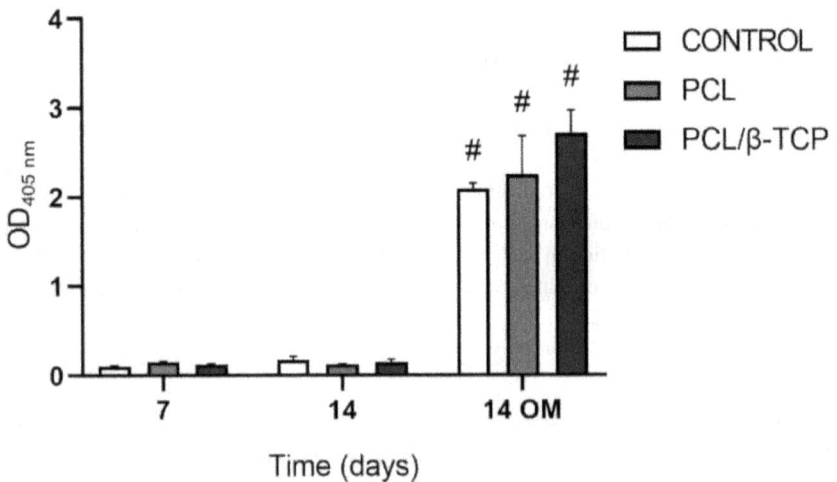

FIGURE 8.7 Comparison of ALP activities of MSCs cultured and differentiated over the PCL and PCL/β-TCP scaffolds in growth media and osteogenic media.

Source: López-gonzález et al. (2021).

construct, and growing condition played a profound role in the differentiation of stem cells to bone cell lineage (Frohlich 2010). The ALP activities of several other scaffolds and implants have been studied as this assay can demonstrate the osteogenic property of the cells growing on the scaffold by the ALP marker genes. Suzuki et al. (2021) developed a porous apatite fibre scaffolds and cultured rat bone marrow cells (RBMCs) over it in a radial flow bioreactor, resulting in a bone construct. By increasing the incubation period the ALP activity was found to be increased in the cultured cells on porous apatite fibre which denoted the osteogenic differentiation of cells (Suzuki et al. 2021).

IMMUNOCYTOCHEMISTRY (ICC) TEST

ICC test is carried out to characterize the osteogenic differentiation marker genes. For this study, cells seeded on the scaffold were isolated and incubated in PBS and Triton x100 solution for 5 min. The constructs were washed with PBS followed by incubation in PBS and glycine solution for 30 min. After adding human anti-rabbit primary osteocalcin antibody, the constructs were incubated at 4°C for 24 hr in cell culture media. After incubation, the samples were rinsed with PBS solution followed by the addition of secondary antibody with 0.1% tween-20 and left for 2 hr. The samples then rinsed properly with PBS solution and were observed under fluorescence microscope at 430–560 nm confirming the presence of osteocalcin in the differentiated cells on the surface of butterfly wings,and thus demonstrated the efficiency of the butterfly wings as scaffold for bone tissue engineering application (Mostofi et al. 2022). In another study, the bone regenerating activity in terms of differentiation of bone marrow derived stem cells to bone cell lineage of the electrospun PCL nanofibrous scaffold was confirmed by the immunofluorescent staining, that exhibited a significant amount of osteoprotegrin and osteocalcin on the cells grown on the surface of scaffold (Ruckh et al. 2010). Frohlich studied the expression of bone sialoprotein (BSP) and osteopontin on hASCs/decellularized bone construct. In this study, the primary and secondary antibodies of the respective proteins were used to evaluate the expressions of BSP and osteopontin on the hASCs/decellularized bone construct. The developed constructs cultured in the osteogenic media showed more expression of BSP as well as osteopontin than in the DMEM media (Frohlich 2010).

IN VITRO ASSESSMENT OF CARTILAGE CONSTRUCTS

Cartilage defects due to accidental injury and degeneration leading to osteoarthritis are one of the major human health issues. About 70% of the population aged above 65 years are affected by osteoarthritis in some way or other (Zhou, Sapowadia, and Chen 2021). Unlike bone tissue, the regeneration of this tissue has a serious limitation as it is an avascular tissue. So, tissue engineers are eyeing on several biomaterials for the fabrication of scaffold that can provide a matrix for faster cartilage tissue regeneration and growth (Kessler and Grande 2008). Similar to bone tissue engineering, prior to clinical or pre-clinical trials, scaffolds or constructs are tested in the laboratory with the conditions appropriate to the body in cartilage tissue engineering (CTE). This *in vitro* laboratory study is the initial assessment of the compatibility of the used scaffold as an artificial ECM or the generated construct by its combination with the cells. In this study, like bone tissue engineering, suitable cells are seeded onto the scaffold in culture media to evaluate the effect of the scaffold towards cellular growth, differentiation, and proliferation. Many experimental assays like cell adhesion, cell proliferation, live dead assay, histological assay, immunohistochemical assay, and biochemical assay, are performed *ex situ* to check the effect or compatibility of the constructs with the chondrocyte or cartilage-specific cells in the host upon transplantation (Chang et al. 2003). A brief review of these *in vitro* assessment for the engineered cartilage graft or cartilage construct is presented below.

CELL ADHESION, CELL PROLIFERATION, AND CELL MORPHOLOGY

In tissue engineering, the assessment of cell adhesion is crucial to understand how cells interact and coordinate their behaviour while combined with the scaffold matrix under the *in vitro* culture condition. Therefore, this is one of the routine tests performed in the cartilage tissue regeneration process. In an *in vitro* study for cartilage tissue regeneration, chondrocyte cells isolated from rabbits were cultured on the developed fibrous chitosan and chitosan-based hyaluronic acid hybrid polymer fibrous scaffolds of 10 mm size loaded with chondrocyte suspensions containing 0.5 $*$ x10 ^{6} cells. The cells were allowed to grow and adhered on the scaffold surface at 37°C and 5% CO_2. After incubation, each sample was washed thoroughly with PBS solution. The chondrocytes which didn't attach to the scaffold were counted by haemocytometer, from which cells attached on the scaffolds were calculated. The chondrocyte cells attached onto different scaffold composition with a varying degree, however, the scaffold containing hyaluronic acid exhibited a significantly higher attachment of chondrocyte cells than the chitosan fibre used as the control (Yamane et al. 2005). In another study, a cartilage construct derived from a decellularized avian articular cartilage scaffold seeded with human chondrocytes was investigated for the articular cartilage regeneration, in which the native cartilage was considered as the control. During the regeneration process, the cell attachment and cell proliferation on the scaffolds were assessed by observing under a phase-contrast microscope. The micrographs revealed that cells were spindle shaped in decellularized scaffold, whereas chondrocytes grown in control group had an elongated shape. Furthermore, an enhanced cell proliferation was achieved with decellularized scaffold construct than the construct made with control, signifying that the former is an ideal matrix for articular cartilage regeneration (Figure 8.8) (Ayariga, Huang, and Dean 2022).

There was also difference in chondrocyte morphology found in cells seeded in decellularized scaffold construct and native cartilage constructs. Chondrocytes seeded on the decellularized scaffold were of elongated shape, with a long proboscis spreading over the scaffold. The chondrocytes were seemed to leaving most of their cytoplasmic body outside the scaffold as indicated in Figure 8.9(A). On day 3, cells were appeared to fill the pores of decellularized scaffold (Figure 8.9(B). As reported at the early stage of culturing chondrocytes spread their pseudopodia into the scaffold while leaving their main body outside, thereby confirming the compatibility of the cells with the scaffold, which was exhibited by the decellularized scaffold. In later stage, the stretchy appearance of chondrocytes due to the smaller

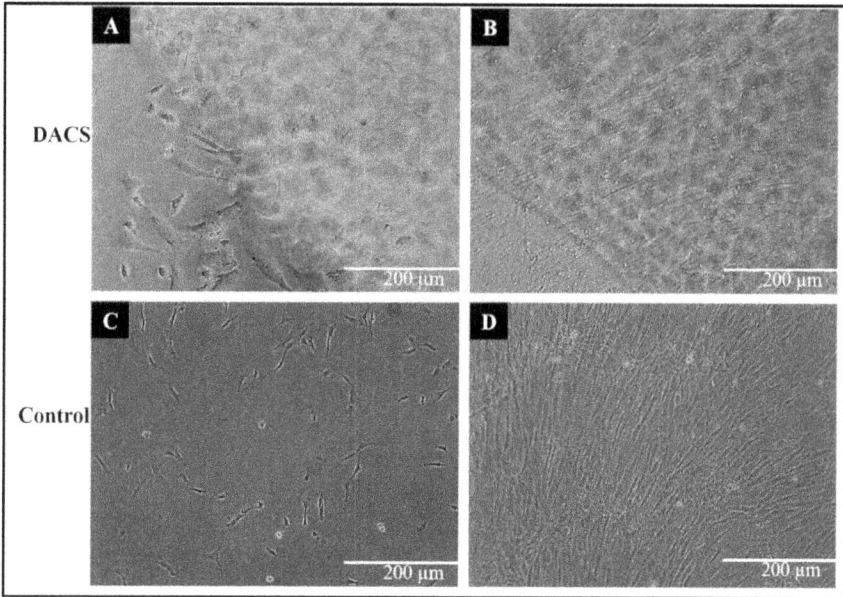

FIGURE 8.8 Attachment and proliferation of chondrocyte cells cultured over the decellularized avian articular scaffold construct (DACS) and native cartilage treated as a control during15 days of culture. The phase-contrast microscopic images revealed the cells were of spindle shape in decellularized scaffold construct, whereas elongated shape was shown in the control group. An enhanced cell proliferation was achieved with decellularized scaffold construct compared to the control.

Source: Ayariga, Huang, and Dean (2022).

size pores of decellularized scaffold was observed. On the 15th day, the cells were completely spread on the scaffold surface after invasion as shown in Figure 8.9(C). The developed cell-seeded scaffold constructs were stained with DAPI at day 5 and the formation of colony was observed under phase-contrast microscope as evident from Figure 8.9(D). The performed phallodin staining showed the stretched actin filaments of chondrocytes, which indicated the strong cell attachment on the scaffold (Figure 8.9(E)). Figure 8.9(F) showed the stretching behaviour of actin filament on scaffold stained by phallodin and DAPI. In native cartilage (control), due to the presence of monolayer of cells, less number of chondrocytes were able to attach on the scaffold surface. Furthermore, there was no change in morphology of chondrocytes seeded on the native cartilage (Figure 8.9(G–L)) (Ayariga, Huang, and Dean 2022).

CELL VIABILITY ASSAY

Maintaining cell viability within engineered 3D scaffolds is a vital step. The evaluation of cell viability in 3D scaffolds is necessary to monitor and optimize in vitro generation of engineered tissue constructs Cell viability is an important

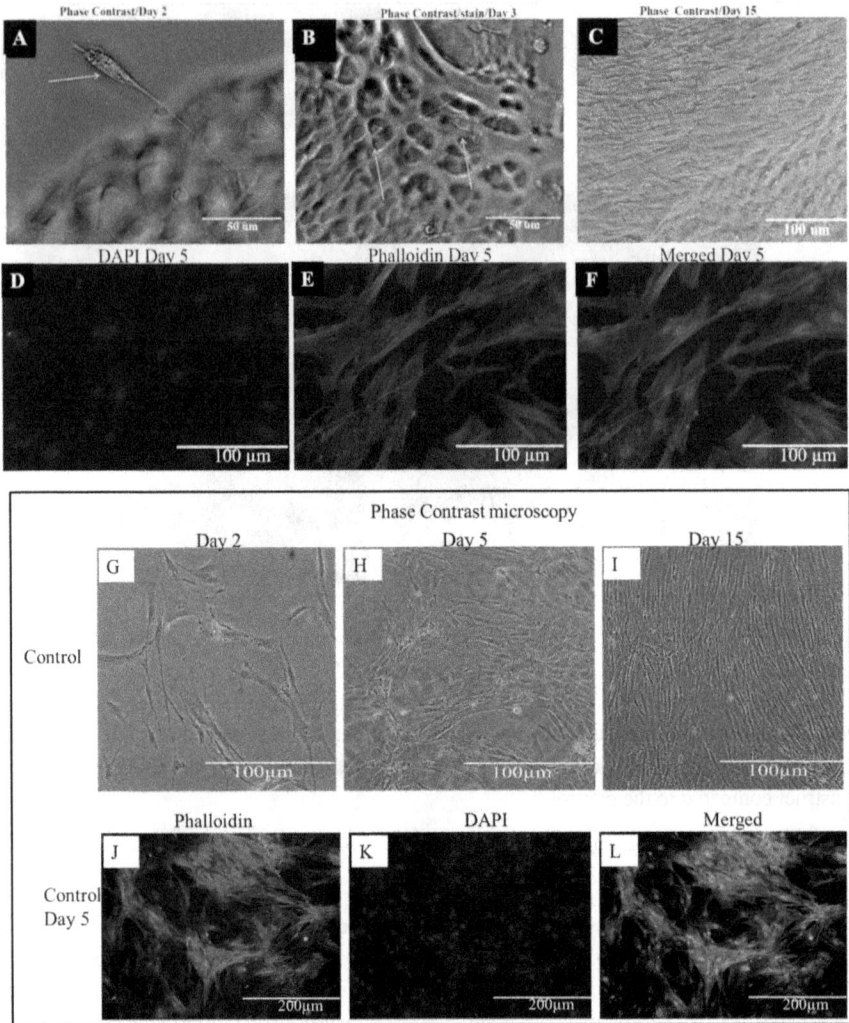

FIGURE 8.9 Attachment and proliferation of the chondrocyte cells on decellularized avian articular scaffold construct (DACS) and native cartilage. (A-B) Cell attachment with different morphology on decellularized scaffold at different incubation time intervals. In figure 8.9C the chondrocytes are shaped like spear-shaped with distinct long pseudopodia in DACS. (D) DAPI staining of colony of chondrocyte on decellularized scaffold. (E) The actin cytoskeleton in chondrocytes-seeded scaffold constructs. (F) Micrograph showing the proliferation and stretching of actin filaments by phallodin and DAPI staining. (G–I) Attachment and proliferation of chondrocytes on native cartilage (control) at different incubation periods. (J) The phallodin staining of actin filament of native cartilage-seeded chondrocytes. (K) Phase-contrast micrograph of DAPI staining of chondrocytes seeded on the control scaffold. (L) Micrograph revealing the proliferation and actin filament of chondrocyte on native cartilage.

Source: Ayariga, Huang, and Dean (2022).

routine test in CTE which is usually performed by MTT assay similar to the BTE. Hong et al. (2008) performed MTT assay with chondrocyte cell-seeded collagen-coated polylactide microcarriers/chitosan hydrogel scaffold construct. At the initial days of chondrocyte cell seeding over the scaffold, the number of viable cells were low due to the cell seeding, encapsulation, and gelation. After 1 week of culture, cells became more viable and formed a cluster over the scaffold surface. Chondrocytes were grown as cluster over the surface of the scaffold, which showed the compatibility of cells with the scaffold (Hong et al. 2008). In another study, MTT assay of electrospun fibrous scaffold and 3D-printed scaffold of gelatin/poly (lactic-*co*-glycolic acid) (PLGA) were seeded with chondrocytes to investigate the cartilage regenerating activity of the scaffolds. Cell viability study revealed that the scaffold was suitable for cartilage growth and regeneration (Chen et al. 2019). Bryant and Anseth (2001) encapsulated chondrocytes with poly(ethylene oxide) hydrogels of different thicknesses to match the defect site in cartilage. The live/dead assay of the cell-seeded scaffold was done by using calcein AM and ethidium homodimer. The former is permeable to live cell membrane, whereas, ethidium homodimer is not permeable. After 2 weeks of culture, the cell-seeded scaffold was observed under the fluorescence microscope. The viable cells were found to be profusely present throughout the scaffold, with an insignificant number of dead cells confirming the appropriate pore size of the hydrogel for efficient transfer of nutrients irrespective of the height of the scaffold demonstrating the its significant cartilage proliferation activity (Bryant and Anseth 2001). In a study, hydrogel prepared from the decellularized human umbilical cord tissue was used as a 3D scaffold for the growth of the umbilical cord-derived MSCs. The cell viability on the hydrogels with varying concentrations was evaluated by calcein AM stain at different incubation periods. The stained samples observed under a fluorescent microscope showed that the spindle-shaped cells were progressively grown on the scaffold with time representing the nontoxic and cell supportive nature of the scaffold. The proliferation rate of MSCs on the scaffold was analysed by alamar blue assay. Alamar blue reagent was added into each well and left for 4 hr of incubation. Then, the absorbance of the samples was taken to know the proliferation rate of the cells on decellularised hydrogel scaffold and the result is shown in Figure 8.10. As indicated, the proliferation of MSCs on the scaffold was enhanced by increasing the incubation period (Ramzan et al. 2022).

In an *in vitro* cartilage tissue engineering research, a hybrid hydrogel scaffold consisting of hyaluronic acid methacryloyl (HAMA), gelatin methacryloyl (GelMA), and acrylate-functionalized nano-silica (AFnSi) crosslinker was developed. The ASCs were grown on the scaffolds with different compositions such as hyaluronic acid (HA) hydrogel, HAMA-GelMA (HG) (hydrogel), HG+0.5%AFnSi, and HG+1%AFnSi for a period of 5 days in a culture media. The cell viability in the construct evaluated by MTT assay revealed that the viability of cells in the various cell-scaffold constructs was comparable to the HA hydrogel scaffold used as a control as shown in Figure 8.11. The cross-linking of AFnSi didn't affect the cell viability on HG hydrogels and the cell proliferation rate increased with the progress of the culture. The cell viabilities of the cell-seeded hydrogel constructs were further assessed by observation under a fluorescence microscope. The results indicated the maximum

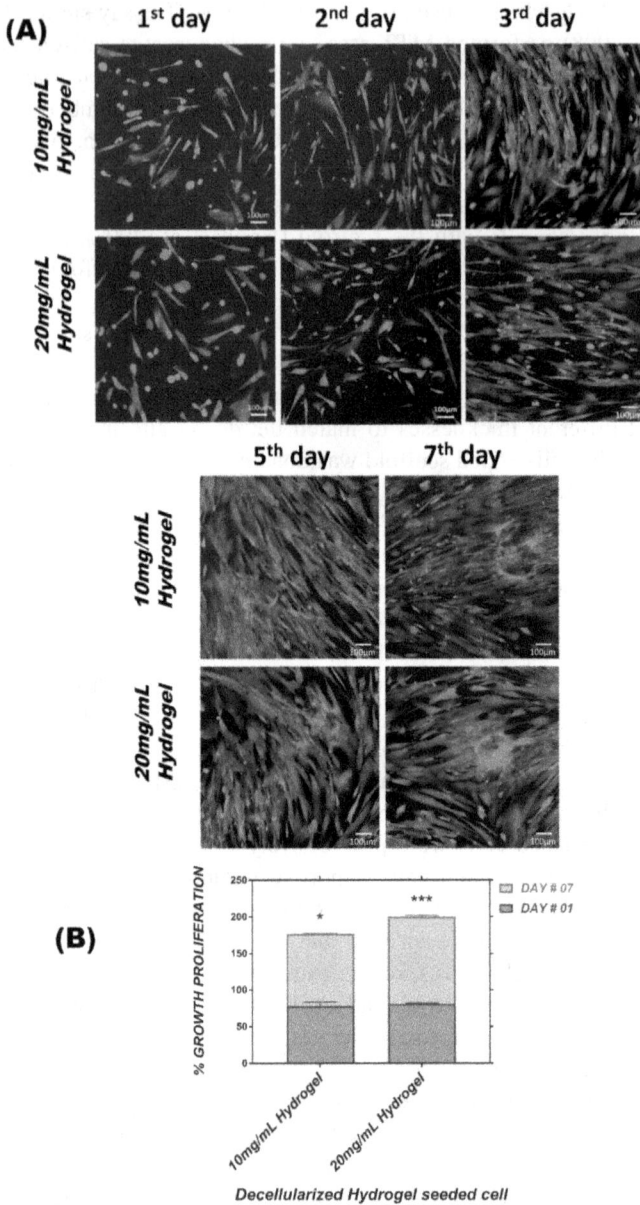

FIGURE 8.10 Proliferation and viability of MSCs seeded on the decellularized human umbilical cord tissue-derived hydrogel scaffold were assessed by calcein-AM staining and alamar blue assay. (A) Fluorescent microscopic images of MSCs-seeded decellularized hydrogel stained by calcein-AM dye. (B) The bar graph represents the proliferation rate of cells on decellularized hydrogel scaffold, evaluated by alamar blue assay.

Source: Ramzan et al. (2022).

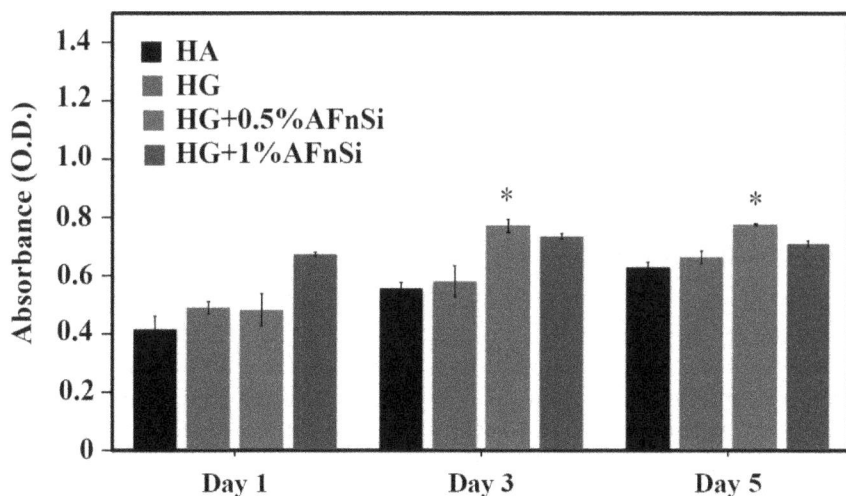

FIGURE 8.11   MTT assay of adipose-derived stem cells (ADSCs) grown on the HA hydrogel, HG hydrogel, and HG hydrogel cross-linked with AFnSi.

Source: Nedunchezian et al. (2022).

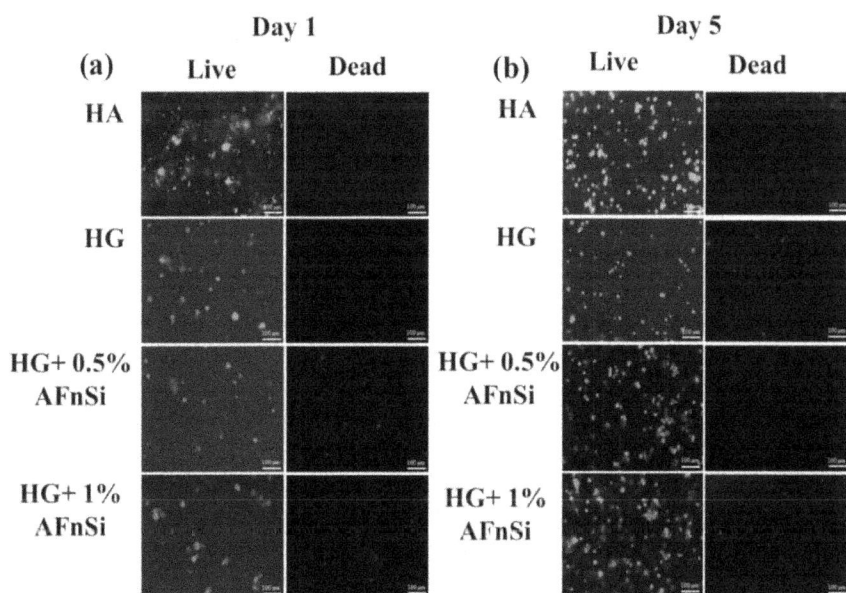

FIGURE 8.12   Cytotoxicity study of ADSCs seeded and cultured on different hydrogels (HA, HG, HG+0.5%AFnSi, and HG+1%AFnSi).

Source: Nedunchezian et al. (2022).

number of live cells with only a few dead cells on each set of scaffolds (Figure 8.12). So far as cell morphology is concerned, cells were spherical in shape with aggregated in nature on 5th day of culture. The study further revealed that the cross-linking of AFnSi didn't have any effect on the cell viability. However, HG+0.5%AFnSi had more pronounced effect on cell viability than the other hydrogel scaffolds (Nedunchezian et al. 2022).

HISTOLOGICAL EVALUATION

Histological study of the cell-seeded scaffold is done to assess the cell organelles as well as the cell morphology by using different staining dyes. A scaffold made up of gelatin/PLGA was fabricated by the combined techniques of 3D printing and freeze-drying. Chondrocytes were allowed to grow on PLGA matrix for appropriate incubation periods. After incubation of 4 weeks, the chondrocyte cells seeded in the scaffold were fixed with 4% paraformaldehyde and the samples were investigated for the structure and mineralization deposition. The samples were then stained with haematoxylin and eosin (H&E) and safranin-O. The glycosaminoglycan (GAG) contents of the samples was quantified using the Alcian blue method. The scaffolds showed cartilage-like growths after seeded with chondrocytes and provided appropriate environment for the growth and proliferation of chondrocytes. The ECM produced by chondrocytes on the surface of both the scaffolds was clearly visible (Chen et al. 2019). In another study, chondrocytes-encapsulated PEO hydrogels after culturing in media were sectioned transversely in 2-mm-thick sections. The specimens were fixed in formalin overnight, followed by staining with different stains like safranin O (stain GAG), Fast Green (stain nucleus and GAG), and Masson trichrome technique (stain nuclei and collagen). Safranin O generally stains the GAG for its positive charge and counterstaining with Fast Green stains nucleus in black and GAG in orange/red color. In Masson trichrome staining, nucleus and collagen are stained blue black and blue, respectively. The results revealed the uniform distribution of GAGs throughout the scaffold irrespective of the thickness of the hydrogel. The collagen was also profused uniformly in all the scaffolds (Bryant and Anseth 2001). Li et al. (2005) developed a cell-seeded scaffold constructed by culturing MSCs on a developed PCL-based nanofibrous scaffold with the addition of transforming growth factor-β (TGF-β). The morphology of the cultured cells was examined by H&E and Alcian blue staining. Three different morphologies of the cells were observed in the cell-seeded scaffold constructs. Flat fibroblast cells formed sheath covering the fibres of the scaffold, whereas large and round chondrocyte-like cells were found in the middle region of the fibrous construct. At the lower portion of the fibre, small flat cells were found to be surrounded by the ECM. Strong alcian blue staining revealed that the ECM surrounding the cells was rich in sulphated proteoglycans (Li et al. 2005). Liao et al. (2010) fabricated an electrospun acellular PCL/ECM scaffold to assess its chondrogenic differentiating activity. In the study, MSCs were cultured on the scaffold in serum-free media with and without incorporation of TGF-β in a perfusion bioreactor. The resulting constructs were fixed with neutral buffered formalin (10%) and submerged in ethanol solution and the fixed samples were used for the histological study by staining with haematoxylin and safranin O. Generally haematoxylin

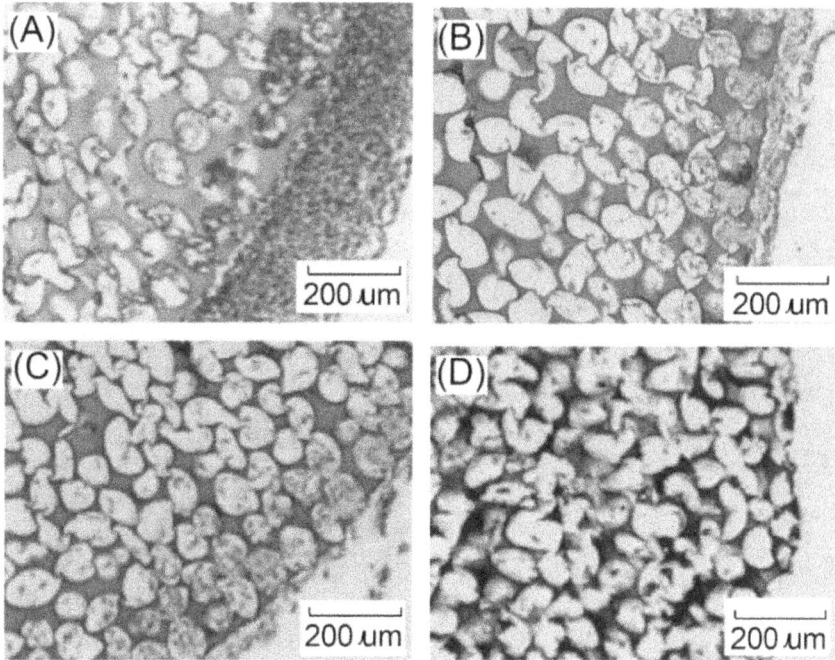

FIGURE 8.13 Histological analysis of the constructs comprising of chondrocytes-laden the gelation-based porous scaffolds in tidal bioreactor using haematoxylin and eosin staining with varying incubation periods: (A) 7 days, (B)14 days, (C) 21 days, and (D) 28 days in tidal bioreactor.

Source: Liu et al. (2022).

and safranin O dyes are used to assess the distribution of cells and cartilaginous ECM deposition, respectively. From the SEM micrographs shown, cells were evenly distributed throughout the scaffold and a proper cartilaginous matrix was formed over the scaffold surface (Liao et al. 2010). Using a microfluidic 3D foaming technology a gelatin-based hydrogel was fabricated for cartilage tissue engineering. Articular chondrocyte cells isolated from the rabbit knee joint were cultured on this fabricated hydrogel in both static and dynamic tidal bioreactor for 4 weeks. After incubation, the generated constructs were subjected to histological study by staining with H&E. The results showed that the chondrocytes were properly distributed throughout the scaffold in dynamic culture and the rate of cell proliferation increased by increasing the incubation period. The cytoplasm and intercellular substances were clearly visible in the image (Figure 8.13). The Alcian blue stained nuclei and GAG of the construct as shown in Figure 8.14. After 7 days of dynamic culture, chondrocytes were profusely distributed throughout the hydrogel and the proliferation rate of cells was more pronounced (Liu et al. 2022).

Yang et al. (2018) developed cell-seeded scaffolds comprising the 3D bioprinted sodium alginate/collagen (SA/COL) and sodium alginate/agarose (SA/AG) scaffolds

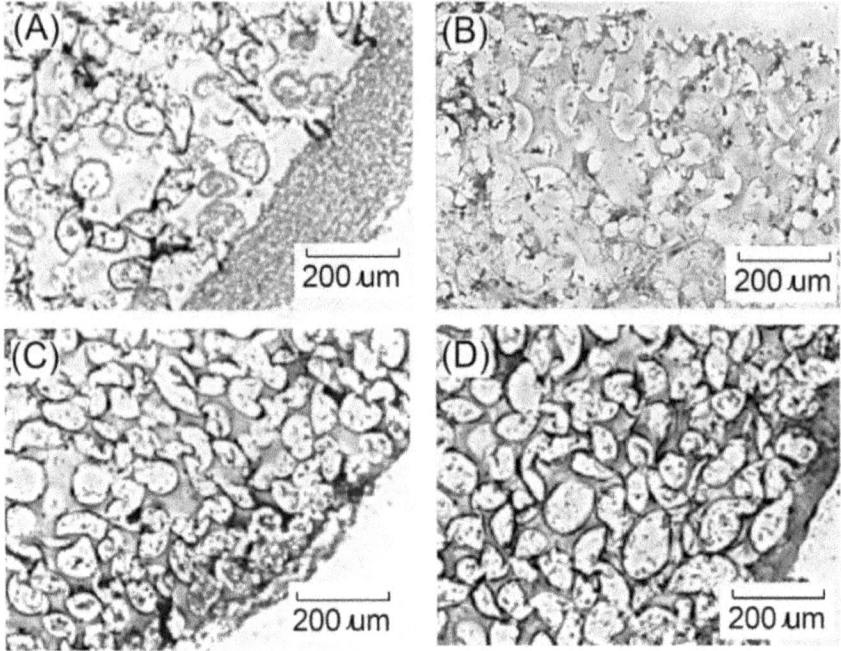

FIGURE 8.14 Histological study of chondrocyte cells-seeded on the gelation-based porous scaffold in tidal bioreactor using Alcian blue staining method at different culture periods. (A) 7 days, (B) 14 days, (C) 21 days, and (D) 28 days. The figure displaying the glycosaminoglycan and nucleus formation on hydrogel.

Source: Liu et al. (2022).

seeded with chondrocyte cells. A histological study performed with the constructs by H&E staining revealed that the cell proliferation rate was higher in SA/COL scaffold than that observed with SA/AG (Yang et al. 2018).

Immunohistochemical Assay

Immunohistochemistry is an essential assay to check the expressions of specific genes in specific tissue using monoclonal as well as polyclonal antibodies. Bhardwaj et al. (2011) examined the deposition of collagen on a porous silk fibroin/chitosan scaffold seeded with chondrocyte cells. After 2 weeks of *in vitro* culture the immunohistochemical staining for collagen was done with the cell-seeded scaffold construct using mouse monoclonal primary and secondary antibodies. The results showed the presence of collagen II in the construct and no collagen I was noticed (Bhardwaj et al. 2011). Li et al. (2005) studied the immunohistochemical assay on PCL nanofibrous scaffold seeded with MSCs in chondrogenic media with and without

TGF-β growth factor. After 21 days of culture, the cell-seeded scaffold with TGF-β exhibited a positive staining response for chondrogenic specific molecules like ECM, aggrecan, collagen type II, and link protein. However, no staining was found in the construct when it was cultured without TGF-β (Li et al. 2005). Liu et al. (2022) developed a highly porous gelatin hydrogel by microfluidic 3D foaming technology and cultured articular chondrocytes in a tidal bioreactor for 28 days. To study the expression of specific proteins on the chondrocyte-seeded gelation-based hydrogels, an indirect immunofluorescence staining was performed for specific proteins like collagen type II, matrix metalloproteinase 13 (MMP13), Sox 9, and aggrecan. The constructed cell-seeded scaffold was treated with the primary antibody of the specific proteins including collagen type II, MMP13, Sox 9, and aggrecan followed by the removal of excess antibodies through washing. Fluorescein-conjugated secondary antibodies were added to the sample for detection of specific proteins. As observed from Figure 8.15 (a and b), the expression of type II collagen was gradually increased from 21 to 28 days of culture indicating the differentiation of chondrocyte cells on the scaffold. The fluorescence images as shown in Figure 8.15 (c and d) revealed that the expression of MMP13 increased with culture time. Furthermore, the expressions of Sox 9 and aggrecan were observed to be maintained during the progression of culturing (Figure 8.15(e–h)). The results concluded that the gelatin-based hydrogel is a potential artificial ECM for cartilage regeneration by promoting the culturing and differentiating the chondrocyte-like cells with maintained chondrocyte property without dedifferentiation (Liu et al. 2022).

BIOCHEMICAL ASSAY

A biochemical assay is an *in vitro* procedure used to detect, quantify, and/or study a biological molecule, such as an enzyme. In tissue engineering, biochemical assays are performed to quantify the different matrix components and analyze the quality of engineered tissues. For example, proteoglycans and type II collagen are quantified by biochemical assays and thus the quality of tissue-engineered cartilage is ensured. In an *in vitro* study, the chondrocyte-seeded scaffold was dried and digested with papain solution. GAG in chondrocytes-encapsulated PEO (Polyethylene oxide) hydrogel was quantified by using dimethylmethylene blue dye and collagen was quantified by measuring the hydroxyproline content. The results showed that there is no significant change in the GAG content of the constructs comprising scaffolds with different thicknesses, whereas the collagen content was slightly higher in the construct containing scaffold with higher thickness. It was concluded that encapsulated chondrocytes in the hydrogel can easily cross the thickness of articular cartilage (Bryant and Anseth 2001). Yang et al. (2018) developed 3D bioprinted scaffolds from SA/COL and SA/AG which were seeded with chondrocyte cells by culturing, thereby producing cell-seeded scaffold constructs. In this study, the production of GAG was detected by 1,9-dimethylmethylene blue and the formation of GAG was high in SA/COL scaffold as compared to the SA/AG scaffold during the 14 days of culture period (Yang et al. 2018).

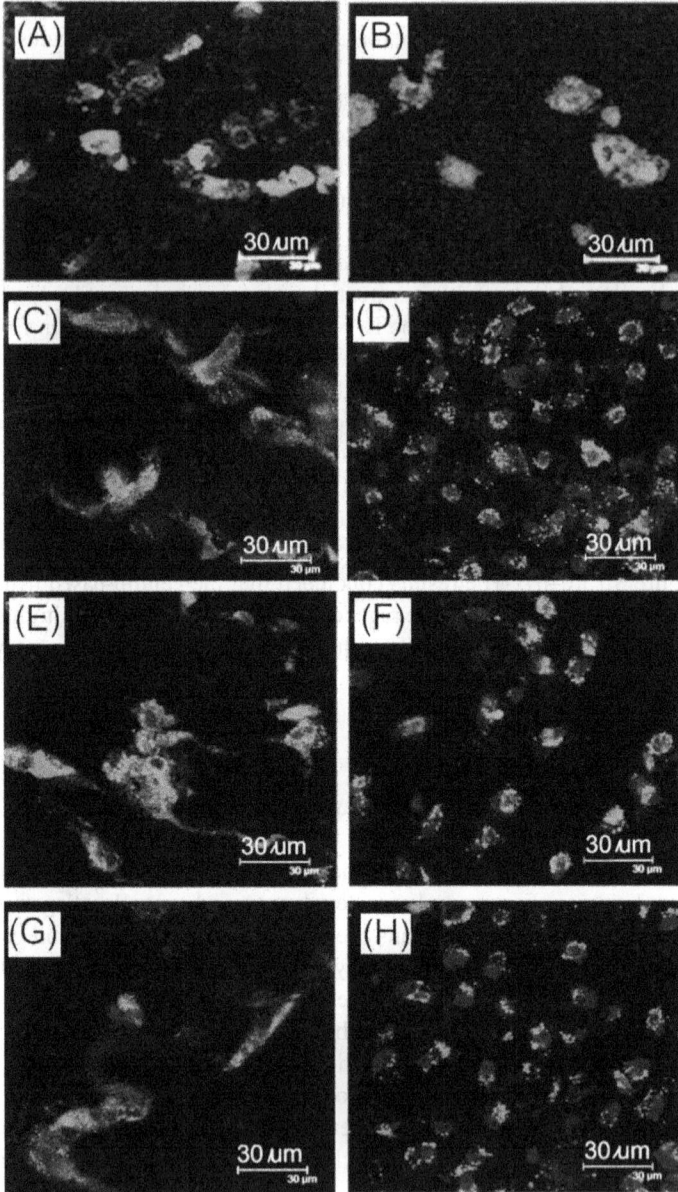

FIGURE 8.15 Immunohistochemical staining of chondrocytes seeded on gelatin-based hydrogel scaffold in tidal bioreactor for collagen type II (A) after 21 days and (B) after 28 days; for MMP13 (C) after 21 days and (D) after 28 days; sox9 (E) after 21 days and (F) after 28 days; and aggrecan (G) after 21 days and (H) after 28 days.

Source: Liu et al. (2022).

EXERCISE

1. What is MTT assay?
2. Which type of cells are used in bone tissue engineering scaffold?
3. What is the importance of Alizarin Red-S staining bone tissue engineering?
4. Which chemicals are used for the cell viability study in bone tissue engineering?
5. What are bone-specific marker genes?
6. Which types of genes are involved in bone cell differentiation?
7. Discuss the importance of *in vitro* study?
8. What different types of dyes are used for in the histochemical study of the bone constructs?
9. What are cartilage specific genes?
10. Give a brief account of in vitro assessment of bone tissue constructs.
11. Give a brief account of in vitro assessment of bone tissue constructs.
12. In which type of construct ALP activity is measured: bone tissue scaffold or cartilage scaffold?
13. What is the importance of immunohistochemical study in bone and cartilage tissue engineering?
14. Explain different methods which can be used to assess osteogenic differentiation?
15. What is the purpose of measuring biomineralization activity during bone tissue regeneration process
16. Which reagent is used to stain Actin filament?
17. What is the need of staining of actin filament in *in vitro* study?
18. Explain how biochemical assays are important for evaluating engineered cartilage construct with example.
19. How do you detect glycosaminoglycan in *in vitro* study?
20. What is ALP? Write the importance method of ALP assessment in bone tissue construct.
21. What are the different types of cartilage markers have you come across for gene expression study?
22. What are the various staining methods employed in the assessment of engineered bone and cartilage constructs.
23. Which chemical is used fix cells on cell seeded scaffold?
24. Describe the procedure of fixing cells on cell seeded scaffold construct?
25. What does Alamar blue detect?
26. Give a brief account of different microscopic assessment performed in evaluating bone and cartilage tissue constructs.

REFERENCES

Ayariga, J. A., H. Huang, and D. Dean. 2022. "Decellularized avian cartilage, a promising alternative for human cartilage tissue regeneration." Materials (Basel). 2022 Mar 7;15(5): 1–34.

Baek, J. W., Park, H., Kim, K. S., Chun, S. K., & Kim, B. S. 2022. "Marine plankton-derived whitlockite powder-based 3D-printed porous scaffold for bone tissue engineering." *Materials* 15(10): 3413.

Bhardwaj, N., and S. C. Kundu. 2012. "Chondrogenic differentiation of rat MSCs on porous scaffolds of silk fibroin/chitosan blends." *Biomaterials* 33 (10): 2848–2857. https://doi.org/10.1016/j.biomaterials.2011.12.028

Bhardwaj, N., Q. T. Nguyen, A. C. Chen, D. L. Kaplan, R. L. Sah, and S. C. Kundu. 2011. "Potential of 3-D tissue constructs engineered from bovine chondrocytes/silk fibroin-chitosan for in vitro cartilage tissue engineering." *Biomaterials* 32 (25): 5773–5781. https://doi.org/10.1016/j.biomaterials.2011.04.061

Bryant, S. J., and K. S. Anseth. 2001. "The effects of scaffold thickness on tissue engineered cartilage in photocrosslinked poly(ethylene oxide) hydrogels." *Biomaterials* 22 (6): 619–626. https://doi.org/10.1016/S0142-9612(00)00225-8

Chang, C. H., H. C. Liu, C. C. Lin, C. H. Chou, and F. H. Lin. 2003. "Gelatin-Chondroitin-Hyaluronan Tri-Copolymer scaffold for cartilage tissue engineering." *Biomaterials* 24 (26): 4853–4858. https://doi.org/10.1016/S0142-9612(03)00383-1

Chen, H., Y. Liu, Z. Jiang, W. Chen, Y. Yu, and Q. Hu. 2014. "Cell-Scaffold interaction within engineered tissue." *Experimental Cell Research* 323 (2): 346–351. https://doi.org/10.1016/j.yexcr.2014.02.028

Chen, W., Y. Xu, Y. Liu, Z. Wang, Y. Li, G. Jiang, X. Mo, and G. Zhou. 2019. "Three-Dimensional printed electrospun fiber-based scaffold for cartilage regeneration." *Materials and Design* 179: 107886. https://doi.org/10.1016/j.matdes.2019.107886

Chuenjitkuntaworn, B., T. Osathanon, N. Nowwarote, P. Supaphol, and P. Pavasant. 2016. "The Efficacy of polycaprolactone/hydroxyapatite scaffold in combination with mesenchymal stem cells for bone tissue engineering." *Journal of Biomedical Materials Research – Part A* 104 (1): 264–271. https://doi.org/10.1002/jbm.a.35558

Csaba Matta, Csilla Szűcs-Somogyi, Elizaveta Kon Dror Robinson, Tova Neufeld, Nir Altschulere, Agnes Berta, László Hangody, Zoltán Veréb, Róza Zákány, Osteogenic differentiation of human bone marrow-derived mesenchymal stem cells is enhanced by an aragonite scaffold, Differentiation Volume 107, May–June 2019, Pages 24-34

Frohlich, M.. 2010. "Bone grafts engineered from human adipose-derived." *Tissue Engineering Part A* 16 (1): 179–189.

Hong, Y., Y. Gong, C. Gao, and J. Shen. 2008. "Collagen-Coated polylactide microcarriers/chitosan hydrogel composite: Injectable scaffold for cartilage regeneration." *Journal of Biomedical Materials Research – Part A* 85 (3): 628–637. https://doi.org/10.1002/jbm.a.31603

Ju, J., X. Peng, K. Huang, L. Li, X. Liu, C. Chitrakar, L. Chang, Z. Gu, and T. Kuang. 2019. "High-performance porous PLLA-Based scaffolds for bone tissue engineering: preparation, characterization, and in vitro and in vivo evaluation." *Polymer* 180 (August): 121707. https://doi.org/10.1016/j.polymer.2019.121707

Kang, S. W., W. G. La, J. M. Kang, J. H. Park, and B. S. Kim. 2008. "Bone morphogenetic protein-2 enhances bone regeneration mediated by transplantation of osteogenically undifferentiated bone marrow-derived mesenchymal stem cells." *Biotechnology Letters* 30 (7): 1163–1168. https://doi.org/10.1007/s10529-008-9675-8

Kessler, M. W., and D. A. Grande. 2008. "Tissue engineering and cartilage." *Organogenesis* 4 (1): 28–32. https://doi.org/10.4161/org.6116

Khalili, A. A., and M. R. Ahmad. 2015. "A review of cell adhesion studies for biomedical and biological applications." *International Journal of Molecular Sciences* 16 (8): 18149–18184. https://doi.org/10.3390/ijms160818149

Kim, Y. B., and G. Kim. 2012. "Functionally graded PCL/β-TCP biocomposites in a multi-layered structure for bone tissue regeneration." *Applied Physics A: Materials Science and Processing* 108 (4): 949–959. https://doi.org/10.1007/s00339-012-7004-5

Li, W. J., R. Tuli, C. Okafor, A. Derfoul, K. G. Danielson, D. J. Hall, and R. S. Tuan. 2005. "A three-dimensional nanofibrous scaffold for cartilage tissue engineering using human mesenchymal stem cells." *Biomaterials* 26 (6): 599–609. https://doi.org/10.1016/j.biomaterials.2004.03.005

Liao, J., Xuan Guo, K. J. G.-A., F. K. Kasper, and A. G. Mikos. 2010. "Bioactive polymer/extracellular matrix scaffolds fabricated with a flow perfusion bioreactor for cartilage tissue engineering." *Biomaterials* 31 (34): 8911–8920. https://doi.org/10.1016/j.biomaterials.2010.07.110

Liu, H.-W., W.-T. Su, C.-Y. Liu, and C.-C. Huang. 2022. "Highly organized porous gelatin-based scaffold by microfluidic 3D-foaming technology and dynamic culture for cartilage tissue engineering." *International Journal of Molecular Sciences.* 2022 Jul 30; 23 (15): 8449.

Logeart-Avramoglou, D., F. Anagnostou, R. Bizios, and H. Petite. 2005. "Engineering bone: Challenges and obstacles." *Journal of Cellular and Molecular Medicine* 9 (1): 72–84. https://doi.org/10.1111/j.1582-4934.2005.tb00338.x

López-gonzález, I., C. Zamora-ledezma, M. I. Sanchez-lorencio, E. T. Barrenechea, J. A. Gabaldón-hernández, and L. Meseguer-olmo. 2021. "Modifications in gene expression in the process of osteoblastic differentiation of multipotent bone marrow-derived human mesenchymal stem cells induced by a novel osteoinductive porous medical-grade 3d-printed Poly(E-caprolactone)/B-tricalcium Phosphate C." *International Journal of Molecular Sciences* 22 (20): 1–21. https://doi.org/10.3390/ijms222011216

Mostofi, F., M. Mostofi, B. Niroomand, S. Hosseini, and A. Alipour. 2022. "Crossing phylums: Butterfly wing as a natural perfusable three-dimensional (3D) bioconstruct for bone tissue engineering." Journal of Functional Biomaterials. 2022 Jun 1; 13 (2): 68.

Motamedian, S. R.. 2015. "Smart scaffolds in bone tissue engineering: A systematic review of literature." *World Journal of Stem Cells* 7 (3): 657. https://doi.org/10.4252/wjsc.v7.i3.657

Murphy, C. M., M. G. Haugh, and F. J. O'Brien. 2010. "The effect of mean pore size on cell attachment, proliferation and migration in collagen-glycosaminoglycan scaffolds for bone tissue engineering." *Biomaterials* 31 (3): 461–466. https://doi.org/10.1016/j.biomaterials.2009.09.063

Nedunchezian, S., C. W. Wu, S. C. Wu, C. H. Chen, J. K. Chang, and C. K. Wang. 2022. "Characteristic and chondrogenic differentiation analysis of hybrid hydrogels comprised of hyaluronic acid methacryloyl (HAMA), gelatin methacryloyl (GelMA), and the acrylate-functionalized nano-silica crosslinker." *Polymers* 14 (10). https://doi.org/10.3390/polym14102003

Nöth, U., R. Tuli, A. M. Osyczka, K. G. Danielson, and R. S. Tuan. 2002. "In vitro engineered cartilage constructs produced by press-coating biodegradable polymer with human mesenchymal stem cells." *Tissue Engineering* 8 (1): 131–144. https://doi.org/10.1089/107632702753503126

Oliveira, J. M., S. S. Silva, P. B. Malafaya, M. T. Rodrigues, N. Kotobuki, M. Hirose, M. E. Gomes, J. F. Mano, H. Ohgushi, and R. L. Reis. 2009. "Macroporous hydroxyapatite scaffolds for bone tissue engineering applications: Physicochemical characterization and assessment of rat bone marrow stromal cell viability." *Journal of Biomedical Materials Research – Part A* 91 (1): 175–186. https://doi.org/10.1002/jbm.a.32213

Park, S. A., S. H. Lee, and W. D. Kim. 2011. "Fabrication of porous polycaprolactone/hydroxyapatite (PCL/HA) blend scaffolds using a 3D plotting system for bone tissue engineering." *Bioprocess and Biosystems Engineering* 34 (4): 505–513. https://doi.org/10.1007/s00449-010-0499-2

Polyethylene, N., and G. Scaffolds. 2021. "The development of polylactic acid / multi-wall carbon." *Polymers* 2021,13 (11): 1–18.

Przekora, A. 2019. "The summary of the most important cell-biomaterial interactions that need to be considered during in vitro biocompatibility testing of bone scaffolds for tissue engineering applications." *Materials Science and Engineering C* 97 (March 2018): 1036–1051. https://doi.org/10.1016/j.msec.2019.01.061

Ramzan, F., S. Ekram, T. Frazier, A. Salim, O. A. Mohiuddin, and I. Khan. 2022. "Decellularized human umbilical tissue-derived hydrogels promote proliferation and chondrogenic differentiation of mesenchymal stem cells." *Bioengineering* 9 (6): 239. https://doi.org/10.3390/bioengineering9060239

Rhee, S., J. L. Puetzer, B. N. Mason, C. A. Reinhart-King, and L. J. Bonassar. 2016. "3D bioprinting of spatially heterogeneous collagen constructs for cartilage tissue engineering." *ACS Biomaterials Science and Engineering* 2 (10): 1800–1805. https://doi.org/10.1021/acsbiomaterials.6b00288

Rodrigues, C. V. M., P. Serricella, A. B. R. Linhares, R. M. Guerdes, R. Borojevic, M. A. Rossi, M. E. L. Duarte, and M. Farina. 2003. "Characterization of a bovine collagen-hydroxyapatite composite scaffold for bone tissue engineering." *Biomaterials* 24 (27): 4987–4997. https://doi.org/10.1016/S0142-9612(03)00410-1

Rogina, A., M. Antunović, L. Pribolšan, K. C. Mihalić, A. Vukasović, A. Ivković, I. Marijanović, G. G. Ferrer, M. Ivanković, and H. Ivanković. 2017. "Human mesenchymal stem cells differentiation regulated by hydroxyapatite content within chitosan-based scaffolds under perfusion conditions." *Polymers* 9 (9): 1–17. https://doi.org/10.3390/polym9090387

Rouwkema, J., Jan De Boer, and C. A. Van Blitterswijk. 2006. "Endothelial cells assemble into a 3-dimensional prevascular network in a bone tissue engineering construct." *Tissue Engineering* 12 (9): 2685–2693. https://doi.org/10.1089/ten.2006.12.2685

Ruckh, T. T., K. Kumar, M. J. Kipper, and K. C. Popat. 2010. "Osteogenic differentiation of bone marrow stromal cells on poly(ε-caprolactone) nanofiber scaffolds." *Acta Biomaterialia* 6 (8): 2949–2959. https://doi.org/10.1016/j.actbio.2010.02.006

Shalumon, K. T., K. H. Anulekha, K. P. Chennazhi, H. Tamura, S. V. Nair, and R. Jayakumar. 2011. "Fabrication of chitosan/poly(caprolactone) nanofibrous scaffold for bone and skin tissue engineering." *International Journal of Biological Macromolecules* 48 (4): 571–576. https://doi.org/10.1016/j.ijbiomac.2011.01.020

Shin, M., H. Yoshimoto, and J. P. Vacanti. 2004. "In vivo bone tissue engineering using mesenchymal stem cells on a novel electrospun nanofibrous scaffold." *Tissue Engineering* 10 (1–2): 33–41. https://doi.org/10.1089/107632704322791673

Soumya, S., K. M. Sajesh, R. Jayakumar, S. V. Nair, and K. P. Chennazhi. 2012. "Development of a phytochemical scaffold for bone tissue engineering using cissus quadrangularis extract." *Carbohydrate Polymers* 87 (2): 1787–1795. https://doi.org/10.1016/j.carbpol.2011.09.094

Suzuki, K., J. Fukasawa, M. Miura, P. N. Lim, M. Honda, T. Matsuura, and M. Aizawa. 2021. "Influence of culture period on osteoblast differentiation of tissue-engineered bone constructed by apatite-fiber scaffolds using radial-flow bioreactor." *International Journal of Molecular Sciences* 22 (23). https://doi.org/10.3390/ijms222313080

Thein-Han, W. W., and R. D.K. Misra. 2009. "Biomimetic chitosan-nanohydroxyapatite composite scaffolds for bone tissue engineering." *Acta Biomaterialia* 5 (4): 1182–1197. https://doi.org/10.1016/j.actbio.2008.11.025

Wang, W., G. Caetano, W. S. Ambler, J. J. Blaker, M. A. Frade, P. Mandal, C. Diver, and P. Bártolo. 2016. "Enhancing the hydrophilicity and cell attachment of 3D printed PCL/ graphene scaffolds for bone tissue engineering." *Materials* 9 (12): 992. https://doi.org/ 10.3390/ma9120992

Woodfield, T. B. F., J. Malda, J. De Wijn, F. Péters, J. Riesle, and C. A. Van Blitterswijk. 2004. "Design of porous scaffolds for cartilage tissue engineering using a three-dimensional fiber-deposition technique." *Biomaterials* 25 (18): 4149–4161. https://doi.org/10.1016/ j.biomaterials.2003.10.056

Xie, J., C. Peng, Q. Zhao, X. Wang, H. Yuan, L. Yang, K. Li, X. Lou, and Y. Zhang. 2016. "Osteogenic differentiation and bone regeneration of IPSC-MSCs supported by a biomimetic nanofibrous scaffold." *Acta Biomaterialia* 29: 365–379. https://doi.org/ 10.1016/j.actbio.2015.10.007

Yamane, S., N. Iwasaki, T. Majima, T. Funakoshi, T. Masuko, K. Harada, A. Minami, K. Monde, and S. I. Nishimura. 2005. "Feasibility of chitosan-based hyaluronic acid hybrid biomaterial for a novel scaffold in cartilage tissue engineering." *Biomaterials* 26 (6): 611–619. https://doi.org/10.1016/j.biomaterials.2004.03.013

Yang, X., Z. Lu, H. Wu, W. Li, L. Zheng, and J. Zhao. 2018. "Collagen-Alginate as bioink for three-dimensional (3D) cell printing based cartilage tissue engineering." *Materials Science and Engineering C* 83 (June 2017): 195–201. https://doi.org/10.1016/ j.msec.2017.09.002

Yang, Y., A. Kulkarni, G. D. Soraru, J. M. Pearce, and A. Motta. 2021. "3D printed sioc(N) ceramic scaffolds for bone tissue regeneration: Improved osteogenic differentiation of human bone marrow-derived mesenchymal stem cells." *International Journal of Molecular Sciences* 22 (24): 13676. https://doi.org/10.3390/ijms222413676

Yang, Z., Y. Wu, C. Li, T. Zhang, Y. Zou, J. H. P. Hui, Z. Ge, and E. H. Lee. 2012. "Improved mesenchymal stem cells attachment and in vitro cartilage tissue formation on chitosan-modified poly(l-Lactide-Co-Epsilon-Caprolactone) scaffold." *Tissue Engineering – Part A* 18 (3–4): 242–251. https://doi.org/10.1089/ten.tea.2011.0315

Zhou, L., A. Sapowadia, and Y. Chen. 2021. "Cartilage tissue engineering." *Musculoskeletal Tissue Engineering*, 41–66. https://doi.org/10.1016/B978-0-12-823893-6.00009-7

9 In Vivo Assessment of Regenerated Bone, Cartilage, and Joint Tissue

INTRODUCTION

After successful in vitro assessment, the evaluation of the safety and efficacy of the newly developed engineered tissue constructs and tissue grafts for the treatment of defect bone, cartilage, and their more complex form, for example, osteochondral defects by in vivo study, is the next crucial step for their application point of view. The acquisition of pre-clinical immunocompetent animal study information before entering into the clinical study is vital to assess the suitability of use of any engineered tissue in clinical setting. While *in vitro* studies usually provide prior information regarding the biocompatibility and stability, *in vivo* studies demonstrate the proof-of-concept, efficacy of the engineered tissue products, and the risks associated with them, including the tumourigenicity, toxicology, etc.

These *in vivo* studies involve the use of animal models which are also referred to as pre-clinical studies that are done prior to the clinical trials. The use of animals is justified because of their anatomical and physiological similarity to humans and the human diseases to a large extent. The experiments using animals are well recognized as the critical translational models which are helpful for developing effective treatments for bone and cartilage damage. Keeping this in view, animal study has widely been performed with these tissue engineered products predominantly by using small animals like mice model. Animal experiments, which are considered as the critical translational models, are helpful for developing effective treatments for cartilage injuries (Chu, Szczodry and Bruno 2010). Like cartilage tissue engineering, a number of protocols for *in vivo* animal experiments have been evolved to validate the engineered bone and related tissue products. *In vivo* study actually involves two steps-animal testing and further clinical trials. The animal study of engineered tissue products is carried out usually at subcutaneous implantation sites, and it is performed prior to clinical trials. The intense pre-clinical experiment is essential for getting the Food and Drug Administration (FDA) authorization for their actual use and ethical consideration. The *in vivo* experimental parameters eventually measure the efficacy of the engineered tissue grafts. The various *in vivo* parameters are evaluated in terms of morphology, histology, biochemical and biomechanical characteristics following different procedures. This chapter reviews and discusses different in vivo assessment

DOI: 10.1201/9781003245353-9

methods of bone, cartilage, and osteochondral tissue-engineered products based on animal studies, which have been reported by the researchers.

ASSESSMENT OF CARTILAGE AND RELATED TISSUE CONSTRUCTS OR TISSUE GRAFTS

In cartilage tissue engineering (CTE) approaches, numerous *in vivo* animal models using mice, rats, rabbits, pigs, sheeps, dogs, and even horses have been used for the validation of cartilage and related tissue grafts. Although, it is quite difficult to make a comparison of the different animal models used by the researchers worldwide as too many factors influence the pre-clinical animal study results (Ahern et al. 2009) an attempt has been made to present some of the methods that have widely been used for *in vivo* studies of the cartilage tissue grafts.

MORPHOLOGICAL ASSESSMENT

Micro-Computed Tomography (micro-CT or μ-CT), Scanning Electron Microscopy, and Magnetic Resonance Imaging (MRI) techniques have been used to assess the microstructure of the cartilage grafts. In an *in vivo* study, the micro-architecture of osteochondral complex comprising bone, cartilage, and their interface (cartilage–bone transition) in a human knee joint and conjunctions of the osteochondral complex has been evaluated by μ-CT analysis (Bian et al. 2016). Multi-layered chitosan-gelatin scaffolds have been seeded with MSCs which were derived from bone marrow of the knee joints of rabbits. The cell-seeded scaffolds (constructs) were tested *in vivo* in 4-month-old male New Zealand white rabbits. It is evident from gross appearance that the defects were fully filled with glossy white tissue that was closely integrated with the surrounding allogenic chondrocyte and the macroscopic observation did not display any inflammatory outcome (Rajagopal et al. 2020). In another study involving a rodent cartilage defect, an osteochondral defect with dimension 1.5 × 1.5 diameter × height was made in the knee joint and the implanted construct consisting of size-sorted zonal chondrocytes and bi-layer 3D fibrin hydrogel facilitated the repair of the defect with mechanically improved cartilage. The spatial distribution of cells in the 3D construct was observed by levelling the cells of superficial zone with PKH26 fluorescence and, middle and deep zone cells with a carboxyfluorescein diacetate cell tracer before implantation and neotissues formed at the defect site of the cartilage in the distal femurs were imaged using fluorescent microscope (Yin et al. 2018). The functionalities of the decellularized coastal cartilage grafts for rhinoplasty prostheses were investigated *in vivo* by implanting the graft in the created cavity of 24 male New Zealand white rabbits. At 3 and 6 months post-implantation, the size, morphology, and relationship between the regenerated cartilage and the surrounding tissue were assessed by MRI (Lin et al. 2021). In another study, the construct comprising hADSCs-seeded with TGF-β3 PLGA microspheres implanted in rabbits (osteoarthritis model) promoted regeneration of articular cartilage. After 6 and 12 weeks post-operation, for the gross morphological characteristics, certain scores were assigned as grade I to IV representing the normal to severely abnormal following the International

Cartilage Repair Society (ICRS) norms for the evaluation of cartilage repair system on the basis of the observed femoral and tibia plateaus, structure of the intra-articular cartilage and the surrounding joint tissues (Sun et al. 2018). In a chemically induced osteoarthritis (OA) mice model, tri-layer porous scaffolds comprising chitosan and collagen incorporated with Etanercept which acts as a resister of pro-inflammatory cytokines were implanted in the knees of mice. Micro-CT scan was performed using a SkyScan 1076 Micro-CT scanner and the CT scan images of the mice legs were used to assess the neocartilage formation in the OA site. The obtained near-infrared imaging data were analysed using the IMPULSE software, which depicted the degradation behaviour of the implant (Figure 9.1) (Campos et al. 2022).

In another experiment of cartilage regeneration involving a zonal construct comprised of chondrocyte-seeded upper layer for inducing hyaline cartilage and MSCs-seeded bottom layer for inducing calcified cartilage of a hydrogel-filled PCL-constructs was implanted in a minipig model to repair cartilage defect. After 6 months, the observation of the defect site by macroscopic studies did not display any visible sign of inflammation or deterioration. The defect site treated with PCL-hydrogel construct exhibited similar white cartilage tissue, mostly located at the edge of the defects. A significant bone loss was revealed by the µCT analysis and the implants were observed to be pushed into the subchondral bone. In an *in vivo* study, the gross morphology of the hADMSCs-microrobot was investigated during targeting and after 1 week of targeting in rabbit knee joint. It was observed that hADMSCs-microrobots were mostly found in the defect sites that were filled by targeting with Electromagnetic actuation (EMA) system and fixed using the magnet in comparison to the hADMSC-microrobots that were inserted without targeting and fixing by EMA system (Go et al. 2020). After implanting the human nasal chondrocyte-seeded 3D-printed aqueous counter collision–bacterial nanocellulose (ACC–BNC) construct and ACC–BNC as control in nude mice for 1 and 2 months, respectively, the mice were euthanized and the harvested explants were subjected to morphological and biochemical evaluation (Apelgren et al. 2019). For morphological analysis, the tissue sections were deparaffinized and stained by the Alcian blue and van Gieson staining. The stained tissue sections were scanned by a fluorescence microscope. The analysis of the captured fluorescence images revealed that the constructs were rapidly well-integrated retaing 3D structure. Moreover, the harvested explants generated from the implanted 3D-bioprinted constructs were found to be white, shiny, and elastic with excellent mechanical properties (Apelgren et al. 2019). In an another study, the regenerated cartilage explants obtained after sacrificing the New Zealand white rabbits bearing a construct comprising oriented cartilage ECM-derived 3D scaffold and bone MSCs for repairing full thickness articular cartilage were subjected to morphological study using a desktop microcomputer tomography. The micro-CT study was performed with a regenerated cartilage obtained from *in vivo* study in a rabbit model bearing cell–scaffold construct with 360° scan at 80 kV, 80 µA, and 2960 ms exposure time. The recorded CT data set was used to analyse the cylindrical region of interest corresponding to the originally created defect site and made a 3D reconstruction. The scanning showed the cartilage as well as subchondral bone formation at the periphery of the defect areas, developing both tissues further towards the centre

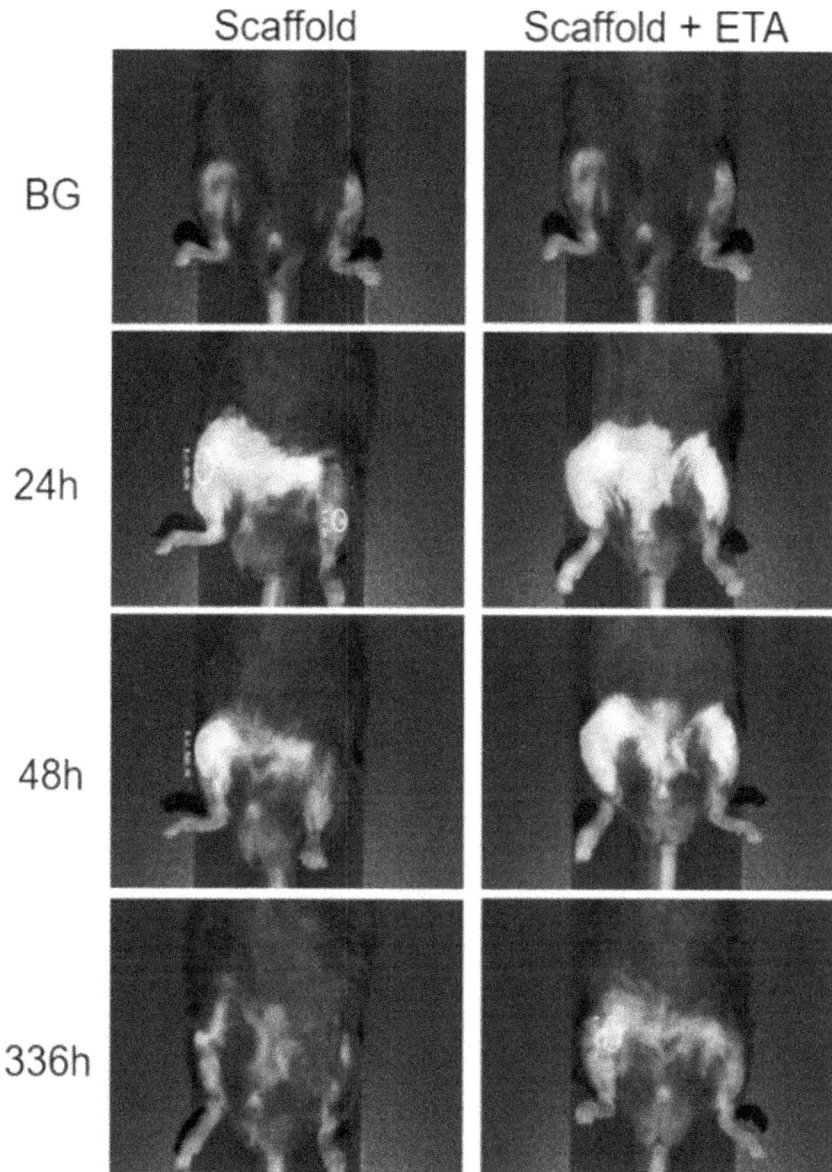

FIGURE 9.1   The captured near infrared images of *in vivo* implanted scaffold with and without etanercept implanted in the defect knee joint of mice with osteoarthritis.

Source: Campos et al. (2022).

of the full thickness articular cartilage defect (Jia et al. 2015). After 6 months of post-implantation, a smooth and flat surface of the regenerated cartilage in an oriented cartilage construct was found with an interface formed between the newly generated cartilage and the surrounding tissue that was almost indistinguishable. Furthermore, the total histomorphological score was higher with the oriented scaffold constructs than that with the random and negative control scaffold constructs groups.

In yet another *in vivo* study with a rabbit model carrying a novel xenogeneic costal cartilage, the gross morphology and inflammation of the harvested explants were examined by subjecting the randomly selected tissue at both low (10×10) and high (10×40) magnifications. The number of inflammatory cells and their average value were determined (Lin et al. 2021). The morphological study of the harvested neocartilage tissue from an *in vivo* animal model was grafted with the autologous dorsal onlay grafts and it showed diffuse calcium deposition at the defect area as visualized by microtomography analyses (Kushnaryov et al. 2014). In a study, aptamer-functionalized silk fibroin sponge was embedded into a hydrogel consisting of silk fibroin/hyaluronic acid–tyramine composite which was used to repair cartilage and osteochondral defects in the trochlear grooves of rabbit knees through aptamer-introduced homing of joint-resident MSCs. The regenerated tissues were evaluated based on gross examination and further histological, and immunohistochemical analysis. The results did not show any sort of infection or inflammatory response and the regenerated tissues were like the surrounding original cartilage with respect to colour, representing the formation of hyaline cartilage-like tissue. The average ICRS score corroborated the macroscopic assessment results (Wang et al. 2019).

Histological and Immunohistochemical Assessment

The histological analysis of the tissue constructs or tissue grafts includes immunohistochemical analysis that depicts the cartilage markers expression including type II collagen, aggrecan, Sox 9, and Matrilin-1. Various staining methods employed in these analyses such as haematoxylin and eosin (H&E), Alcian blue, safranin O/Fast Green (which indicates the presence of GAG), and von Kossa staining (which determines the presence of mineralized matrix, etc.). An *in vivo* study in the New Zealand white rabbit model to repair osteochondral defect by implanted BM-MSC-seeded chitosan–gelatin scaffold constructs was performed. The safranin O staining (SO) demonstrated the development of smooth hyaline cartilage in the defect site which was found to be well-integrated with the surrounding allogeneic cartilage, subchondral bone, and trabecular bone volume beneath the neo-cartilage. The GAG synthesis was also estimated by SO. The amount of cartilaginous repair was evaluated by O'Driscoll scoring system. Immunohistochemistry analysis of the light micro-scopic images revealed that the regenerated tissue was stained positively for type II collagen and negatively for type X collagen, thereby confirming hyaline cartilage formation and the absence of hypertrophic cartilage in the defect area (Rajagopal et al. 2020). In another study relating to a rodent cartilage defect in the knee joint, the implanted construct comprising the size-sorted zonal chondrocyte-laden bi-layer 3D fibrin hydrogel promoted cartilage repair with the mechanically enhanced cartilage.

The efficacy of the construct was also evaluated by performing a histological test. For this purpose, the operated distal femurs in knee joints harvested after 6 weeks of implantation were subjected to immunohistochemical analysis. The performed Alcian blue and collagen II immunostaining revealed the formation of cartilage-ECM throughout the defect site of the knee and collagen II-hyaline cartilage tissue was predominant with significantly lower type I collagen. Higher cartilage regeneration in the rat knees was further evident from the histologic scoring than the other group used in the study. Furthermore, the quality of cartilage repair was evaluated by a modified O' Driscoll histologic grading system (Yin et al. 2018). When a zonal construct made of hydrogel-filled PCL scaffold-seeded chondrocyte at the upper layer and the bottom layer seeded with MSCs was implanted in a minipig model for repairing cartilage defect *in vivo*, important tissue heterogeneities were observed, but with lower modified O'Driscoll-score than that obtained with defect without filling with the construct (control). This result signifies the occurrence of induced bone erosion during the joint loading and dislocation of the regenerated tissues *in vivo* impeding sufficient permanent alignment of the zones than the surrounding native cartilage (Bothe et al. 2019). In an *in vivo* nude mice experiment, the implanted human nasal chondrocytes-loaded ACC–BNC construct promoted the human collagen type II synthesis as assessed by the immunohistochemical analysis with the harvested explant, indicating the neocartilage tissue regeneration at the defect site (Apelgren et al. 2019). The quality of cartilage repair by culturing construct derived from size-sorted zonal chondrocytes-seeded in bi-layered hydrogel was investigated by the modified O' Driscoll histologic grading system that involved three blinded independent observers for different parameters such as cell morphology, surface and structural integrity, deposited ECM staining and its thickness, bonding, and freedom from degenerative cellular alternations. In a study performed with New Zealand white rabbits, autologous bone MSC-seeded oriented scaffold constructs were inserted for repairing defects of full-thickness articular cartilage. The harvested neotissue specimens were subjected to histological and immunohistochemical analyses (Jia et al. 2015). The regenerated tissue samples were sectioned and stained with H&E, Toluidine blue, and Safranin O staining, according to the prescribed protocols (Jia et al. 2012). Cartilage regeneration was also evaluated by the modified O'Driscoll grading scale through semi-quantitative histomorphological analysis involving two blinded observers (Huang et al. 2007), Collagen type II was identified by immunohistochemical study, using monoclonal anti-collagen type II antibodies, as per the method described elsewhere (Dai et al. 2010). After euthanizing the rabbits at 6 months post-surgery, the grafts containing the decellularized xenogeneic costal cartilage and the adjoining tissues were harvested. A small number of inflammatory cells were observed to be located on the surface of the regenerated graft without showing any significant degradation in the combination method-based decellularized costal cartilage (CDCC) group as evident from the H&E staining results, whereas a drastic reduction in inflammatory cell numbers in the CDCC group was observed showing lesser number of this cell than that was seen in the sodium deoxycholate-based decellularized costal cartilage (SDCC) group as confirmed by the inflammatory cell count analysis (Lin et al. 2021). The immunohistochemistry study results obtained by safranin O staining and quantifying GAGs and type II collagen were used to assess the changes in compositions of formed tissue grafts prior and post *in vivo* implantation. These were helpful in determining the degradation and absorption pattern of the grafts. The safranin O staining also exhibited higher GAGs synthesis specifically in the superficial zone of CDCC group, whereas the SDCC grafts displayed poor staining because of their degradation. Almost intact collagen structure of the graft belonging to CDCC group and the presence of a very small quantity of neocollagen in the superficial area were confirmed by the immunohistochemical staining of type II collagen (Lin et al. 2021). In another study, after harvesting the hMSC-ECM constructs as well as the control consisting of chondrocyte cell sheet constructs from the mice, the explants were harvested following standard procedure. The histological sections of 7 μm thickness were subjected to safranin O staining for the detection of sGAG using Fast Green as a counterstain. A higher intensity of safranin O staining of sGAG with the cell-laden ECM constructs was noticed than that shown in the cell sheet constructs (Yang et al. 2018). The histology, histochemistry and immunohistochemistry studies were performed in the sturgeon cartilage substitutes such as decellularized cartilage disks (DCD) and recellularized cartilage disks (RCD), which were implanted subcutaneously in the dorsal area of male immunodeficient athymic Nude-Foxn1nu mice of 6 weeks old. The grafted constructs and the surrounding tissues were subjected to histological analysis at 60 days of post-surgery. The harvested sectionized tissue specimens were rehydrated followed by H&E staining to assess their structure, or stained with 4',6-diamidino-2-phenylindole (DAPI), to identify the cell nuclei. SEM analysis was performed by fixing DCD in 2.5% glutaraldehyde and then sequentially dried, gold sputter-coated, and analysed (Ortiz-Arrabal et al. 2021).

Type II collagen, KI-67, Caspase 7, CD 4, CD 8, and CD 206 as well as unspecific sites were detected by immunohistochemistry analysis performed with the harvested tissue sections by treating with specific primary antibodies and the negative controls with PBS. The specimens were stained with Harry's haematoxylin and the obtained microscopic images were analysed using Image J software. Immunohistochemical assays showed a significant increase of type II collagen in all types of the grafts compared to non-grafted DCD and sturgeon cartilage (Ortiz-Arrabal et al. 2021). The neocartilage constructs from the autologous dorsal onlay grafts were evaluated for histological and immunohistochemical analyses (Kushnaryov et al. 2014). The histologic examination performed with the harvested neocartilage sections exhibited the distribution of chondrocytes in void space within the generated ECM, which is typically of the native cartilage. The immunohistochemistry study performed with the explants using Vectastain Elite ABC kit, a peroxidase-based detection system, and stained with one of the antibodies like anti-type I or anti-type II collagen, or a mouse nonspecific IgG as a negative control. The tissue sections were counterstained with methyl green nuclear stain. The neocartilage showed intense staining for both collagen types I and II than the nonspecific IgG control and the explants had an enlarged spaces with huge clusters of cells (Kushnaryov et al. 2014).

3D engineered cartilage gel (ECG) was developed from 3 and 15 days cartilage sheets by culturing goat-derived chondrocytes in chondrogenic media for 3 and 15 days and were seeded into the decalcified bone matrix (DBM), resulting in

ECG–DBM constructs. The 3-day and 5-day cultured ECG–DBM constructs were able to successfully regenerate feasible 3D cartilage having characteristics of typical natural cartilage in nude mice model as well as autologous goat model (Ci et al. 2021). Four different implants such as non-woven fleece of polyglactin (F), non-woven fleece of polyglactin immersed in alginate suspension (FA), non-woven fleece of polyglactin seeded with chondrocytes (FC) and non-woven fleece of polyglactin seeded with chondrocytes suspended in alginate suspension (FAC) were implanted in the subcutaneous dorsal pockets of athymic mice to investigate the effect of alginate in chondrogenesis. Macroscopic analysis revealed that after 8 weeks of implantation, in the defect site, fat and fibrous tissues were formed instead of cartilage in F implanted group, whereas in FA implanted group naïve cartilage was formed in less areas. In FC implanted group, the grafts were shrunk and coiled. FAC implants remained intact after 8 weeks of implantation and cartilage was prominently formed at the defect site. So, from the above study it is clearly observed that alginate based scaffold can accelerate the chondrogenesis process in defect site. For more conformation of the study, histological analysis of the grafts were done by the Alcian Blue for glycosaminoglycans staining and collagen type-II antibodies for collagen. In F implanted group no staining for glycosaminoglycans and collagen type II were found, whereas in FA graft small patches of alcian blue staining with islets stained positive for collagen type II were observed. In FC construct, due to the unequal distribution of chondrocytes uneven alacin blue staining with positive stained collagen type II antibodies were observed. In FAC construct chondrocytes were evenly distributed throughout the surface. These obervations demonstrated that alginate helped in retention of shape of the graft (Marijnissen et al. 2002).

In an *in vivo* rat model experiment, osteochondral defects of critical size were created. The defects were implanted with the constructs made of chondrogenic predifferentiated and undifferentiated human umbilical cord blood-derived MSCs seeded with hyaluronic acid hydrogels into the defects in the right knees and into the left knees, respectively, for cartilage repair. After 16 weeks of post-implantation, the immunohistochemical staining with safranin O and type II collagen depicted colour similar to that of the natural articular cartilage in the undifferentiated-MSCs group. This was further confirmed by the histological scores revealing the superior cartilage ECM formation shown by undifferentiated MSCs than chondrogenic differentiated MSCs (Park et al. 2019). In another study, the regenerated cartilage obtained after sacrificing the New Zealand white rabbits bearing the autologous BMSCs-scaffold constructs was examined through histological and immunohistological assessment. The explants harvested following standard protocol from the defect site were sectioned with 5-μm thickness each, followed by staining with H&E, toluidine blue, and safranin O stains. In immunohistochemical study, monoclonal anti-collagen type II antibodies were used for detecting type II collagen (Jia et al. 2015). Toluidine blue and safranin O staining depicted that the repair of cartilage defect was associated with the formation of both fibrocartilage and fibrous tissue in the oriented scaffold groups and only fibrous tissue was formed in the random scaffold, without the cartilage formation.

In an *in vivo* experiment rabbits with articular cartilage knee defect was transplanted with hypoxia preconditioned buccal fat pad stem cells-seeded bilayer chitosan-based hydrogel constructs. The regenerated cartilage was assessed by immunohistological and histological staining analyses by the use of Alcian blue and H&E staining. The Alcian blue stained images depicted an intense Alcian blue staining with the regenerated ECM deposition indicating the presence of proteoglycans. Collagen type II was determined by immunohistochemistry study. The harvested neotissue was preincubated in the 5% normal goat serum followed by incubation by adding primary anti-COLII (Collage II) antibody. The regenerated tissue samples were further incubated with FITC (Fluorescein isothiocyanate)-conjugated antibody against rabbit IgG followed by staining of the cell nuclei with DAPI and were sectioned. The tissue sections were observed under a microscope. All these analyses showed an increased collagen type II and proteoglycans expressions, the former being the predominant one (Nazhvani, Amirabad et al. 2021). In another *in vivo* study, cell-seeded scaffold constructs developed by culturing canine tracheal epithelial cells and canine yolk sac endothelial progenitor cells over the canine decellularized tracheal matrices were subcutaneously implanted in BALB (Bagg Albino)-c nude mice. The explants harvested after 45 days post-surgery were subjected to H&E and Gömori trichrome staining analyses and the immunohistochemistry studies by using Dako EnVision™ FLEX detection system (de Sá Schiavo Matias et al. 2022).

A cell- free collagen I-based scaffold (S) was developed to repair the damaged articular cartilage lesions (ACL). For implantation of this scaffold, lesions were created in the articular cartilage region of the femoropatellar groove in rat knees. The developed scaffolds were implanted into the defect site of the rats (ACL-S) groups. The group of rats in which scaffolds were not used in the defect site was referred to as the ACL group. After 4 -16 weeks of post-implantation of scaffold, the level of cartilage regeneration was evaluated by histological analysis. For this analysis, the regenerated samples were stained with Alcian blue staining and then subjected to the computerized densitometric measurement and image analysis. The regeneration of cartilage was also evaluated by indirect method of deposition of GAG. The deposition of sulphated GAG in different groups was stained by Alcian blue staining as shown in Figure 9.2. In Figure 9.2(a), the control group showed the prominent GAG layer. ACL group (Figure 9.2(b, c, d)) at 4 weeks showed the deposition of GAG as stained in blue colour which was reduced remarkably by increasing the incubation periods. ACL-S group had a strong Alcian blue staining, demonstrating the deposition of GAG, and the staining was progressive by increasing the incubation periods from 8 weeks to 16 weeks (Figure 9.2(e, f, g)). The study showed the potentiality of the acellular collagen scaffold as a matrix for articular cartilage formation (Szychlinska et al. 2020).

The H&E staining depicted the microscopic morphology of the femoral articular cartilage in both the ACL-S and ACL groups. The micrographs of the control (normal articular cartilage) group showed the normal cartilage cytoarchitecture. The cells on upper layer were flat and small, whereas the middle and lower layer chondrocytes were arranged columnary with proper tidemark (Figure 9.3(a)). In ACL group articular cartilage, the normal tissue architecture was completely changed owing to

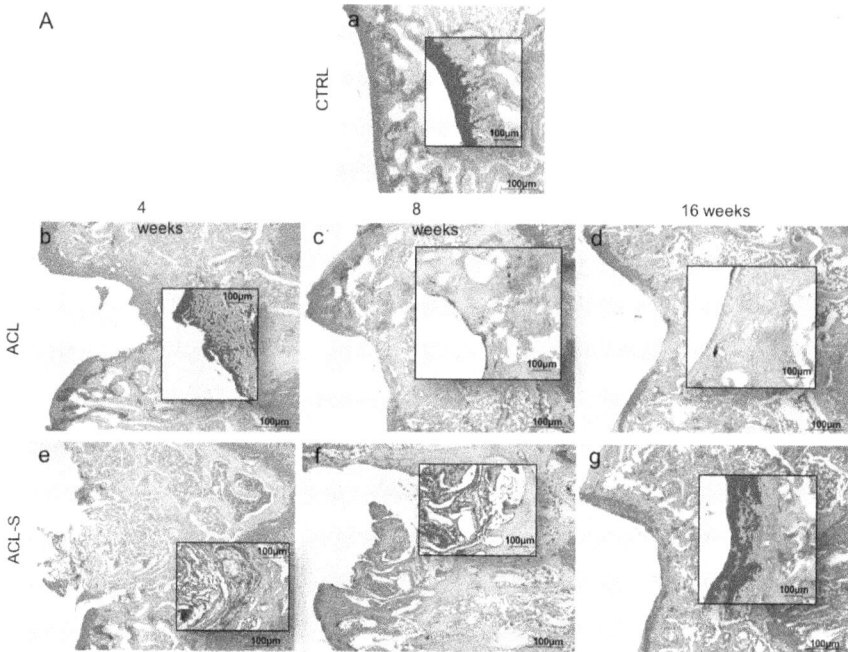

FIGURE 9.2 Histochemical study of synthesis of sGAGs in the defect femoral articular cartilage of rat knees in normal articular cartilage (control) (a), without scaffold (ACL) (b,c,d), and collagen-I-based scaffold (ACL-S groups) (e,f,g) after 4-, 8-, and 16-weeks post-implantation. The neocartilage samples were stained with Alcian blue and were evaluated by computerized densitometric measurements and image analysis.

Source: Szychlinska et al. (2020).

the defect induction. The superficial, middle, and deep zones, as well as the tide-mark, were not visible at all the incubation periods in the ACL group (Figure 9.3(b)). At 4 weeks in the ACL group fibrous tissues were formed at the superficial zone of subchondral bone at the defect site. After 8 and 16 weeks of implantation, the fibrous scar tissue was replaced by a tissue that appeared to be calcified with poor proteoglycans deposits (Figure 9.3(c, d)). In ACL-S group at 4 weeks the histological study revealed the existence of regenerated tissue in between the subchondral bone and collagen scaffold (Figure 9.3(e)). At 8 weeks, the efficiency of the scaffold was to attract host cells that invaded, attached, and proliferated within the ACL-S scaffold (Figure 9.3(f)). At 16 weeks, a progressive integration and replacement of the degradable collagen scaffold with the regenerated cartilage-like tissue were observed (Figure 9.3g) (Szychlinska et al. 2020).

The histologic analysis of chondral and osteochondral regenerative tissue generated in the defect site of rabbit knees by the aptamer-functionalized silk fibroin-based scaffold was performed by H&E staining and safranin O staining. These staining results showed clear distinction between the repaired and the

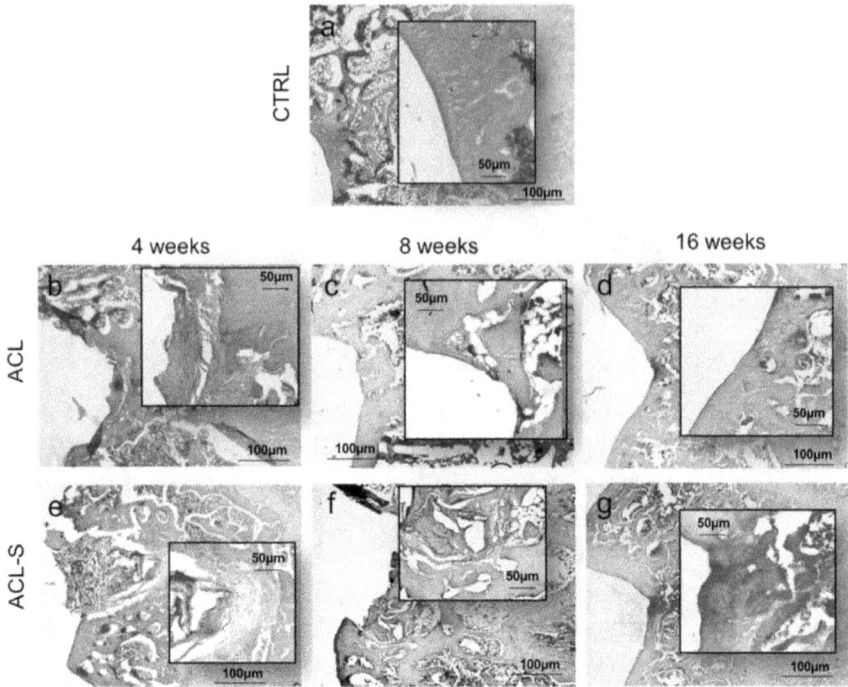

FIGURE 9.3 Histological studies of femoral articular cartilage of a normal articular cartilage (control), ACL group, and ACL-S group were done. Haematoxylin and eosin (H&E) staining of the sample showed the normal cartilage cytoarchitecture in control group (a). In ACL group, scar tissue was developed at an early stage and in later stage, tissues were calcified with little proteoglycan deposition (b–d). Micrographs of the ACL-S group (e–g) revealed the newly formed tissue in between the subchondral bone and collagen scaffold as well as the progressive migration of native cell towards the defect site.

Source: Szychlinska et al. (2020).

surrounding tissues. Nonetheless, the newly formed cartilage matrix was shallow in comparison to the native cartilage matrix after 6 weeks of implantation. The defects were found to maintain concave shape, with a smooth surface for an extended period of time. The aptamer-functionalized constructs exhibited superior cartilage repair than the controls. The analysis of immunohistochemical staining analysis showing the expression of collagen types II, I, and X indicated the maximum ECM synthesis with uniform texture obtained with the aptamer-functionalized constructs (Wang et al. 2019). The histological examination of the OA using New Zealand white rabbit model bearing human adipose-derived stem cells (hADSCs)-seeded TGF-β3 PLGA microspheres as constructs was found to be consistent with the ICRS scores. It was evident from the toluidine blue staining, that the superficial region of the defect cartilage was found to be repaired by the regenerated hyaline-like cartilage tissue with the hADSCs/PLGA microspheres group after 6 and 12 weeks of post-implantation.

At 12 weeks post-surgery, the hADSCs/PLGA microspheres exhibited an original cartilage and maintained a normal subchondral bone in comparison to the control, in which the disappearance of the cartilage portion and deterioration of the subchondral bone were observed, the latter being filled with the fibrous tissue (Sun et al. 2018). In an *in vivo* animal experiment for repairing focal chondral lesions, the rabbits bearing rabbit bone marrow-derived MSCs encapsulated in the photopolymerizable cartilage mimetic hydrogel were euthanized at 6 months post-surgery. The tissue quality was evaluated in the harvested explant with 5-mm-thick sections by safranin-O and immunofluroscence for type II collagen staining and microscopic images were analysed. The histological sections were graded as per the modified O'Driscoll score, wherein the total point values were ranged from 0 representing no sign of cartilage repair to 28 depicting as high cartilage repair (Pascual-Garrido et al. 2019).

BIOMECHANICAL ASSESSMENT

Biomechanical assessment is important to understand the mechanical behavior of the 3D engineered tissue grafts to prevent graft failure in vivo due to and it is a crucial aspect in bone, cartilage and complex tissue constructs. In an *in vivo* rat model with knee osteochondral defect, the distal femurs after 6 weeks post-surgery were subjected to compressional assessment using a mechanical tester of Instron make (model 5567). An enhanced compressive strength of the cartilage ECM resulted using the construct derived from the size-sorted zonal chondrocytes seeded with a bilayered 3D fibrin hydrogel compared to the control and other groups (Yin et al. 2018). In an another animal study (Jia et al. 2015), the regenerated cartilage harvested from the defect site of the full thickness articular cartilage in rabbit filled with a construct derived from bone mesenchymal stem cell (MSCs)-seeded scaffold was kept in a stainless steel plate containing PBS solution and then biomechanical analysis of the sample was performed by unconfined compression test using a universal material testing machine following the method described elsewhere (Hoenig et al. 2011). The regenerated cartilage specimen height was measured by applying a compressive force with threshold value of 0.05N, whereas the Young's modulus was measured from the recorded load and displacement data following the method described previously (Jia et al. 2012). An *in vivo* nude mice and autologous goat model was investigated for cartilage regeneration using a construct made from engineered chondrocyte cartilage gel–decalcified bone matrix (DBM). The harvested explants were tested for mechanical strength using a mechanical analyser Instron make of model No. 5542 operated at a constant compressive strain at 0.5 mm/min speed. The strength of the regenerated cartilage sheet was found to reach the favourable level. The generated stress–strain curves were used to calculate the Young's modulus (Ci et al. 2021). In an *in vivo* study, nasal septal defects created in the female New Zealand white rabbit were used as animal models, which were implanted with septal cartilage constructs. After 30 or 60 days post-implantation, the regenerated cartilages harvested from the autologous dorsal only grafts were subjected to confined compression tests, thereby measuring their aggregate modulus and hydraulic permeability. The results indicated a significant enhancement in mechanical stiffness of the neocartilage. The mechanical stiffness was also increased with an increase in the *in vivo* incubation period (Kushnaryov et al. 2014). To repair focal chondral lesions, an *in vivo* rabbit model carrying a construct developed from rabbit bone marrow-derived MSCs seeded in a photopolymerizable cartilage mimetic hydrogel was used. At 6 months of post-surgery, the compressive modulus was measured to assess the cartilage ECM deposition from the generated stress–strain curve using a mechanical testing machine.

BIOCHEMICAL ASSESSMENT

The biochemical characterization of cartilage tissue constructs or tissue grafts generated in *in vivo* animal study includes the total DNA content, GAG content collagen content, and calcium content. An *in vivo* study using mice model, transplanted with human nasal chondrocyte-loaded ACC–BNC construct, promoted cartilage formation as characterized by biochemical analysis with the harvested tissue section showing an increased proliferation of chondrocytes and glycosaminoglycan deposition from day 30 to 60 days (Apelgren et al. 2019). The fluorescence *in situ* hybridization analysis of the explant harvested from the euthanized mice further confirmed the presence of GAG positive cells in the regenerated tissue and that they are of human origin and were stained positive for both human X and Y chromosomes representing their male origin, that is, they are derived from chondrocytes (Apelgren et al. 2019). In another study, the regenerated cartilage harvested from the defect site in rabbit bearing bone MSCs-laden scaffold constructs (Jia et al. 2015) were subjected to biochemical test for determining the levels of DNA, GAG, and collagen synthesis. The DNA content in the explant was measured by Quant-iT™ PicoGreen® dsDNA Assay kit. The GAG deposition and total collagen were estimated using Blyscan™ Sulfated Glycosaminoglycan and Sircol™ Soluble Collagen Assay kits by measuring absorbance at 656 and 555 nm, respectively (Jia et al. 2012).

In an *in vivo* pre-clinical study, the cartilage defect site of rabbits was filled with a novel xenogenic decellularized costal cartilage graft. At post-surgery, the regenerated cartilage was tested for certain biochemical characterization. The estimation of GAGs and collagen type II evaluated the changes in the graft compositions prior to and after *in vivo* transplantation. These were helpful in determining the degradation and absorption pattern of the grafts. Furthermore, quantitative analysis of GAGs synthesis proved an enhanced GAGs content in the combination method-based decellularized costal cartilage group than the sodium deoxycholate-based decellularized costal cartilage groups at 6 months of implantation (Lin et al. 2021). The ability of the hBMSCs-ECM constructs, as well as the chondrocyte cell sheet constructs (control), to form neocartilage *in vivo* by subcutaneous implantation in female severe combined immunodeficient mice of 8–12 weeks old, was investigated by the gene expression levels of the chondrogenic markers like collagen type II and aggrecan. A significantly higher level of type II collagen as well as aggrecan genes was shown in hBMSCs-ECM group than the cell sheet as evident from the results of RT-PCR (Real-time reverse transcriptase-polymerase chain reaction) (Yang et al. 2018). Furthermore, the deposition of cartilage ECM was measured by quantifying the GAG as a function of dsDNA content using dimethylmethylene blue dye-binding assay. dsDNA was also quantified by PicoGreen-based assay (Yang et al. 2018). Similarly, in a study for repairing OA defect of New Zealand rabbit bearing human adipose-derived stem cells-seeded TGF-β3 PLGA microspheres construct, the mRNA expression levels of cartilage-associated genes for both type II collagen and aggrecan were evaluated by RT-PCR analysis. These gene expression results showed a significant up-regulation in the hADSCs/microspheres group and the results were corroborated with the ICRS scores and histological results (Sun et al. 2018). Several histochemical methods were used to determine the specific ECM components in neocartilage harvested from the defect site of an *in vivo* mice model using male immunodeficient athymic Nude-*Foxn1nu* mice of 6 weeks age grafted with sturgeon cartilage substitutes such as decellularized and recellularized cartilage disks. The toluidine blue and Alcian blue staining identified the cartilage proteoglycans. Picrosirius red staining and Orecein staining were used to detect the mature collagen fibres and the elastic fibres of the regenerated tissue, respectively. GAG deposition was assessed by staining the additional regenerated tissue samples with 0.1% Alcian blue following standard protocol (Ortiz-Arrabal et al. 2021).

Histochemical analysis of neocartilage tissue harvested from the defect site of *in vivo* animal models implanted with the autologous dorsal onlay grafts showed the deposition of sGAG in the defect site. The incubation of the neocartilage constructs *in vivo* resulted in the diffused calcium deposition as revealed by the analysis of Alizarin Red S staining images and the result was consistent with the microtomography analyses (Kushnaryov et al. 2014). The synthesis of the total GAG and total collagen content in the regenerated 3D cartilage sheet having characteristics of a typical natural cartilage in nude mice and autologous goats was performed by the Alcian blue staining method and hydroxyproline assay, the results of which were consistent with that determined by histological staining (Ci et al. 2021). These analyses demonstrated that the GAG deposition and the total collagen content in the newly formed cartilage reached the desired levels.

An electrospun PCL fibre was functionalized with ozone functional group and TGF-β3 protein loaded in scaffold for better compatibility with the human muscle-derived stem cells (hMDSCs). In this study, both ozonized (O) and non-ozonized (NO) cartilage scaffolds with or without TGF-β3 were investigated by conducting *in vitro* and *in vivo* experiments. For *in vivo* study, 14 CB17SCID female mice of 6–7 weeks of age were used. After 4 and 8 weeks of implantation, the mice were sacrificed and the regenerated cartilage was taken out from the defect area followed by fixing with 4% paraformaldehyde. The safranin O staining of the harvested explant revealed the formation of GAGs in the regenerated ECM. Scaffolds with loaded TGFβ3 and hMDSCs showed more prominent GAG-deposited area than the hMDSC-seeded scaffolds without TGFβ3. The human chondrocyte-seeded scaffold exhibited more abundant O-positive staining after 4 weeks; however, it was slightly decreased after 8 weeks post-injection. No GAG deposition in the scaffolds without containing cell was noticed (Figure 9.4). Although there was a significant increase in the synthesis of GAG in O scaffold having TGF-β3 and hMDSCs, no significant difference in GAG formation in O as well as NO scaffolds seeded with human chondrocytes was observed at 4 weeks of post-implantation. The staining area in both the scaffold groups containing hMDSCs was reduced, but it was remarkably high in scaffold containing TGF-β3 in

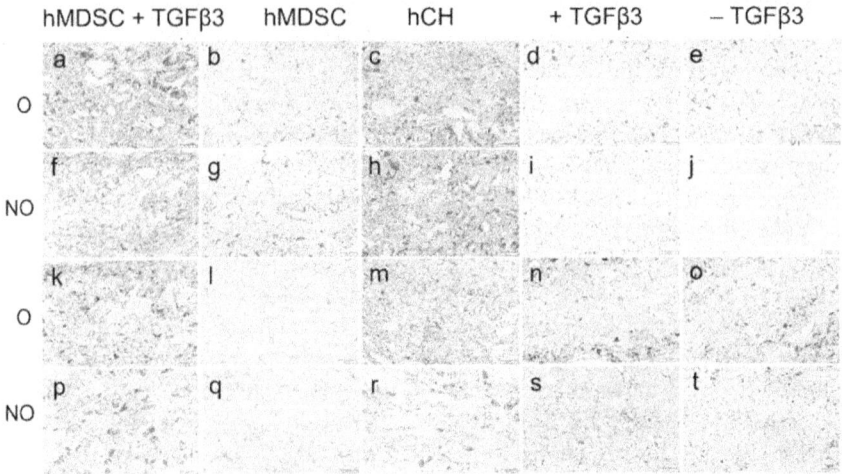

FIGURE 9.4   Deposition of GAG in the ozonized (O) and non-ozonized (NO) scaffolds with or without TGF-β3 protein-seeded human muscle-derived stem cell (hMDSCs) constructs implanted in the subcutaneous region of female mice was revealed by the safranin O staining after 4 weeks (a–j) and 8 weeks (k–t) of implantation.

Source: Jankauskaite et al. (2022).

comparison to the scaffolds without protein at 8 weeks of implantation. The staining area was same in ozonized scaffolds seeded with human chondrocytes and ozonized scaffolds containing TGF-β3 and seeded with hMDSCs. A lesser staining area was exhibited in the non-ozonized-seeded human chondrocyte construct. In cell-free scaffolds, the safranin O- stained area detected was not much significant. The study demonstrated that the ozonized positive scaffolds loaded and seeded with the TGF-β3 and hMDSCs, respectively, showed the potential construct for GAG deposition, and hence can promote cartilage regeneration (Jankauskaite et al. 2022).

Biochemical evaluation was carried out with a small portion of the neocartilage construct generated in an *in vivo* study using rabbit models with the created nasal septal defects. The construct specimen was digested with proteinase K in phosphate-buffered EDTA and the digests were used for the estimation of sGAG and total collagen (Kushnaryov et al. 2014). The sGAG content was measured by the dimethyl-methylene blue reaction following a reported method (Farndale, Buttle and Barrett 1986). The amount of total collagen in the digests was measured by the total collagen hydroxyproline assay and the DNA content was determined by the PicoGreen DNA assay (McGowan et al. 2002).

ELECTROMAGNETIC ACTUATION SYSTEM

In an experimental *in vivo* study, a microrobot system was proposed to regenerate the cartilage in the knee defect created in the rabbit and the hADMSCs cultured on the microrobot. Both hADMSCs and the microrobot were targeted by positioning in the electromagnetic actuation system workspace and were delivered depending on the flow of injected PBS. The magnetic targeting by using this system can be applied both in the liquid and in the air-filled environment, as well as within the joint space. The hADMSC-microrobot was subsequently fixed by attaching one magnet to the outer femur with a double-sided tape depending on the defect area, and the self-adherent wrap was bordered by the legs and waist of the rabbit, and thereby the magnet was prevented from fleeing (Go et al. 2020).

ASSESSMENT OF ENGINEERED BONE AND RELATED TISSUE CONSTRUCTS OR GRAFTS

Bone, a highly vascular connective tissue, is the second most commonly and widely transplanted tissue following blood (Fragogeorgi et al. 2019). Although bone can heal and remodel on its own, it loses its regenerative capacity during tumour resection, traumatic bone loss, or osteoporotic fractures. Bone tissue-engineered grafts or bone substitutes with desired properties like osteoinduction, osteoconduction, and osteointegration enable new bone growth and development, as well as ensure its proper integration with the host bone tissue for reconstruction of the bone defects pre-clinically (Amini et al. 2012). The evaluation of the safety and efficacy of these bone grafts and constructs is of utmost important prior to their application. For this, numerous protocols for *in vivo* animal experiments have been reported to validate the engineered bone and related tissue grafts, which are described in the following section.

MORPHOLOGICAL ASSESSMENT

The quality and consistency of the regenerated bone tissue are evaluated morphologically by various methods, such as macroscopic observation, gross analysis, scanning electron microscopy analysis, X-ray analysis, radiological evaluation, micro-computed tomography, and cone beam computed tomography. An *in vivo* study was performed using six-week old Dawley rats for bone repair. The rats were implanted with a construct comprising a biphasic calcium sulfate and hydroxyapatite composite scaffold combined with recombinant human bone morphogenic protein-2 (rhBMP-2) that acts as a bone inducer, and zoledronic acid (ZA) that can control early resorption of the scaffold. The gross analysis performed with the harvested tissue specimen showed the largest dimension and hard in appearance when scaffolds were loaded with rhBMP-2 and zoledronic acid. The X-ray radiographic analysis of the harvested implant depicted that the biphasic scaffold combined with rhBMP-2 protein and ZA was dimensionally larger and denser than the biphasic material alone after 4 weeks of implantation. SEM images indicated the formation of apatite in the form of apatite particles and typical trabecular bone formation on the scaffold containing rhBMP-2 and ZA. The μ-CT analysis of the harvested explants exhibited higher amount of mineralized volume in comparison to the control as confirmed by both 3D and 2D imaging of the specimen slides (Raina et al. 2016). In another *in vivo* animal experiment, the radiographs of the femur bone taken sequentially at regular time intervals during days 0 to 3 months postoperatively assessed the status of the construct implanted and the level of interaction between the host bone tissue and the implant material.

An aligned electrospun cellulose/cellulose nanocrystals (CNCs) nanocomposite incorporated with rhBMP-2 as a promoter for osteogenic differentiation was inserted into the square-sized (5×5 mm) cranial defect area of female New Zealand white rabbits. For the study scaffolds were divided into six different groups like negative control (without scaffold), positive control (without surgery), aligned scaffold with and without BMP-2, and random scaffold with and without BMP-2. The μ-CT performed at 100 kV, 500 mA, and 6 μm resolution assessed the structure, bone regeneration, and mineralization in the defect region. After 12 weeks of surgery, 2D micro-CT images of the defect area showed a slight new bone formation in negative control group (Figure 9.5(a)), whereas the positive control groups (Figure 9.5(b)) exhibited normal cranial bone. A significant spongy bone was formed at the endocardium side as observed with the aligned and random scaffold groups containing BMP-2, as indicated in Figure 9.5(c) and Figure 9.5(d), respectively. Both aligned and random scaffolds without BMP-2 groups showed more bone formation than the negative control group, as evident from Figure 9.5(e) and Figure 9.5(f), respectively. The aligned scaffold group loaded with BMP-2 had more bone volume (Figure 9.5(g)) and bone mineral density (Figure 9.5(h)) than the other groups except the positive control group. The random scaffold group with BMP-2 showed greater bone density as well as mineral deposition than the two groups without BMP-2 (Zhang et al. 2019).

In an *in vivo* animal experiment involving New Zealand white rabbits, gelatin/chitosan-composite scaffolds fabricated with bioactive ceramic nanoparticles such as hydroxyapatite (HAp) (H), β-tricalcium phosphate (β-TCP) (T), and bioglass (B) containing 30 wt% each were inserted into the defect femur. The analyses of the radiographs of the defect sites obtained using X-ray at 0 to 3 months post-operation were used to evaluate the femur bone regeneration (Figure 9.6) in terms of bone volume and bone mineral density. After 1 and 3 months, the radio density of the implant was little bit reduced at the defect site. At 1 month, a lower radio density with insignificant gap between the bone and scaffold representing the initiation of bone formation at the defect site was observed, as indicated in Figure 9.6(a). The radio density of the implant was mixed with the bone at 3 months of implantation, which indicates satisfactory healing (Figure 9.6(b)). Radiographs of the implanted GCT30 scaffold at 1 month showed progressive bone healing with decrease in shape, size, and radio density (Figure 9.6(c)). By increasing the incubation period from 0 to 1 month, the reduction in radio density demonstrated the new bone formation. At 3 months GCB30 was not clearly visible, which indicates the satisfactory amount of new formation at the defect site (Figure 9.6(d)) (Dasgupta, Maji and Nandi 2019).

In the fluorochrome assay, the new bone and old bone areas were flourished in different colors like bright golden yellow and deep sea green fluorescence, respectively. After 1 month of incubation GCB30 implant exhibited more intense golden yellow fluorescence in new bone formation compared to other implants (Figure 9.7).

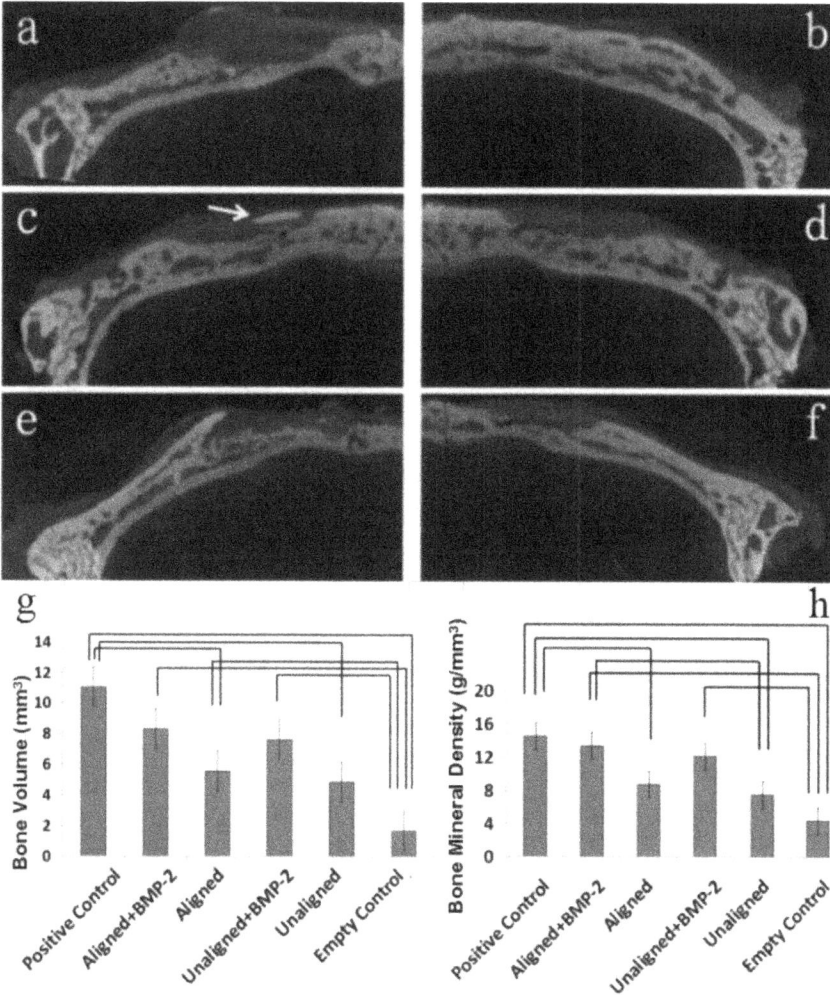

FIGURE 9.5 Representative micro-CT images and their analysis for the evaluation of bone formation and mineralization in the cranial defect area of female New Zealand white rabbits with different scaffold implanted groups like (a) Negative control, (b) Positive control, (c) Aligned scaffold with BMP-2, (d) Random scaffold with BMP-2, (e) Aligned scaffold without BMP-2, (f) Random scaffold without BMP-2. (g) Bone volume and (h) bone mineral density were quantified.

Source: Zhang et al. (2019).

At 3 months, control samples showed a few patches of new bone (Figure 9.7a) representing insignificant new bone formation at the defect site. In GCH30, a higher level of bone regeneration than the control group was occured (Figure 9.7b). The implanted region of GCT30 depicted wider new bone synthesis which reflects the

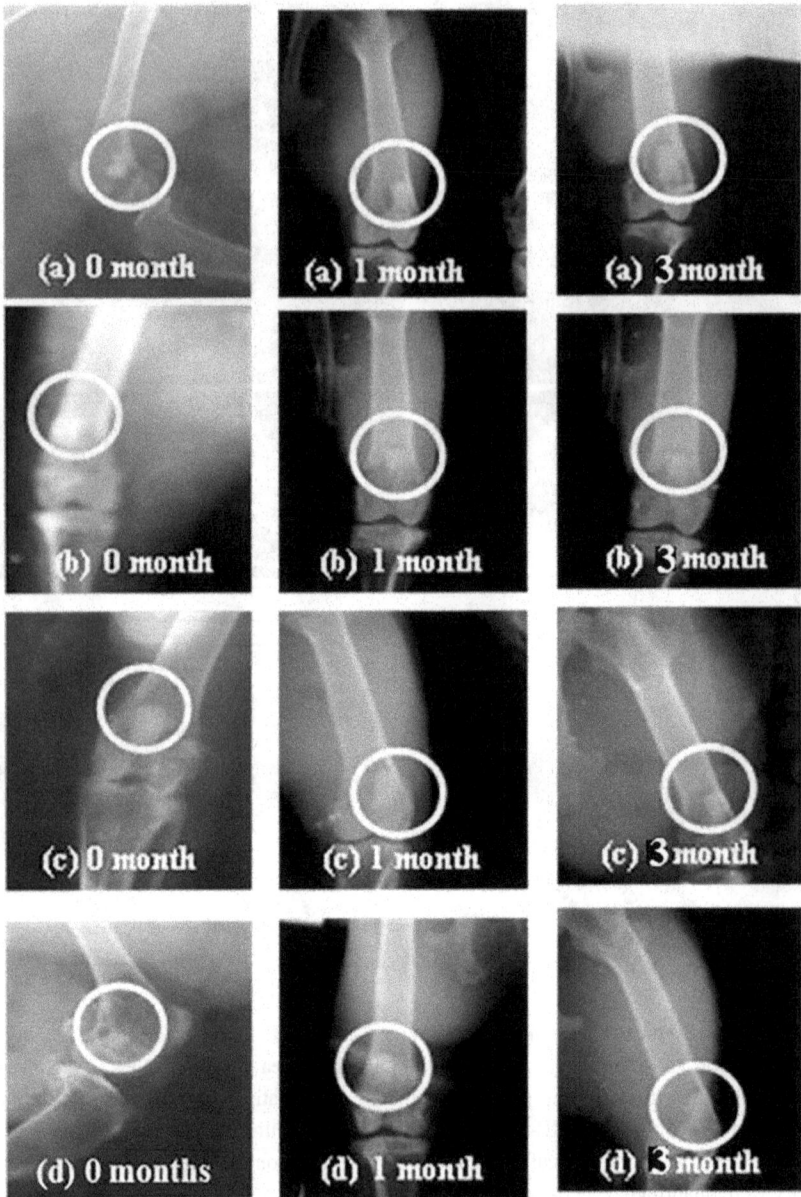

FIGURE 9.6 Radiographic images of the defect site of the femur of the New Zealand white rabbits implanted with different scaffolds, captured at 0 to 3 months post-operation: (a) gelatin/chitosan, (b) gelatin/chitosan/HAP, (c) gelatin/chitosan (β-TCP), and (d) gelatin/chitosan/bioglass implant exhibited the bone formation. License Number 5362990491260.

Source: Dasgupta et al. (2019).

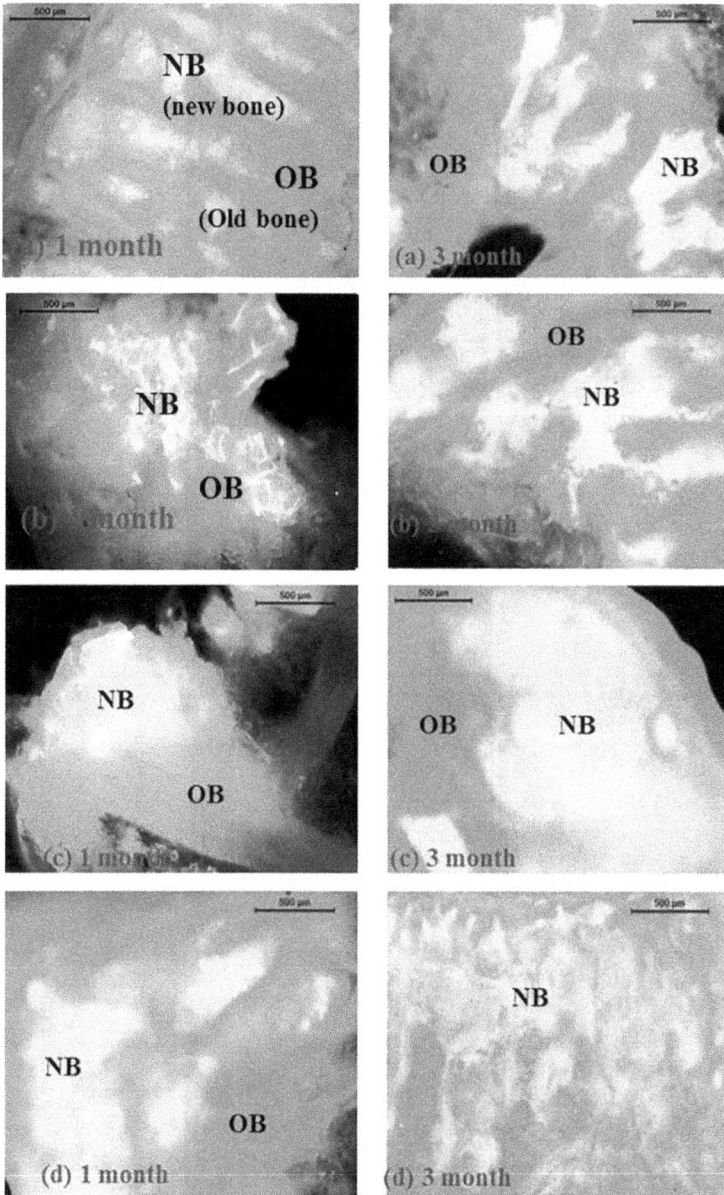

FIGURE 9.7 Flurochrome labelling images taken after 1 and 3 months implantation of the (a) gelatin/chitosan, (b) gelatin/chitosan-hydroxyapatite, (c) gelatin/chitosan/β-TCP, and (d) gelatin/chitosan/bioglass in defect site of the femur of the New Zealand white rabbits. The images exhibited the new bone formtion and the old bone zone. At 3 months, gelatin/chitosan/bioglass-implanted region showed the highest new bone formation throughout the section which was patchy in nature.

Source: Dasgupta et al. (2019).

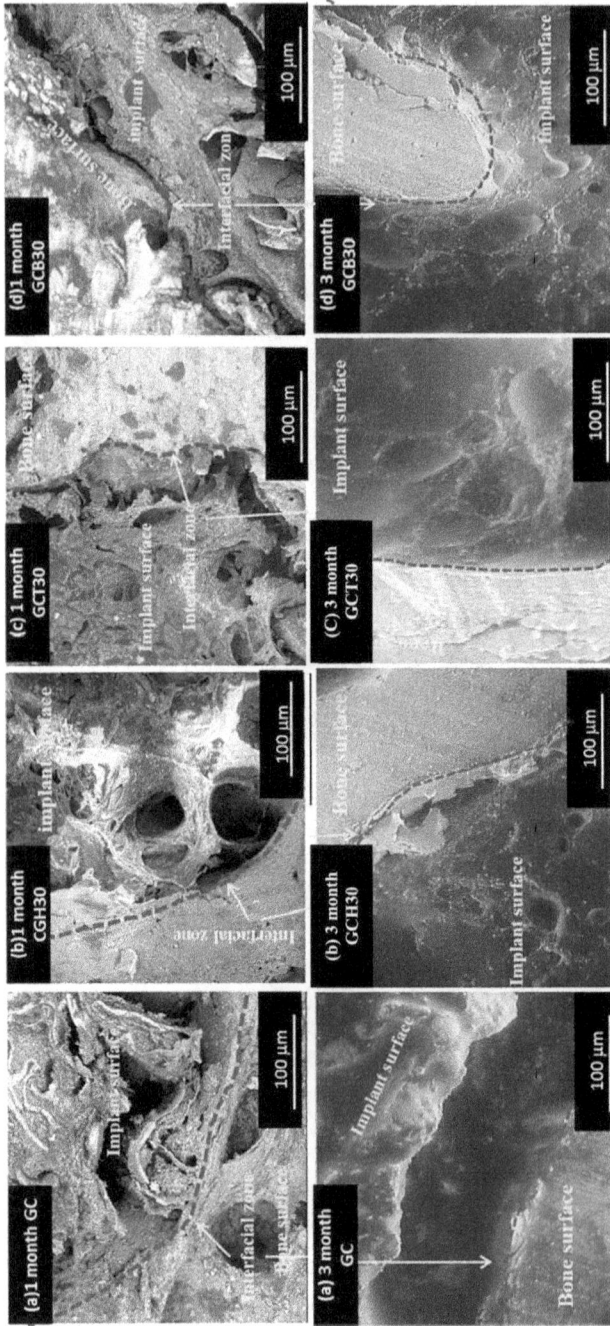

FIGURE 9.8 E-SEM micrographs of the host implant interface in (a) gelatin/chitosan (GC), (b) gelatin/chitosan/β-TCP(GCT30), and (d) gelatin/chitosan/bioglass (GCB30) scaffolds after 1 month (above) and 3 months (below) of implantation. A significant osseous ingrowth and deposition of ECM occurred in the scaffold groups (b–d). The interfacial zones of GCT30 and GCB30 implants were collapsed at 3 months of implantation. The formation of scaffold–bone tissue interface is seen in GCB30 with densified ECM.

Source: Dasgupta et al. (2019).

more rapid bone tissue regeneration in this group (Figure 9.7c). At 3 months, GCB30 implanted region showed the highest new bone formation throughout the section which was patchy in nature (Figure 9.7d) (Dasgupta et al. 2019).

The ESEM images depicted the osseous ingrowth inside and interfacial regions of the scaffolds. A considerable interfacial gap with insignificant bone tissue growth was occurred at the host tissue graft interface of GC-implanted sample (Figure 9.8(a)), whereas a significant osseous ingrowth and deposition of ECM occurred in the other scaffold groups (Figure 9.8(b–d)). The interfacial zones of GCT30 and GCB30 implants were collapsed in 3 months of implantation. In GCB30 both sites of implant were densified with ECM which led to the formation of scaffold–bone tissue interface (Dasgupta et al. 2019).

In an *in vivo* sinus lift model, experiment conducted in adult sheep carrying a polysaccharide-hydroxyapatite composite matrix was evaluated for new bone formation. The harvested bone tissue samples at 3 or 6 months post-implantation were subjected to macroscopic observations, which revealed the presence of the polymer-HAp composite matrix implanted inside the sinus cavity of all the sheep and no adverse response such as infection or formation of granulation tissue was elicited by any specimen. Furthermore, the formation of a vascular tissue network was detected macroscopically in some explants in the mucosa after 3 months post-operation and mineralized tissues were found with the sample containing matrix-HAp in the sinus area which was almost filled with the mineralized tissue after 6 months of implantation. Cone beam computed tomography (CBCT) images were used to assess the mineralization of bone explants by calculating the mineralized volume over total grafted volume for the explants after 3 and 6 months of implantation and the CBCT analysis of the images of bone regenerated by the autologous BM-MSCs-laden gel foam scaffolds demonstrated its potentiality to speed up the regeneration in the mandibular distraction site. Furthermore, the SEM images of the newly regenerated bone tissue were found to be more organized and differentiated with the newly synthesized network of dense osteocytes in direct contact with numerous zones and blood vessels in matrix-HAp group (Fricain et al. 2018). In another *in vivo* study, a construct comprising a biomimetic simvastatin-incorporated calcium phosphate (BioCaP) granules seeded with human adipose-derived stem cells was implanted subcutaneously in the nude mice to repair bone defect. The X-ray image analysis of the explant revealed the bone-like tissue formation in the defect site (Zhang et al. 2018). Micro-CT, a nondestructive and suitable method, is employed for assessing 3D microstructural bone properties. The micro-CT test was performed to assess how the ECM structure for both the aligned and random scaffolds loaded with rhBMP-2 mimics *in vivo* for the growth of stem cells and generates aligned collagen and cortical bone (Zhang et al. 2019). In an *in vivo* test, male New Zealand white rabbits carrying a construct generated by culturing mesenchymal stem cells obtained from rabbit bone marrow over the silk-nano calcium phosphate composite scaffold was investigated for the regeneration of tissue for the critical size osteochondral defect in the knee. After 4 weeks of post-implantation, the macroscopic images of the harvested explants showed proper integration of the regenerated implant with the host knee joint tissue and no infection was noticed. The micro-CT analysis was performed in wet state to create a cylindrical model area with dimension 4×4 mm^2 and the top 2 mm and the next

2 mm regions were considered as cartilage and subchondral bone domain, respectively. The μ-CT result displayed the regular morphology and the subchondral bone ingrowths and cartilage regeneration, thereby filling the defect (Yan et al. 2015). In another *in vivo* animal study, the obtained μ-CT images were used for the assessment of bone regeneration in the defect sites (Sun et al. 2013). New Zealand rabbits were transplanted with an MSCs-seeded β-TCP construct for bone defect repair. The SEM images of the harvested explant revealed that the mesenchymal stem cells filled the pores and surfaces of the constructs with a significant bone regeneration. Similarly, in an animal testing, the μ-CT and MRI displayed the formation of artificial lamina of the vertebral arch (Dong, Chen and Hong 2013).

The efficacy of the BMP-hBMSCs-laden constructs intramuscularly implanted in a severe combined immunodeficient mice model was investigated towards bone regeneration. The construct exhibited rapid bone formation in the defect area as evident from the micro-CT imaging data of the implant harvested from the defect site at 14 days post-implantation (Lin et al. 2019). In an *in vivo* experiment, xenogeneic grafts had shown its ability to substitute autogenous bone tissue grafts in dental bone defects. The experiment was conducted in male adult New Zealand white rabbits with calvarial critical-size defects by implanting a procine graft developed from collagen scaffold. The explants images obtained by micro-CT scanning revealed superior performance of the porcine collagen graft in new bone regeneration (Salamanca et al. 2018). The efficiency of a nanosynthetic silicated calcium phosphate putty was evaluated for postero-lateral intertransverse process of spinal fusion in a rabbit model. The nanosynthetic graft exhibited a development of fusion between 6 and 12 weeks, which had similarity with the autograft alone. After 26 weeks of post-implantation, an excellent fusion outcome, bone regeneration, and graft resorption were achieved. The fusion success was assessed by subjecting the sample to a nondestructive range of motion testing like manual palpation, radiographic analysis, and micro-CT imaging techniques (Conway et al. 2021). In another study, electrospun PCL nanofibrous structures either blended with non-mulberry silk fibroin (NSF) before electrospinning or implanting NSF onto PCL structures were evaluated by comparing the introductory methods into the structures. The matrices were inserted into the defect site in distal metaphysis area of the rabbit femurs and subsequently tested for the host tissue immuno-compatibility. Further, the formation of bone tissue by the matrices was confirmed by radiological assessment, fluorochrome labelling, and SEM micrographs analysis. The bone regeneration activity was found to be significantly better for NSF-grafted matrices over blended matrices that represents the potentiality of NSF/PCL nanofibrous structure for bone repair and bone regrowth than the blended matrices (Bhattacharjee et al. 2016). In another animal study involving male Wistar rats having critical bone defect, hydroxyapatite (HAp) /PLGA scaffold was implanted into the defect site. The micro-CT analysis with the explant harvested from the defect site depicted an enhanced bone regeneration activity on the PLA/HAp, matrix and the formation of an excellent neo-vessel (Tayton et al. 2014).

In a study using New Zealand white rabbits of 3.5 to 4.5 kg weight, chitosan-nano hydroxyapatite scaffold was transplanted into the bone defect site. The specimens harvested after post-implantation were subjected to scanning using a high-resolution micro-CT system. The μ-CT image analysis revealed bone formation in the defect

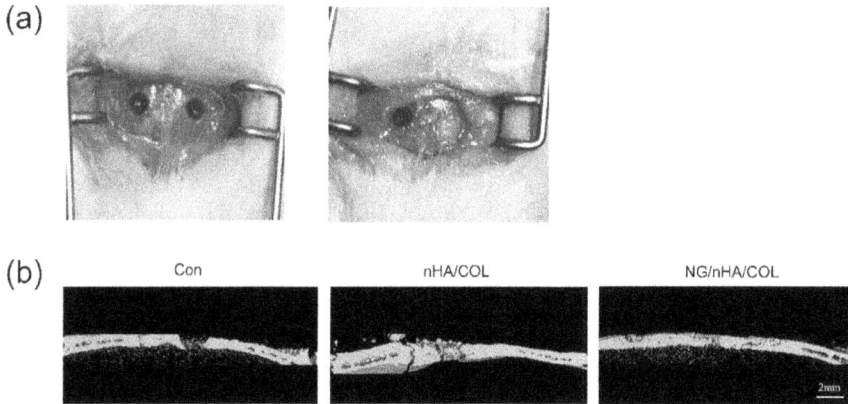

FIGURE 9.9 Micro-CT images representing the *in vivo* bone regeneration by the implanted nano-hydroxyapatite/collagen (nHA/ COL) and nano-hydroxyapatite/collagen/naringin (NG/nHA/COL) scaffolds in skull cranial parietal of rat model. Figure (a) nHA/COL and NG/nHA/COL scaffolds were implanted to the skull defect areas of rats. Figure (b) μCT scan image of tested groups Here HAp is represented as HA].

Source: Zuo et al. (2022).

area as evident from the measurement of the total bone volume, bone volume and its percentage, bone surface density, trabecular patterns in terms of trabecular number and its thickness, and trabecular separation and its quality. Furthermore, the process of bone regeneration was monitored by a radiographic study (Lee et al. 2014). Environmental scanning electron microscopic images were used to assess the osseous ingrowth processes within the different gelatin-chitosan and gelatin chitosan-bioceramics composite scaffolds as well as across the interfacial areas after 1 and 3 months post-implantation. The gelatin-chitosan/HAp30, gelatin-chitosan/bioglass 30, and gelatin-chitosan/β-TCP 30 scaffolds exhibited excellent bone mineralization and bone ECM formation at the scaffold–bone tissue interfacial area as evident by the significant decrease in the interfacial gap and substantial osseous ingrowth. Among the composite scaffolds, gelation-chitosan/bioglass showed the densification of bone ECM, thereby strengthening the scaffold–bone tissue interface (Dasgupta et al. 2019). Zuo et al. (2022) developed a nano-hydroxyapatite/collagen (nHAp/COL) and nano-hydroxyapatite/collagen/naringin (NG/nHAp/COL) scaffold by using the freeze-drying method. A critical bone defect was created in skull cranial parietal of rat model. Both the scaffolds were imbedded in the defect site of the tested model. After 4 weeks of implantation of scaffolds in defect sites, μ-CT scan was done to evaluate the cranial parietal defect in the skull. In the control group no scaffold was implanted into the defect site. A higher bone density mass and speedy recovery were observed in NG/nHAp/COL tested group than the nHA/COL tested group (Figure 9.9).

A 3D-printed silica-based bioglass scaffold was developed and inoculated into the defect site of the 1-year-old matured male rabbit's femoral diaphysis region. 3D scaffolds and bioactive glass powder (control) were incorporated at the femoral

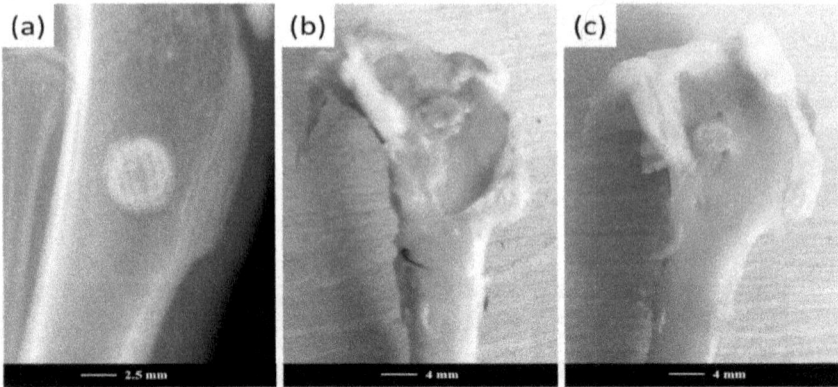

FIGURE 9.10 Represented X-ray images of the defect filled with implant after surgery completion (a), extracted femurs after 3 months (b), and extracted femurs after 6 months of implantation (c). The analysis of the images revealed that scaffold-incorporated group exhibited skin or rose-coloured tissue surrounding the implant representing the integration between the regenerated bone and the scaffold.

Source: Tulyaganov et al. (2022).

defect site for 3 months and 6 months. After the incubation periods, the control and the tested implants groups were sacrificed by immediate decapitation followed by the extraction of the femurs. The X-ray study of the femurs of the groups showed that scaffold-incorporated group had skin or rose coloured tissue surround the scaffold, representing the integration between the regenerated bone and the scaffold (Figure 9.10) (Tulyaganov et al. 2022).

Histological and Immunohistochemical Assessment

Histology is one of the important microscopic studies that can provide information about the progressive cellular events of bone remodelling such as the osteoblast proliferation, angiogenesis, and osteoclastic activity that occur during the bone regeneration process at the implanted site (Mukherjee, Nandi et al. 2016). In a study involving New Zealand white rabbit models, the animals were implanted with chitosan-nano hydroxyapatite scaffold for bone defect repair. The newly formed bone tissues isolated from the defect rabbit tibia fixed in PBS solution were stained by H&E and Masson-trichrome staining methods followed by histologic observation using a light microscope. The staining results revealed the filling up of the bone defect area implanted with the composite scaffold and degenerated cells and further the important role of nHAp in the bone ossification (Lee, Baek et al. 2014). Similarly in a 3-month animal study, histological assessment of explants harvested from the defect bone site of the adult male and female New Zealand white rabbits of weight between 2.5 and 3 kg was performed. The *in vivo* rabbit model consisted of freeze-dried 3D scaffold derived from gelatin-chitosan-based composite biomaterials developed with different bioceramic materials, namely HAp, TCP, and bioactive glass. For histological ana-lysis, the decalcified new tissues were subjected to H&E staining to evaluate the bone matrix deposition using an optical microscope. The results revealed the forma-tion of trabecular structure consisting of osteoblast, osteocyte, and minimal fibrous tissue and medulla containing large amounts of red blood cells, osteoblast cells, and fibrinous deposits, angiogenesis, and some relatively avascular medullary cavities. Furthermore, good osteoblast proliferation was also observed. The bone remodelling activity at the defect site filled with scaffold-containing bioglass was evident from the presence of osteoblastic and osteoclastic activity (Dasgupta et al. 2019).

For an *in vivo* experiment, bilayer scaffolds comprising silk fibroin layers integrated with silk-nano calcium phosphate layer were developed and were subcutaneously implanted in a critical size osteochondral (OCD) knee defect rabbit for osteochondral tissue regeneration. Histological evaluation performed by the H&E staining of the explants harvested from the defect knee area depicted de-novo bone infiltration in the subchondral region, signifying the well integration between the scaffolds and the host tissue with a stable structure. Furthermore, the captured images of Masson's trichome staining with high magnification revealed that the chondrocytes exhibited with usual round phenotype and grew in the interior of the scaffold silk layer in the regenerated ECM, whereas in the silk-nano CaP layer, the new bone growth and new blood vessels were detected (Yan et al. 2015). The immunohistochemical staining of the harvested explant using mouse anti-rabbit collagen II alpha 1 and biotinylated Sambucus nigra bark lectin showed the formation of neocartilage tissue within the silk layer, showing the positive staining for collagen II. The GAG formation in the defect area was assessed by the histological study using safranin O staining method, whereas immunohistochemical staining using SNA-lectin angiogenic marker exhibited the enlarged image of the SNA-lectin staining, representing the formation of endothelial cells colony abundantly inside the silk-nanoCaP layer, and identified the new bone as well as the blood vessel formation.

In an *in vivo* bone regeneration study, cranial defect model was formed in the adult female New Zealand white rabbits, in which aligned electrospun cellulose/ cellu-lose nanocrystals (CNCs) nanofibrous composite seeded with BMP-2 was implanted for bone defect repair. The explants were stained with H&E and Masson trichrome staining for the evaluation of cortical bone regeneration by histological analysis. The obtained histological images were scanned by a virtual microscopic solution and visualized by an Image Scope viewing software. The results demonstrated the formation of bone ECM and distribution of regenerated aligned collagen fibres that were integrated with the host bone tissues (Zhang et al. 2019). In another *in vivo* histological study of explants using Masson Goldner technique, bone formation was observed in the polysaccharide-hydroxyapatite composite matrix group after 3 months post-implantation. An increased bone regeneration was observed with an increased post-implantation period. The epifluorescence microscopic analysis exhibited the lamellar bone structures in the area of the newly formed bone juxtaposing optical microscopy (Fricain et al. 2018). In another study, the implantation of the constructs made by culturing human foetal mesenchymal stem cells on the apatite microcarriers subcutaneously in a mouse model was investigated for bone tissue regeneration. The harvested explants were subjected to three histological studies by using H&E,

Masson's trichrome, and von Kossa staining methods to assess the morphology of the neobone tissue, the type of regenerated bone, and the level of mineralized bone tissue, respectively, whereas immunohistochemistry assay of osteopontin confirmed the active bone formation by the cell-seeded scaffold construct (Lim et al. 2017). The ability of the artificial lamina of vertebral arch was evaluated in a rabbit model with decompressive laminectomy. After the segmental defects with dimension 20 mm × 8 mm created in the adult New Zealand rabbits by laminectomy, they were filled with mesenchymal stem cells-seeded beta-tricalcium phosphates bioceramics constructs. The histological examination of the harvested explants using H&E and Masson trichrome staining assessed the artificial laminae of the vertebral arch. The immunohistochemistry results revealed that the implanted construct promoted the bone morphogenetic protein expression and hence the bone regeneration outcome *in vivo* (Dong et al. 2013). The ability of a dissociated mucosa soft tissue suspension as a substitute for bone graft was evaluated in an *in vivo* study involving male Wistar rats of 12 weeks old. The defects were filled with the dissociated mucosa soft tissue suspension and hydrogel in combination. The new bone formation with significantly greater bone volume was confirmed by histological analysis by staining of the harvested explants with H&E stain after 1 and 2 weeks post-implantation (Kawakami et al. 2021).

In a study, the subcutaneous implantation of a construct generated from the rabbit bone marrow-derived mesenchymal stem cells loaded onto the novel bilayered silk/silk-nanoCaP scaffolds promoted the regeneration of critical size osteochondral defects in the knee of the rabbit. There was neither any acute inflammation found in any of the explants nor was there any indication of collapse of the adjacent tissues in the defects filled with scaffolds. The histological study on the regenerated osteochondral tissue explants by H&E and Masson's trichrome staining depicted the formation of neocartilage in the upper layer (silk layer) and the subchondral bone tissue growth in the silk-nanoCaP layer in the bottom domain. The immunohistochemical staining using mouse anti-rabbit collagen II alpha 1 and biotinylated Sambucus nigra bark lectin was visualized under a fluorescence microscope. The results revealed the presence of collagen II positive cartilage and GAG deposition in the silk layer, whereas the bone ingrowths and the blood vessel formation in the silk-nanoCaP layer (Lin et al. 2019). The incorporation of bone marrow concentrate into glass-reinforced HAp composite in a new microporous pellet formulation promoted an early bone regeneration and bone healing. The efficacy of this construct was evaluated in an *in vivo* ovine model, wherein a total of 90 non-critical sized bone defects were made in the femurs of nine Merino breed sheep. The defects were filled with composite pellets combined with autologous bone marrow concentrate. At 3, 6, and 12 weeks post-implantation, the explants were undergone histological analysis by staining with haematoxylin/eosin and Solochrome cyanine R, and the stained newly formed bone specimens were assessed by digital camera. The histomorphometric analysis with the sample revealed the osteointegration, bone apposition, as well as bone ECM formation in the defect area following a reported method (Atayde et al. 2014; Torres et al. 2017).

An *in vivo* study was conducted in the female New Zealand white rabbit spinal fusion model to determine the efficacy of an implanted bone graft comprising the engineered nanosynthetic silicated calcium phosphate putty in combination with autograft. The regenerated spine specimens were processed for decalcified paraffin histology to evaluate the tissue response and bone ECM deposition using H&E and Tetrachrome or staining method or undecalcified polymethyl methacrylate histology by staining with methylene blue and basic fuchsin to quantify the regenerated bone tissue and graft resorption on the basis of the performed histomorphometric analysis. The results exhibited an excellent spinal fusion outcome, bone regeneration and graft resorption at 26 weeks post-implantation by using the model excluding the need of excessive autograft and thereby promote their effective use in surgery (Conway et al. 2021). Electrospun PCL matrices blended with non-mulberry silk fibroin (NSF) before electrospinning and implanting silk fibroin onto the nanofibrous PCL matrices showed bone regenerating property at the bone defect area created in distal metaphysis region of the rabbits' femur. Further, formation of bone tissue for both implant varieties was confirmed using radiological examinations along with fluorochrome labelling and scanning electron microscopy. Bone formation was found to be significantly better for NSF-grafted matrices than for blended matrices. From the cumulative results of the *in vivo* tests, it was confirmed that NSF-grafted PCL nanofibrous matrices are suitable as an ECM for bone repair and regrowth than the blended matrices (Bhattacharjee et al. 2016). In an *in vivo* experiment involving a canine mandibular critical-size defect model in 12–15-month-old male beagle dogs with average weight of 12.1±0.5 kg was implanted with nano-hydroxyapatite/coralline blocks which was prevascularized or coated with recombinant human vascular endothelial growth factor. The histological analysis using H&E staining and Masson trichrome quantified the total scaffold area by Image-Pro Plus software, and the per cent of neobone fill. The immunohistological study performed in a rabbit antidog vWF primary antibody and biotinylated anti-rabbit immunoglobulin G and counterstaining with haematoxylin was used to assess the blood vessel formation and calculate the blood vessel density by the same software. These analyses exhibited the large amount of regenerated bone with significant neovascular density at the periphery and cores of the implanted constructs at 3 and 8 weeks post-implantation, respectively (Du et al. 2015).

In an *in vivo* female sprague–dawley rat model, simulated body fluid-coated chitosan-gelatin cryogel cylindrical discs were transplanted. The explants harvested from the defect area were sectioned with 5- μm thickness. The specimen was then histologically analysed by staining with H&E and the stained image was taken using a light microscope. The histopathological evaluation of the explants was done for bone and muscle tissues individually to assess the host tissue response. The results did not show any necrotic tissue present in the abdominal or thoracic region, inflammation or degeneration in the bone and muscle tissues. The irritation scores determined that the implanted cryogel scaffold exhibited minimum irritant to muscle tissue and did not show any irritation for bone tissue, which were decided according to the irritation classification of ISO 10993-6:2016 protocol (Öfkeli, Demir and Bölgen 2021). In an *in vivo* adolescent domestic pigs model, constructs made of autologous stem cells seeded with the developed gelfoam scaffolds were transplanted into the mandibular distraction sites. After post-surgery, bone mineralization at the distraction area was evaluated by histological analysis by staining with fluorescent dyes calcein and alizarin-3-methyliminodiacetic acid. The undecalcified histological sections were assessed for mineralization at the defect area after fixing the regenerated specimen, followed by dehydration and embedding in the microbed resin solution. The sectioned tissues were observed under fluorescent microscope to visualise the regenerated and old bones (Sun et al. 2013).

An aligned electrospun cellulose/cellulose nanocrystals (CNCs) nanocomposite containing rhBMP-2 was inserted into the square-sized cranial defect area of adult female New Zealand white rabbits (Figure 9.11). Different groups like negative control (without scaffold), positive control (without surgery), aligned scaffolds with and without rhBMP-2, and random scaffolds with and without rhBMP-2 were used.

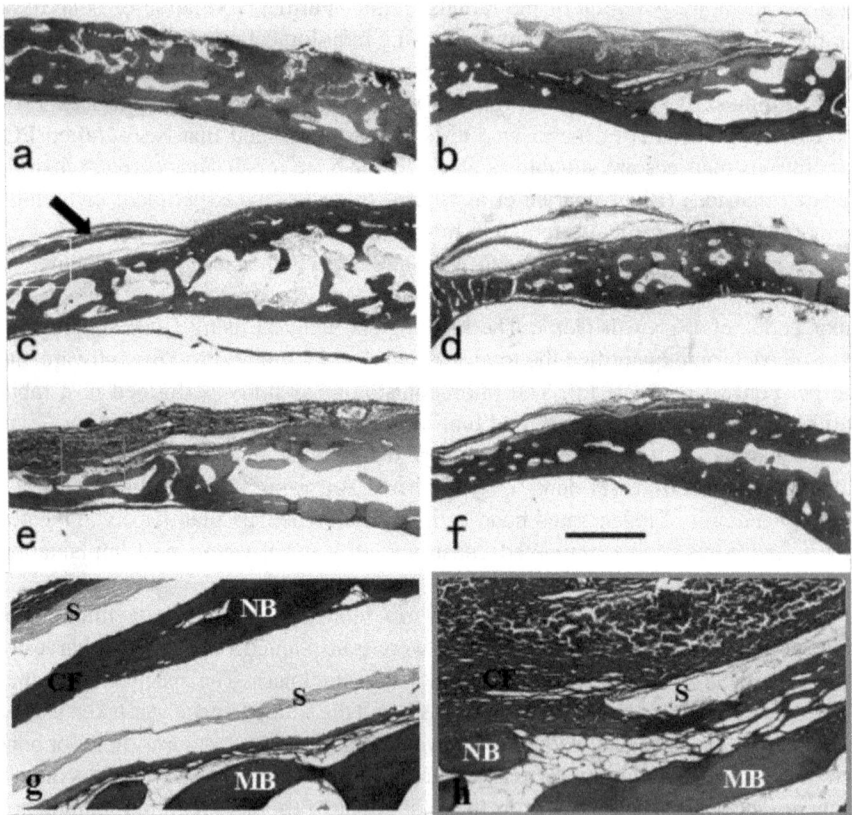

FIGURE 9.11   Cranial defect area of New Zealand white rabbits implanted with different groups like, (a) positive control, (b) negative control, (c) aligned scaffold with BMP-2 group, (d) aligned scaffold without BMP-2 group, (e) random scaffold with BMP-2 group, and (f) random scaffold without BMP-2 group showed Masson's trichrome staining. In these images osteoid and new bone formation are found by (Masson's trichrome staining. (g) Synthesis of aligned collagen fibres and (h) random collagen fibres are found. Labels indicate: Scaffold (S), new bone (NB), mature bone (MB), and collagen fibres (CF).

Source: Zhang et al. (2019).

Under Masson's trichrome staining, old bone, new bone, and collagen fibre are stained red, blue, and red respectively. The positive control sample (Figure 9.11(A)) had normal cranial sample with osteoid and new bone formation. The negative control (Figure 9.11(B)) sample possessed narrow new bone formation region. The aligned electrospun cellulose scaffolds loaded with BMP-2 groups (Figure 9.11(C)) showed cortical bone on the scaffold and the random (Figure 9.11(D)) electrospun cellulose scaffolds loaded with BMP-2 groups showed randomly formed native bone with collagen. Even in the aligned (Figure 9.11(E)) and random (Figure 9.11(F)) groups without BMP-2, some new bone and collagen had been formed at the endocardium side (Zhang et al. 2019).

The histological study of scaffolds, graphene oxide/chitosan/gelatin (GO/CH/GE) and chitosan/gelatin (CH/GE) implanted in the defect region of male Albino-Wistar rats' tibial bone was done to evaluate the formation of new bone. The defects without filled with the scaffold were used as the control group. H&E staining of the sectioned tissue implants revealed higher regeneration of bone in GO/CH/GE groups followed by CH/GE implanted group at the defect site, complying with the results of the radiographic images (Figure 9.12(B)). An enhanced collagen deposition was obtained with the implanted GO/CH/GE as evident from the Masson's trichrome staining results (Figure 9.12(C)) (Saravanan et al. 2017).

In an *in vivo* experiment, a rat model with bone defect was filled with a biphasic scaffold developed from calcium sulphate and HAp combined with recombinant human bone morphogenic protein-2 (rhBMP-2) and zoledronic acid. Histological

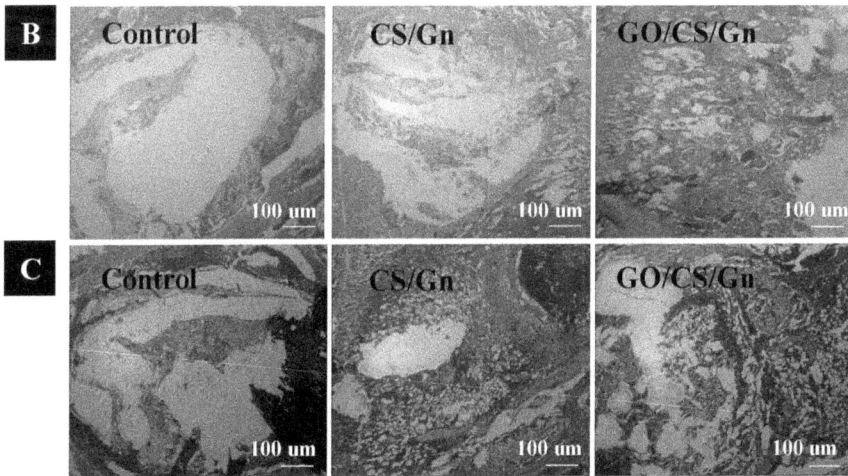

FIGURE 9.12 Representative images of the histological study of chitosan/gelatin (CS/Gn) and graphene oxide/chitosan/gelatin (GO/CS/Gn) scaffolds implanted in rat tibial bone after 2 weeks post-implantation. (B) H&E staining and (C) Masson's trichrome staining of the harvested tissue section. An enhanced bone formation and collagen deposition were resulted in graphene oxide/chitosan/gelatin implanted group.

Source: Chawla et al. (2017).

and histomorphometrical analyses performed with the harvested bone ECM revealed that bone formation in the biphasic material containing the protein and zoledronic acid was considerably higher than the biphasic scaffold containing rhBMP-2 alone (Raina et al. 2016). In another study, combined autografts, allografts, and engineered bone grafts were used to treat the femoral defects created surgically in rabbits. The cell–tissue responses and regeneration of bone tissue were evaluated using histology and histomorphometry by retrieving the explants at 6 weeks at recipient sites. The regenerated tissue samples were subjected to staining using Sanderson's rapid bone stain and counterstaining by van Gieson's picrofuchsin following the method described elsewhere (Magno et al. 2010).

The histological study of a regenerative tissue specimen followed by the analysis of images indicated no sign of inflammation, adverse immune responses, tissue necrosis, osteolysis, and co-integration of the implant with the host tissue and the regenerated bone, whereas, histomorphometric data revealed that the new bone formed by the tricalcium phosphate-based synthetic bone tissue substitute was similar to the allograft as evident from the demineralized bone matrix (Kim et al. 2014). In an another study, the performed fluorochrome labelling evaluated the bone mineralization surrounding the explants harvested after sacrificing the animals implanted with gelatin-chitosan and gelatin-chitosan-nanoceramic composite scaffolds at 1 and 3 months. The various nano-bioceramics used in the scaffold were hydroxyapatite, β-tricalcium phosphate, and bioglass. And tetracycline was used as a bone marker because of its property of deposition at the bone regeneration site (van Gaalen et al. 2010; Kovar et al. 2011). At 1 month post-surgery, the intensity of the golden yellow fluorescence was more in the construct containing the gelatin-chitosan-bioactive glass scaffold than the other cell-scaffold constructs. The similar trend after 3 months post-implantation was observed with the construct containing gelatin-chitosan-nano HAp sample providing a golden yellow fluorescence in wider zone, representing higher level of bone ECM formation than the construct made with the gelatin-chitosan as the control sample (Dasgupta et al. 2019). In an *in vivo* experiment, the subcutaneously implanted cell-scaffold constructs generated by culturing hBMSCs over the mesoporous bioactive glass/silk fibroin and mesoporous bioactive glass/PCL scaffolds into the nude mice were used to evaluate the heterotopic bone formation. The harvested explants after post-operation were tested histologically by staining with Masson tricolour reagent and H&E staining using haematoxylin dye to observe the cell density and cell distribution over the scaffold surface and the formation of collagen. The analysis of the H&E staining images showed the well growth of hBMSCs over the scaffolds. Masson's trichrome staining determined the collagen expression after 8 weeks of implantation. Immunohistochemical analysis was performed with the harvested explants for osteocalcin expression and thereby assessed the bone regeneration by osteogenic differentiation of stem cells. The total RNA collected from the regenerated bone tissue was used for the gene expression analysis using the genetic markers osteocalcin, collagen type I, OPN, and BMP-2 (Du et al. 2019).

BIOMECHANICAL ASSESSMENT

In an *in vivo* animal study, mice model carrying a implant of biphasic calcium sulphate and HAp loaded with recombinant human BMP-2 and zoledronic acid (ZA) at the bone defect site for repair. The mechanical compression test performed with the explants harvested from the defect area after post-implantation revealed the significantly higher stiffness of the biphasic scaffold containing rhBMP-2 (Raina et al. 2016). In another experiment, the biomechanical assessment was performed by measuring the torsional stiffness of the femurs of the different groups (three groups) of rats after 8 weeks of surgery. The statistical analysis of the obtained results indicated the varying degree of torsional stiffness of the femurs among the different groups of the rats tested (Hao et al. 2016). In an another *in vivo* experiment, upon biomechanical stimulation, the umbilical-cord-blood-derived endothelial progenitor cells (EPC) and human foetal messenchymal stem cells (hfMSCs) co-cultured in a biaxial bioreactor exhibited bone mineralization and calcium deposition consistently during the progress of the culturing over 14 days, thereby a cell-seeded scaffold was constructed. The subsequent subcutaneous implantations of these EPC/hfMSC constructs in NOD/SCID mice shown to promote the uniform cellular distribution, vessel infiltration into the scaffold, and an increasing trend of ectopic bone formation, representing an enhanced efficiency and MSCs survival through the early vascularization (Liu

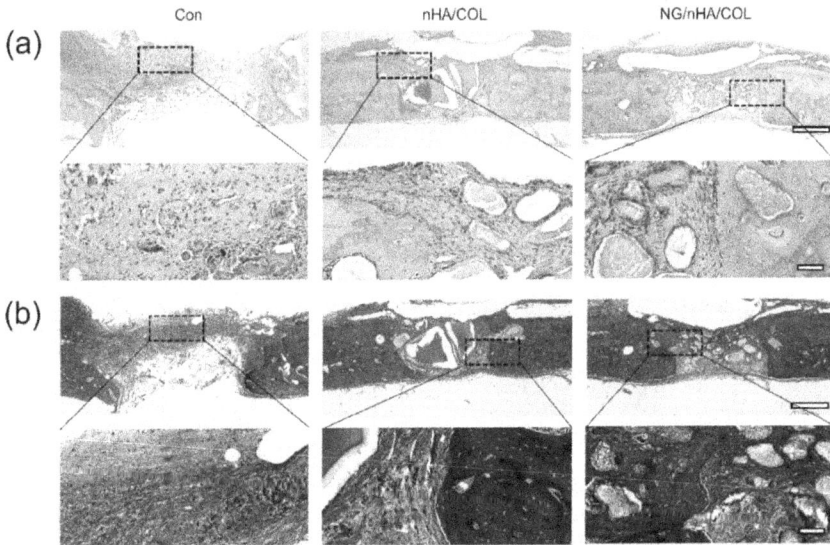

FIGURE 9.13 Captured staining images of the histological study performed in the bone defect site implanted with nano-hydroxyapatite/collagen (nHA/COL) and nano-hydroxyapatite/collagen/naringin (NG/nHA/COL) scaffolds in skull cranial parietal of rat model used in an *in vivo* bone regeneration. (a) H&E staining and (b) Masson's trichrome. The staining results show the bone regeneration in the defect region Here, HAp is represented by HA}.

Source: Zuo et al. (2022).

et al. 2013). An *in vivo* study using female New Zealand white rabbit spinal fusion model was used to evaluate the efficacy of an implanted bone graft comprising the engineered nanosynthetic silicated calcium phosphate putty in combination with autograft. The biomechanical properties of the regenerated spines were evaluated using a nondestructive Denso robot, in axial rotation, flexion-extension, and lateral bending by applying 270 Nmm moments at 33.3 Nmm/sec to a maximum of 300 Nmm for 15 sec with running a 4.5 load–unload cycles in each profile (Conway et al. 2021).

A critical bone defect was created in the skull cranial parietal of rat model, in which nHAp/COL (nano-hydroxyapatite/collagen) and NG/nHAp/ COL (nano-hydroxyapatite/collagen/ Naringin) scaffolds were [e]mbedded in the defect site of the tested model. After 4 weeks of implantation the defect region was tested by the histological study using the Masson's trichrome and H&E staining. The staining results revealed that a good fibrous connective tissue was observed in the control group and a small amount of native bone tissue also formed. The mass of trabeculae bone formation was higher in NG/nHAp/COL group than in nHAp/COL group. The regeneration and reconstruction of bone were high in NG/nHAp/COL scaffold (Figure 9.13). Therefore, naringin is an osteogenic factor that can induce osteogenic property in *in vivo* study (Figure 9.13(b)) (Zuo et al. 2022).

A 3D-printed scaffold was implanted in the matured male rabbit's defect femoral diaphysis region. At 3- and 6-month incubation periods, the harvested regenerated tissue sections were stained with H&E for histological evaluation using optical microscopic images. The bone formation was assessed according to the histological scoring scale ranging from weak osteogenesis to perfect osteogenesis. At 6 months post-operation, the defect area was filled with regenerated bone that is fully composed of osteons, which comprised of concentric lamellae of the bone matrix surrounding a central canal with vascularization and osteocytes.

EXERCISE

1. Explain how *in vivo* animal experiment is important cartilage and bone constructs and their grafts?
2. What are the different tests used for the *in vivo* evaluation of cartilage tissue grafts?
3. What are the different tests used for the *in vivo* evaluation of bone tissue grafts?
4. Write a brief acoount of morphological assessment in *in vivo* study of regenerated cartilage and osteochondral tissue?
5. What are the different staining methods used for the histological study in *in vivo* bone grafts? Explain any two of these methods.
6. What are the marker genes in bone and cartilage tissue?
7. Give two examples of *in vivo* construct for bone tissue and cartilage tissue.
8. Write short notes on the following:
    i.   μ-CT analysis
    ii.   Masson's trichrome staining.
    iii. RT-PCR study
    iv.   Alcian blue and van Gieson staining.

9. Give a brief account of biomechanical tests involved in the assessment of regenerated bone *in vivo*.
10. Explain the various biochemical tests that are performed for the *in vivo* evaluation of bone graft.
11. Explain the importance of biomechanical test involved in the assessment of regenerated cartilage *in vivo*.
12. Explain the various biochemical tests are performed for the *in vivo* evaluation of cartilage graft.
13. Give a brief account of *in vivo* assessment of the regenerated osteochondral tissue for repairing joint defect.
14. Explain in brief the various microscopic methods used in the assessment of regenerated bone and its associated complex tissues.
15. Explain the immunohistological study for the evaluation of cartilage construct.
16. Explain the immunohistological study for the evaluation of bone graft generated *in vivo*.
17. Discuss about the different animals that have been used for *in vivo* study in reference to the engineered bone and cartilage grafts.
18. Explain how large animals are beneficial for *in vivo* study for the subsequent clinical study.
19. Explain the method of harvesting explants from the defect tissue site..
20. Give some examples of animal models that have been used for the assessment of the efficacy of bone tissue and its complex tissue constructs.
21. What is the Electromagnetic Actuation System. Explain the use of this technique for in vivo assessment of joint tissue constructs.

REFERENCES

Ahern, B., J. Parvizi, R. Boston and T. Schaer. 2009. "Preclinical animal models in single site cartilage defect testing: A systematic review." *Osteoarthritis and Cartilage* 17 (6): 705–713.

Amini, A. R., Laurencin, C. T., & Nukavarapu, S. P. 2012. "Bone tissue engineering: recent advances and challenges." *Critical Reviews in Biomedical Engineering*, 40 (5): 363–408.

Apelgren, P., E. Karabulut, M. Amoroso, A. Mantas, H. c. Martínez Ávila, L. Kölby, T. Kondo, G. Toriz and P. Gatenholm. 2019. "In vivo human cartilage formation in three-dimensional bioprinted constructs with a novel bacterial nanocellulose bioink." *ACS Biomaterials Science & Engineering* 5 (5): 2482–2490.

Atayde, L., P. Cortez, T. Pereira, P. Armada-da-Silva, A. Afonso, M. Lopes, J. Santos and A. Maurício. 2014. "A new sheep model with automatized analysis of biomaterial-induced bone tissue regeneration." *Journal of Materials Science: Materials in Medicine* 25 (8): 1885–1901.

Bhattacharjee, P., D. Naskar, T. K. Maiti, D. Bhattacharya, P. Das, S. K. Nandi and S. C. Kundu. 2016. "Potential of non-mulberry silk protein fibroin blended and grafted poly (Є-caprolactone) nanofibrous matrices for in vivo bone regeneration." *Colloids and Surfaces B: Biointerfaces* 143: 431–439.

Bian, W., Q. Lian, D. Li, J. Wang, W. Zhang, Z. Jin and Y. Qiu. 2016. "Morphological characteristics of cartilage-bone transitional structures in the human knee joint and CAD design of an osteochondral scaffold." *BioMedical Engineering OnLine* 15 (1): 1–14.

Bothe, F., A.-K. Deubel, E. Hesse, B. Lotz, J. Groll, C. Werner, W. Richter and S. Hagmann. 2019. "Treatment of focal cartilage defects in minipigs with zonal chondrocyte/

mesenchymal progenitor cell constructs." *International Journal of Molecular Sciences* 20 (3): 653.

Campos, Y., G. Fuentes, A. Almirall, I. Que, T. Schomann, C. K. Chung, C. Jorquera-Cordero, L. Quintanilla, J. C. Rodríguez-Cabello and A. Chan. 2022. "The incorporation of etanercept into a porous tri-layer scaffold for restoring and repairing cartilage tissue." *Pharmaceutics* 14 (2): 282.

Chu, C. R., M. Szczodry and S. Bruno. 2010. "Animal models for cartilage regeneration and repair." *Tissue Engineering Part B: Reviews* 16 (1): 105–115.

Ci, Z., Y. Zhang, Y. Wang, G. Wu, M. Hou, P. Zhang, L. Jia, B. Bai, Y. Cao and Y. Liu. 2021. "3D cartilage regeneration with certain shape and mechanical strength based on engineered cartilage gel and decalcified bone matrix." *Frontiers in Cell and Developmental Biology* 9: 638115.

Conway, J. C., R. A. Oliver, T. Wang, D. J. Wills, J. Herbert, T. Buckland, W. R. Walsh and I. R. Gibson. 2021. "The efficacy of a nanosynthetic bone graft substitute as a bone graft extender in rabbit posterolateral fusion." *The Spine Journal* 21 (11): 1925–1937.

Dai, W., N. Kawazoe, X. Lin, J. Dong and G. Chen. 2010. "The influence of structural design of PLGA/collagen hybrid scaffolds in cartilage tissue engineering." *Biomaterials* 31 (8): 2141–2152.

Dasgupta, S., K. Maji and S. K. Nandi. 2019. "Investigating the mechanical, physiochemical and osteogenic properties in gelatin-chitosan-bioactive nanoceramic composite scaffolds for bone tissue regeneration: In vitro and in vivo." *Materials Science and Engineering: C* 94: 713–728.

de Sá Schiavo Matias, G., A. C. O. Carreira, V. F. Batista, H. J. C. de Carvalho, M. A. Miglino and P. Fratini. 2022. "In vivo biocompatibility analysis of the recellularized canine tracheal scaffolds with canine epithelial and endothelial progenitor cells." *Bioengineered* 13 (2): 3551–3565.

Dong, Y., X. Chen and Y. Hong. 2013. "Tissue-engineered bone formation in vivo for artificial laminae of the vertebral arch using β-Tricalcium phosphate bioceramics seeded with mesenchymal stem cells." *Spine* 38 (21): E1300–E1306.

Du, B., W. Liu, Y. Deng, S. Li, X. Liu, Y. Gao and L. Zhou. 2015. "Angiogenesis and bone regeneration of porous nano-hydroxyapatite/coralline blocks coated with rhVEGF165 in critical-size alveolar bone defects in vivo." *International Journal of Nanomedicine* 10: 2555.

Du, X., D. Wei, L. Huang, M. Zhu, Y. Zhang and Y. Zhu. 2019. "3D printing of mesoporous bioactive glass/silk fibroin composite scaffolds for bone tissue engineering." *Materials Science and Engineering: C* 103: 109731.

Farndale, R. W., D. J. Buttle and A. J. Barrett. 1986. "Improved quantitation and discrimination of sulphated glycosaminoglycans by use of dimethylmethylene blue." *Biochimica et Biophysica Acta (BBA)-General Subjects* 883 (2): 173–177.

Fragogeorgi, Eirini A., Maritina Rouchota, Maria Georgiou, Marisela Velez, Penelope Bouziotis, and George Loudos. "In vivo imaging techniques for bone tissue engineering." *Journal of Tissue Engineering* 10 (2019): 2041731419854586.

Fricain, J., R. Aid, S. Lanouar, D. Maurel, D. Le Nihouannen, S. Delmond, D. Letourneur, J. A. Vilamitjana and S. Catros. 2018. "In-vitro and in-vivo design and validation of an injectable polysaccharide-hydroxyapatite composite material for sinus floor augmentation." *Dental Materials* 34 (7): 1024–1035.

Go, G., S.-G. Jeong, A. Yoo, J. Han, B. Kang, S. Kim, K. T. Nguyen, Z. Jin, C.-S. Kim and Y. R. Seo. 2020. "Human adipose–derived mesenchymal stem cell–based medical microrobot system for knee cartilage regeneration in vivo." *Science Robotics* 5 (38): eaay6626.

Hao, C., Y. Wang, L. Shao, J. Liu, L. Chen and Z. Zhao. 2016. "Local injection of bone mesenchymal stem cells and fibrin glue promotes the repair of bone atrophic nonunion in vivo." *Advances in Therapy* 33 (5): 824–833.

Hoenig, E., T. Winkler, G. Mielke, H. Paetzold, D. Schuettler, C. Goepfert, H.-G. Machens, M. M. Morlock and A. F. Schilling. 2011. "High amplitude direct compressive strain enhances mechanical properties of scaffold-free tissue-engineered cartilage." *Tissue Engineering Part A* 17 (9–10): 1401–1411.

Huang, X., D. Yang, W. Yan, Z. Shi, J. Feng, Y. Gao, W. Weng and S. Yan. 2007. "Osteochondral repair using the combination of fibroblast growth factor and amorphous calcium phosphate/poly (L-lactic acid) hybrid materials." *Biomaterials* 28 (20): 3091–3100.

Jankauskaite, L., M. Malinauskas, L. Aukstikalne, L. Dabasinskaite, A. Rimkunas, T. Mickevicius, A. Pockevičius, E. Krugly, D. Martuzevicius and D. Ciuzas. 2022. "Functionalized electrospun scaffold–human-muscle-derived stem cell construct promotes in vivo neocartilage formation." *Polymers* 14 (12): 2498.

Jia, S., L. Liu, W. Pan, G. Meng, C. Duan, L. Zhang, Z. Xiong and J. Liu. 2012. "Oriented cartilage extracellular matrix-derived scaffold for cartilage tissue engineering." *Journal of Bioscience and Bioengineering* 113 (5): 647–653.

Jia, S., T. Zhang, Z. Xiong, W. Pan, J. Liu and W. Sun. 2015. "In vivo evaluation of a novel oriented scaffold-BMSC construct for enhancing full-thickness articular cartilage repair in a rabbit model." *PLoS One* 10 (12): e0145667.

Kawakami, S., M. Shiota, M. Kon, K. Shimogishi, H. Iijima and S. Kasugai. 2021. "Autologous micrografts from the palatal mucosa for bone regeneration in calvarial defects in rats: a radiological and histological analysis." *International Journal of Implant Dentistry* 7 (1): 1–7.

Kim, J., S. McBride, D. D. Dean, V. L. Sylvia, B. A. Doll and J. O. Hollinger. 2014. "In vivo performance of combinations of autograft, demineralized bone matrix, and tricalcium phosphate in a rabbit femoral defect model." *Biomedical Materials* 9 (3): 035010.

Kovar, J. L., X. Xu, D. Draney, A. Cupp, M. A. Simpson and D. M. Olive. 2011. "Near-infrared-labeled tetracycline derivative is an effective marker of bone deposition in mice." *Analytical Biochemistry* 416 (2): 167–173.

Kushnaryov, A., T. Yamaguchi, K. K. Briggs, V. W. Wong, M. Reuther, M. Neuman, V. Lin, R. L. Sah, K. Masuda and D. Watson. 2014. "Evaluation of autogenous engineered septal cartilage grafts in rabbits: A minimally invasive preclinical model." *Advances in Otolaryngology* 2014: 1–8.

Lee, J. S., S. D. Baek, J. Venkatesan, I. Bhatnagar, H. K. Chang, H. T. Kim and S.-K. Kim. 2014. "In vivo study of chitosan-natural nano hydroxyapatite scaffolds for bone tissue regeneration." *International Journal of Biological Macromolecules* 67: 360–366.

Lim, P. N., J. Feng, Z. Wang, M. Chong, T. Konishi, L. G. Tan, J. Chan and E. S. Thian. 2017. "In-vivo evaluation of subcutaneously implanted cell-loaded apatite microcarriers for osteogenic potency." *Journal of Materials Science: Materials in Medicine* 28 (6): 1–10.

Lin, H., Y. Tang, T. P. Lozito, N. Oyster, B. Wang and R. S. Tuan. 2019. "Efficient in vivo bone formation by BMP-2 engineered human mesenchymal stem cells encapsulated in a projection stereolithographically fabricated hydrogel scaffold." *Stem Cell Research & Therapy* 10 (1): 1–13.

Lin, S., Y. He, M. Tao, A. Wang and Q. Ao. 2021. "Fabrication and evaluation of an optimized xenogenic decellularized costal cartilage graft: Preclinical studies of a novel biocompatible prosthesis for rhinoplasty." *Regenerative Biomaterials* 8 (6): rbab052.

Liu, Y., S.-H. Teoh, M. S. Chong, C.-H. Yeow, R. D. Kamm, M. Choolani and J. K. Chan. 2013. "Contrasting effects of vasculogenic induction upon biaxial bioreactor stimulation of mesenchymal stem cells and endothelial progenitor cells cocultures in three-dimensional scaffolds under in vitro and in vivo paradigms for vascularized bone tissue engineering." *Tissue Engineering Part A* 19 (7–8): 893–904.

Magno, M. H. R., J. Kim, A. Srinivasan, S. McBride, D. Bolikal, A. Darr, J. O. Hollinger and J. Kohn. 2010. "Synthesis, degradation and biocompatibility of tyrosine-derived polycarbonate scaffolds." *Journal of Materials Chemistry* 20 (40): 8885–8893.

Marijnissen, Willem J. C. M., et al. 2002. "Alginate as a chondrocyte-delivery substance in combination with a non-woven scaffold for cartilage tissue engineering." *Biomaterials* 23 (6): 1511–1517.

McGowan, K., M. Kurtis, L. Lottman, D. Watson and R. Sah. 2002. "Biochemical quantification of DNA in human articular and septal cartilage using PicoGreen® and Hoechst 33258." *Osteoarthritis and Cartilage* 10 (7): 580–587.

Mukherjee, S., S. K. Nandi, B. Kundu, A. Chanda, S. Sen and P. K. Das. 2016 "Enhanced bone regeneration with carbon nanotube reinforced hydroxyapatite in animal model." *Journal of the Mechanical Behavior of Biomedical Materials* 60: 243–255.

Nazhvani, F. D., L. M. Amirabad, A. Azari, H. Namazi, S. Hosseinzadeh, R. Samanipour, A. Khojasteh, A. Golchin and S. Hashemi. 2021 "Effects of in vitro low oxygen tension preconditioning of buccal fat pad stem cells on in vivo articular cartilage tissue repair." *Life Sciences* 280: 119728.

Öfkeli, F., D. Demir and N. Bölgen. 2021. "Biomimetic mineralization of chitosan/gelatin cryogels and in vivo biocompatibility assessments for bone tissue engineering." *Journal of Applied Polymer Science* 138 (14): 50337.

Ortiz-Arrabal, O., R. Carmona, Ó. D. García-García, J. Chato-Astrain, D. Sánchez-Porras, A. Domezain, R. I. Oruezabal, V. Carriel, A. Campos and M. Alaminos. 2021. "Generation and evaluation of novel biomaterials based on decellularized sturgeon cartilage for use in tissue engineering." *Biomedicines* 9 (7): 775.

Park, Y. B., C. W. Ha, J. A. Kim, S. Kim and Y. G. Park. 2019. "Comparison of undifferentiated versus chondrogenic predifferentiated mesenchymal stem cells derived from human umbilical cord blood for cartilage repair in a rat model." *American Journal of Sports Medicine* 47 (2): 451–461.

Pascual-Garrido, C., E. A. Aisenbrey, F. Rodriguez-Fontan, K. A. Payne, S. J. Bryant and L. R. Goodrich. 2019. "Photopolymerizable injectable cartilage mimetic hydrogel for the treatment of focal chondral lesions: A proof of concept study in a rabbit animal model." *American Journal of Sports Medicine* 47 (1): 212–221.

Raina, D. B., H. Isaksson, W. Hettwer, A. Kumar, L. Lidgren and M. Tägil. 2016. "A biphasic calcium sulphate/hydroxyapatite carrier containing bone morphogenic protein-2 and zoledronic acid generates bone." *Scientific Reports* 6 (1): 1–13.

Rajagopal, K., S. Ramesh, N. M. Walter, A. Arora, D. S. Katti and V. Madhuri. 2020. "In vivo cartilage regeneration in a multi-layered articular cartilage architecture mimicking scaffold." *Bone & Joint Research* 9 (9): 601–612.

Salamanca, E., C. C. Hsu, H. M. Huang, N. C. Teng, C. T. Lin, Y. H. Pan and W. J. Chang. 2018. "Bone regeneration using a porcine bone substitute collagen composite in vitro and in vivo." *Scientific Reports* 8 (1): 1–8.

Saravanan, S., A. Chawla, M. Vairamani, T. Sastry, K. Subramanian and N. Selvamurugan. 2017. "Scaffolds containing chitosan, gelatin and graphene oxide for bone tissue regeneration in vitro and in vivo." *International Journal of Biological Macromolecules* 104: 1975–1985.

Sun, Q., L. Zhang, T. Xu, J. Ying, B. Xia, H. Jing and P. Tong. 2018. "Combined use of adipose derived stem cells and TGF-β3 microspheres promotes articular cartilage regeneration in vivo." *Biotechnic & Histochemistry* 93 (3): 168–176.

Sun, Z., B. C. Tee, K. S. Kennedy, P. M. Kennedy, D.-G. Kim, S. R. Mallery and H. W. Fields. 2013. "Scaffold-based delivery of autologous mesenchymal stem cells for mandibular distraction osteogenesis: preliminary studies in a porcine model." *PloS One* 8 (9): e74672.

Szychlinska, M. A., G. Calabrese, S. Ravalli, A. Dolcimascolo, P. Castrogiovanni, C. Fabbi, C. Puglisi, G. Lauretta, M. Di Rosa and A. Castorina. 2020. "Evaluation of a cell-free collagen type I-based scaffold for articular cartilage regeneration in an orthotopic rat model." *Materials* 13 (10): 2369.

Tayton, E., M. Purcell, A. Aarvold, J. Smith, A. Briscoe, J. Kanczler, K. Shakesheff, S. Howdle, D. Dunlop and R. Oreffo. 2014. "A comparison of polymer and polymer–hydroxyapatite composite tissue engineered scaffolds for use in bone regeneration. An in vitro and in vivo study." *Journal of Biomedical Materials Research Part A* 102 (8): 2613–2624.

Torres, J., M. Gutierres, L. Atayde, P. Cortez, M. A. Lopes, J. D. Santos, A. T. Cabral and C. F. van Eck. 2017. "The benefit of bone marrow concentrate in addition to a glass-reinforced hydroxyapatite for bone regeneration: An in vivo ovine study." *Journal of Orthopaedic Research* 35 (6): 1176–1182.

Tulyaganov, D. U., E. Fiume, A. Akbarov, N. Ziyadullaeva, S. Murtazaev, A. Rahdar, J. Massera, E. Verné and F. Baino. 2022. "In vivo evaluation of 3D-printed silica-based bioactive glass scaffolds for bone regeneration." *Journal of Functional Biomaterials* 13 (2): 74.

van Gaalen, S. M., M. C. Kruyt, R. E. Geuze, J. D. de Bruijn, J. Alblas and W. J. Dhert. 2010. "Use of fluorochrome labels in in vivo bone tissue engineering research." *Tissue Engineering Part B: Reviews* 16 (2): 209–217.

Wang, X., X. Song, T. Li, J. Chen, G. Cheng, L. Yang and C. Chen. 2019. "Aptamer-functionalized bioscaffold enhances cartilage repair by improving stem cell recruitment in osteochondral defects of rabbit knees." *American Journal of Sports Medicine* 47 (10): 2316–2326.

Yan, L.-P., J. Silva-Correia, M. B. Oliveira, C. Vilela, H. Pereira, R. A. Sousa, J. F. Mano, A. L. Oliveira, J. M. Oliveira and R. L. Reis. 2015. "Bilayered silk/silk-nanoCaP scaffolds for osteochondral tissue engineering: In vitro and in vivo assessment of biological performance." *Acta Biomaterialia* 12: 227–241.

Yang, Y., H. Lin, H. Shen, B. Wang, G. Lei and R. S. Tuan. 2018. "Mesenchymal stem cell-derived extracellular matrix enhances chondrogenic phenotype of and cartilage formation by encapsulated chondrocytes in vitro and in vivo." *Acta Biomaterialia* 69: 71–82.

Yin, L., Y. Wu, Z. Yang, V. Denslin, X. Ren, C. A. Tee, Z. Lai, C. T. Lim, J. Han and E. H. Lee. 2018. "Characterization and application of size-sorted zonal chondrocytes for articular cartilage regeneration." *Biomaterials* 165: 66–78.

Zhang, X., W. Jiang, Y. Liu, P. Zhang, L. Wang, W. Li, G. Wu, Y. Ge and Y. Zhou. 2018. "Human adipose-derived stem cells and simvastatin-functionalized biomimetic calcium phosphate to construct a novel tissue-engineered bone." *Biochemical and Biophysical Research Communications* 495 (1): 1264–1270.

Zhang, X., C. Wang, M. Liao, L. Dai, Y. Tang, H. Zhang, P. Coates, F. Setat, L. Zheng and J. Song. 2019. "Aligned electrospun cellulose scaffolds coated with rhBMP-2 for both in vitro and in vivo bone tissue engineering." *Carbohydrate Polymers* 213: 27–38.

Zuo, Y., Q. Li, Q. Xiong, J. Li, C. Tang, Y. Zhang and D. Wang. 2022. "Naringin release from a nano-hydroxyapatite/collagen scaffold promotes osteogenesis and bone tissue reconstruction." *Polymers* 14 (16): 3260.

10 Translational Approaches and Regulatory Aspects

INTRODUCTION

Translational research is the most vital step that aims to transfer the results obtained from basic research to clinical applications in the area of orthopedic tissue engineering. In spite of tremendous progress has been achieved in this technique over the past few decades, development of a fully functional tissue substitutes that can mimic the structure and function of the natural bone, cartilage, or joint tissue are yet to achieve Significant challenges remain regarding the translation of *in vitro* laboratory cartilage and bone TE results to the clinical application that is so called from bench to bed. Therefore, the challenges in various stages of producing these tissue products that limit their clinical translation need to be addressed. These challenges may be of different categories, including the cell type and their seeding strategy, biomaterial and scaffold design and their manufacturing processes, pre-clinical animal investigation, etc. In many of the cases it is found that *in vivo* clinical trials of the developed tissue products are yet to be performed. For an example related to cell type, chondrocytes are suitable cell for cartilage ECM generation, but their usage is often associated with several disadvantages like difficulty in isolation, generation of secondary injury leading to OA, uncertainty in producing desired cartilage-specific tissue, etc. These limitations can be overcome by the use of mesenchymal stem cells (MSCs) which are becoming attractive for numerous researchers. Because of their excellent differentiation potentiality towards bone and cartilage tissue, MSCs are considered to be the most attractive cell source that will also be helpful in repairing the osteochondral defects. Furthermore, manufacturing of scaffolds with appropriate composition, 3D design and fibrous architecture mimicking the natural bone, cartilage and their complex forms is of great challenge, for which the novel 3D bioprinting technique hold hope in producing targeted engineered tissue products. and thus may pave their clinical translation. With the advancement of this TE field, there is a need for producing tissue-engineered products at large scale to meet their adequate supply and this is important for a successful translation of the bone and related tissue-engineered products. Therefore, the various tissue product formation steps should be scalable and reproducible by adhering to the acceptable manufacturing and clinical practice standards like good manufacturing practice (GMP), good laboratory practice (GLP), etc. It is crucial to follow certain regulatory criteria, including those prescribed by

DOI: 10.1201/9781003245353-10

the organization of human tissue and cells, fabrication in accordance with validated standard operating procedures, in-process controls, ensuring quality control, preservation, and storage of the newly produced engineered tissue products. This chapter reviews the present state of art of translational outcome of cartilage, bone, and joint tissue engineering. The key challenges prevailed in these types of tissue engineering methods in view of cell source, biomaterial and scaffold design, mechanobiology, pre-clinical studies using animal models, and concerns related to regulatory aspects including the requirement of GMP and GLP facility have been described. The chapter also discusses the future direction of research keeping in view the above challenges

CLINICAL STATUS, TRANSLATIONAL CHALLENGES AND FUTURE STRATEGY

ENGINEERED CARTILAGE TISSUE GRAFTS

Cartilage disorders have critical clinical consequences that are growing day by day all over the world and it is presumed to become two fold by 2040. The growth of these disorders is due to the restricted capability to regenerate cartilage tissues. The current repair strategies for cartilage damage are unfavorable and inadequate. There are various cartilage repairing strategies have been evolved in the past decade to treat such lesions. Among these, the recent development in TE has paved the way for the restoration of damaged cartilage tissue function and structure. As for example, a defect in hyaline cartilage of joint carrying living chondrocytes can be repopulated by TE techniques with the hope of boosting its clinical outcomes. These clinical treatments include autologous chondrocyte implantation (ACI), osteochondral allograft transplantation, bone marrow stimulation techniques (BMS), and osteochondral autograft transplantation (Medvedeva et al. 2018).

Among the strategies for bone marrow stimulation, microfracture surgery is the most successful surgery compared to other surgeries and is often referred to as the "gold standard" surgery. It is a comparatively cost-effective surgical procedure. This surgery has shown tremendous clinical improvements in the first few months of surgery, but long-term follow-up studies depicted a reasonable decrease in Tegner activity and International Cartilage Repair Society (ICRS) scores. Tegner activity score is commonly used for assessing patient-administered activity rating of the patient with knee problems; whereas ICRS is used for a macro-level cartilage regeneration assessment (Gudas et al. 2012)]. These issues of reduced activities can be overcome by enhancing the efficiency of the methods of marrow stimulation that utilizes stimulating molecules along with acellular biomembrane to block the loss of cells from the clot (Mirza, Swenson, and Lynch 2015). However, there are no such relevant studies that have proven their efficiency over the conventional microfractures.

Although there are improvements in microfracture, the clinical advantage of ACI is restricted over the conventional microfracture except for the substantial cartilage lesions (>4 cm) because the hyaline-like cartilage produced by ACI technique in humans is not proven by high-quality clinical research. Various cartilages that are engineered for the resconstruction of orthopedic implants have undergone clinical translation and procured access in the market. In spite of tremendous progress in the field of engineered cartilages, there is research aimed at developing a fully functional cartilage that will mimic the structure and function of the original cartilage. In this context, matrix-assisted autologous chondrocyte implantation (MACI) includes the hydrated matrix, in which cells are resuspended has been demonstrated to provide encouraging results in repairing chondral defect in knee. These MACIs were previously injected below the lesion but now are employed for curing the defects in full-thickness cartilage. This incorporation has shown better long-term consequences when compared with ACI, thereby provides increased function of knee joint (Ebert et al. 2015).

Mosaicplasty is an osteochondral autograft transfer that involves obtaining cartilage-bone plugs that are cylindrical in nature from minimal load bearing areas. Femoral condyle is one such an example. This procedure involves the transplantation of the multiple small plugs to the site of injury or defect on the weight-bearing regions (Bartha et al. 2006). This surgical technique used for treating defects of medium size and integrating discrete sizes of grafts. It can attain 95% of filling rate but the availability of graft by this approach is limited. Therefore, other strategies are explored for filling of cartilage defects (Medvedeva et al. 2018). The transplantation of osteochondral allograft involving a single step procedure has shown promising clinical outcome in case of full-thickness joint hyaline articular cartilage defect, but this method suffers from donor site morbidity.

The strategies for the regeneration of tissues like ACI/MACI provides better cure for defects as compared to the native marrow stimulation approach (Gou et al. 2020). But, these treatments anticipate temporary help and there is no definite treatment outcome as the structural coherence in the surface of the tissue is substandard compared to the inherent tissues (Musumeci et al. 2013). A few of recent and crucial clinical applications of cellular based constructs are under clinical trial for articular cartilage repair, which include NOVOCART® 3D. This scaffold has collagen type I as its major component, wherein primary chondrocyte cells are seeded onto it. NOVOCART® 3D is profitably utilized in Europe for treating more than 6,000 subjects from the year 2003 (Niethammer et al. 2014). It is reported that by 2026, 223 patients will undergo for the phase III clinical trial, thereby comparing the effectiveness of NOVOCART® 3D with microfracture surgeries (McCormick et al. 2013). CARTISTEM is another hydrogel scaffold that has hyaluronic acid as its base polymer and umbilical cord blood-derived stem cells are seeded onto this hydrogel. This scaffold construct has shown progressive and steady clinical consequences throughout the study of seven years follow-up (Park et al. 2017). Spherox comprising chondrocyte aggregates, and autologous spheroids, another dignified engineered product designed for treating cartilage injuries, has shown statistically remarkable improvement in Phase II and Phase III clinical trials (Eschen et al. 2020). Many of the advancements have happened in the recent decade in the field of TE technique, although the clinical trials of the developed engineered tissue constructs are yet to be done in most of the cases. Therefore, the accessible proof is not sufficient so far to assert the supremacy of the advanced TE techniques over the currently used clinical techniques to repair the defective or damaged cartilage tissue, thereby restoring the native joint mechanics.

There are several challenges involved in each component of cartilage TE which limit the clinical translation of engineered cartilage tissue products. The different challenges in various stages of CTE clinical application including cell type and their seeding strategy, biomaterial and scaffold design and manufacturing processes, mechanobiology, and pre-clinical animal investigation are discussed here.

There is a gradual increase in the occurrence of osteoarthritis (OA) due to trauma, and degeneration together with the increasing incidence of athletic injury. This has led to major application of engineered cartilage in orthopaedics to repair cartilage defects. The most predominant function for any orthopaedic cartilage is to carry weights of our body. The neocartilages that are engineered should preferably be able to (1) combine the subchondral bone and the adjacent cartilage for mechanotransduction and anchored load distribution and (2) mimic the mechanical strength of the adjoining cartilages in order to avoid the degradation of tissues occurring due to strain inconsistency; (3) be load resistant under motions and large deformations; and (4) review the different zonal architecture in accordance with recreating the structure–function relationship of the innate cartilage tissues. Moreover, the engineered cartilages should avoid and reciprocate the inflammation caused due to their defect.

Chondrocytes are crucial for ECM production and has been derived from cartilage and suitable for cartilage regeneration. Chondrocytes can be derived from various sources, *viz.*, joint surface, non-articular "heterotopic" chondrocytes, nasoseptal chondrocytes, or auricular chondrocytes. OA cartilages that are used often offer several disadvantages, such as difficulty in isolation, may generate secondary injury leading to OA, uncertainty in producing the desired type of cartilage, for example hyaline cartilage (Fahy, Alini, and Stoddart 2018; Frank et al. 2000; Bilgen et al. 2006; Mizuno, Allemann, and Glowacki 2001; Meinert et al. 2017; Pavlovich, Hunsberger, and Atala 2016; Salinas, Hu, and Athanasiou 2018; Butler et al. 2008), dedifferentiation, etc. Furthermore, chondrocytes that are highly expanded may lose their potentiality for re-differentiation (Kurniawan 2019). Moreover, chondrocytes fail to transform into bone tissues in the area of subchondral bone present in an osteochondral defect (Li et al. 2010; Mauck et al. 2007). These limitations of the usage of chondrocytes can be overcome by using MSCs; therefore, MSCs are gently becoming the center of attraction for numerous researchers (Medvedeva et al. 2018). MSCs have the potentiality to be differentiated into bone and cartilage, thereby helping in filling the osteochondral defects by tissue-specific repair (Nicodemus and Bryant 2010; Appelman et al. 2009). MSCs can also be used as a cell source substitute for the repair of articular cartilages, but it has numerous limitations, like requiring careful characterization, low cell number density, presence of numerous cell subpopulations, lengthy and uncontrolled process of chondrogenic differentiation, and unstable chondrogenic phenotypes (Palmoski and Brandt 1984). Besides these, MSCs are reported to engineer various neocartilages that are epigenetically different from autologous cartilages as compared to the neocartilages developed from primary chondrocyte cell lines (Schulz et al. 2008). These restrictions do not allow developing safe regulations to use MSCs in a wide variety of clinical applications.

Biomaterials ideal for manufacturing scaffolds with biomimetic 3D architecture are vital component for cartilage tissue growth. Hydrogels were first used to repair lesions in the focal cartilage region through arthroscopy or injection techniques. These techniques have several advantages such as they display similar swelling, lubricating, and mechanical behaviour of articular cartilage (Lee and Bader 1997). The viscoelastic nature of these hydrogels assists the relocation of mechanical loading (Gou et al. 2020). It also permits the spherical morphology of the cells that are seeded, which is the specific property of any chondrogenic phenotype essential for healthy and resilient cartilage (Hall A C. 2019; Mauck et al. 2000; Lee, Grodzinsky, and Spector 2003). Despite of having unique biocompatibility of hydrogels, their low mechanical properties are the major barrier for cartilage regeneration. Therefore, the strategy is to develop composites by incorporating synthetic or natural fibers in the hydrogel formulation thereby achieving enhanced mechanical performance and constructs with superior mimicking cartilage architecture. In another approach, Cell-hydrogel constructs are substantially used as bioinks for developing cartilage by 3D bioprinting techniques having structure and function that mimic the native tissues (Wernike et al. 2008; Savadipour et al. 2022). There are also advancements since the past two decades for developing hydrogels which have thermoresponsive (Mollon et al. 2013; Santoro et al. 2010), photosensitive (Hall 1999; Smith et al. 1996; Salinas et al. 2020), or self-assembling characteristics (Savadipour et al. 2022), or the hydrogels that offer the release of chondroprotective drugs (Lee, Grodzinsky, and Spector 2003) or chondroinductive factors (Smith et al. 1996) in a controlled manner and their combination with other types of scaffolds, etc. (Lee, Grodzinsky, and Spector 2003). However, novel hydrogels are designed by focusing on definite material property, mostly these hydrogels are incapable of replicating the native chondrogenic niche due to its complexities in structure and function. Hence, the formation of hydrogels with required electrical conductivity, biocompatibility, degradation rate, mechanical properties, and chondroinductive properties is of paramount importance. The amalgamation of 3D bioprinting with novel hydrogels is also highly encouraging (Hall 1999).

Scaffolds derived from natural and synthetic polymers are used to construct cartilage for repair of substantial and uncontained defects, and for this reason they have attracted the interests of researchers. Among these, collagen sponge possessing biological signalling cues is the most extensively used scaffold for the modification or repair of defective cartilages clinically. Synthetic PGA polymer has been shown to be an excellent scaffold for engineering cartilages both *in vitro* and *in vivo* by employing various types of cells for meniscus reconstruction or repair of articular cartilage lesion (Li et al. 2010). The major drawback of these scaffolds is the need of multi-phasic scaffolds that are necessary especially to repair complex tissue defect like osteochondral defects (Mollon et al. 2013). The efficacy of these advanced biomaterials and the developed engineered tissue constructs or tissue grafts using such biomaterials required to be proven by conducting long-term pre-clinical large-animal study to ensure their use in clinical trials. Over the past two decades, osteochondral or cartilage defects in pigs were investigated (Fahy, Alini, and Stoddart 2018; Savadipour et al. 2022). Hence, there should be proper standardization of various study designs and outcome parameters, such as biochemical, histological, and biomechanical assessments (Hall 1999). Furthermore, most of the defects developed in a large animal model are generally fresh wounds. But in case of clinical settings, the defects are chronic and have a disrupted local environment that is distinct from the environment present in freshly generated wounds (Lee and Bader 1997).

Mechanical stress is an important factor that has an influence on particular cellular responses such as its differentiation, phenotype, apoptosis, growth, etc., which should be taken into consideration. The mechanical stimuli remarkably influence the development of cartilage structure and function (Fahy, Alini, and Stoddart 2018). The framework developed with the help of mechanical loading mechanism in cartilage homeostasis from a mechano-biological perspective led to the creation of innovative bioreactor systems, which provide the required tools for researching chondrocyte mechanotransduction. Numerous types of shear bioreactors (such as contact shear, fluid shear, perfusion bioreactor, low shear bioreactor) are inspected for cartilage TE (Frank et al. 2000; Mizuno, Allemann, and Glowacki 2001). It has been demonstrated that by applying intermittent biaxial stimulation at a period of 14 days alternately to cartilage constructs encompassing therapeutically apt cells and biomaterials can increase matrix formation, producing cartilage constructs with better, natural-looking biomechanical attributes (Meinert et al. 2017). Although, these strategies help in generating constructs that are relevant for clinical trials, still there are numerous hurdles that need to be looked into (Pavlovich, Hunsberger, and Atala 2016).

One of the most difficult tasks is to create expandable tissue-engineered constructs that mimic the structure, function, and natural architecture of native tissues, like cartilage. However, advances in engineering methods, specifically the incorporation of biophysical cues (such as topography, stiffness, porosity, pore size, and stress relaxation), have enabled the development of more functional biomimetic constructs (Salinas, Hu, and Athanasiou 2018; Butler et al. 2008).

Mechanobiology has encouraged the incorporation of several types of stimuli in current TE techniques due to the importance of the biomechanical and physical interaction between cells and its environment for tissue growth and maintenance (Kurniawan 2019). Numerous studies have shown that uniaxial compression has positive impacts on chondrogenesis, both in terms of gene expression levels (Li et al. 2010; Mauck et al. 2007) and deposition of matrix on the 3D scaffolds (Nicodemus and Bryant 2010). Additionally, it has been demonstrated that dynamic compressive loading improves the mechanical performance of the final constructs by raising its compressive modulus (Appelman et al. 2009). More specifically, tissue engineers can use certain mechanobiological responses to pinpoint the role of biomechanical factors for the maintenance of tissues, regulating tissue development, and fine-tuning the biosynthetic potential of the constructs.

Biophysical and biomechanical cues have critical roles in the cellular growth and regeneration of cartilage tissue. Hyaline cartilage can give rise to several mechanical factors, despite the fact that the precise methods by which these forces are transmitted are not yet fully understood. However, studies have shown that particular forms of stimulation have a positive impact on cartilage formation and remodelling. The essential element of typical stimulation within the knee joint is compression loading. In several studies static as well as dynamic compressions has been applied to produce cartilage *in vitro* (Palmoski and Brandt 1984; Schulz et al. 2008). In a study, the levels of glycosaminoglycan were increased under the compression of 15% at a frequency of 1 Hz in chondrocytes encapsulated in agarose scaffolds (Lee and Bader 1997). In comparison to free-swelling structures, cell-seeded scaffolds produce more collagen with a higher equilibrium modulus (Mauck et al. 2000). In another study, dynamic compressive loading caused chondrocytes to produce more proteoglycan, but static stimulation led to less matrix deposition (Lee, Grodzinsky, and Spector 2003). In addition to regulating the chondrogenic phenotype, they boosted deposition of GAGs and collagen type II expression in the designed constructs (Wernike et al. 2008).

Hydrostatic pressure is also applied to chondrocytes followed by the cartilage's compressive stimulation. The chondrocyte matrix deposition is enhanced by hydrostatic pressure at a physiological level of 5–15 MPa, by altering some particular chondrocyte transporters (Savadipour et al. 2022; Hall 1999). After being exposed to a static pressure of 10 MPa for 4 hours, monolayer chondrocytes produced significantly more proteoglycan (aggrecan) (Smith et al. 1996). A 2021 study reported that the transient receptor potential channels could mechanotransduce the hydrostatic pressure and thereby promote the development of the matrix (Savadipour et al. 2022). The genes encoding into primary cilia are polycystin I and II. These genes have exhibited strong upregulation in response to shear in chondrocytes (Salinas et al. 2020).

As discussed above, CTE principles has clinical applications primarily seen in ACI or other related methods (Mollon et al. 2013). Cartilage tissue-engineered products like Hyalograft® C and Carticel® are available for treating defective cartilage lesions in clinical trials. However, the ACI-based technologies do not show remarkable clinical outcome over the conventional methods like microfractures, with an exception for larger lesions (Mollon et al. 2013), where microfractures don't have enough potential to treat large defects such as OA (Santoro et al. 2010), and to reconstruct the whole structural unit like a meniscus or joint head. Therefore, advanced research has been undertaken with the aim of developing large-scale cartilage constructs that are cost-effective, safe, and have a good GMP compliance (Santoro et al. 2010). However, most of these new developments are yet to translate into clinical application (Mollon et al. 2013).

Overall, after two decades of uninterrupted development, CTE has accomplished certain remarkable progress which has led to increasing number of clinical studies that offer great prospects to this field. At the same time, there are growing difficulties associated with converting the research of proof-of-concept onto pre-clinical or clinical trials. Integration into the synthetic cartilage along with subchondral bone and the surrounding cartilages is a significant hurdle for orthopaedic therapeutic applications. To impart short- and long-term function of load-bearing properties, the mechanical characteristics of the designed cartilage should really match those with the surrounding tissues. In order to prevent the subcutaneous or intramuscular implantation sites from experiencing an initial immune response, the synthesized cartilage should be strictly biocompatible. The synthetic cartilage should also precisely mimic the structural and functional characteristics of the tissue that is being rebuilt. To achieve the desired clinical outcome, it is essential that surgeons, policymakers, and specialists in cell biology, developmental biology, and material science work closely together so that the field of study can be efficiently developed into practical application (Mollon et al. 2013).

ENGINEERED BONE TISSUE GRAFTS

Large-scale production of tissue-engineered products is one of the major challenges for a successful translation of such tissue products. In this respect, the various stages of tissue production processes should be scalable and reproducible, adhered to acceptable manufacturing and clinical practice standards, secured for patients, and financially viable. In this context, bioprinting techniques can provide tissue constructs with reproducible and appropriate design. However, these techniques offer only a small-scale manufacturing of constructs. The extrusion methods yielding structures with an elevated resolution than the conventional inkjet-based printing are appropriate to be used clinically. When internal pore architecture is a crucial component of computer-aided design, the STL file format that controls bioprinters is not feasible. Furthermore, mechanical forces are crucial in the remodeling of bones. The fluid shear stress, microgravity, mechanical cyclical stretching and compression influence cell differentiation and proliferation associated with bone remodelling. Studying the impact of biomechanical forces on remodelling of bone may be made possible for creating porous models using medical imaging data (Wang, Jia et al. 2018).

In vivo animal models provide many appropriate data for bone repair procedures that can be used for testing the efficacy of 3D bioprinted bone constructs; however, the use of huge number of animals raises ethical issues and is not economical. The use of *in vitro* organ cultures and chick chorioallantoic membranes in *in silico* predictive models have facilitated the reduction in the numbers of animal subjects used for the research related to bone repair. The long-term *in vitro* and *in vivo* evaluation of biofabricated bone constructs lacks comparative data despite all these advancements. The use of many high-resolution microscopic imaging technique has the advantage of being non-destructive for the analysis of tissue constructs. However, a significant drawback of most commonly used microscopy techniques is their poor penetration, which make it difficult to image cells within scaffolds and tissue grafts. 3D reconstruction and slice-wise optical sectioning of these engineered constructs have been made possible by the development of multi-photon microscopy and micro-computed tomography, which has helped to overcome some of the restrictions. However, massive requirement of computing power and storage space is the limitation of these techniques (Santoro et al. 2010).

Biofabrication offers an attractive approach for bone tissue generation. In order to enhance osteogenesis and osseointegration, there are still substantial problems with this technology for the production of therapeutically relevant bone constructs associated with obtaining adequate vascularization of the constructs and spatiotemporal biochemical and mechanical stimulation. The bioprinting platforms are also not flexible in handling multiple bioinks or biomaterials for fabricating tissue-engineered substitutes which should have structural integrity and must be clinically relevant. A therapy is clinically relevant if it provides a positive benefit from a patient's perspective. Kang et al. (2016) created one tissue-organ printer and successfully produced various tissue types *in vivo*, paving the way for the practical application of this technology, even though there are still obstacles to overcome (Kang, Lee et al. 2016).

Therefore, it is essential to make advancements in biomaterial and scaffold development, medical imaging and microscopy technology, computational modelling, and bioreactor design in order to address challenges and raise the currently low cost-effectiveness of biofabricated bone for clinical therapy. Additionally, appropriate cell selection is necessary for a successful clinical outcome (Iaquinta et al. 2019).

TISSUE ENGINEERED GRAFT FOR OSTEOARTHRITIS: A CASE STUDY

Osteoarthritis is an ageing-related disorder that affects more than 528 million people worldwide and the numbers are anticipated to increase with an increase in population. Osteoarthritis is caused when chondrocytes possess low mitotic index and therefore lack the ability for congruent regeneration (Benedek 2006). The symptoms of osteo-arthritis include several structural changes in synovial joints like articular cartilage degradation, joint inflammation, chondrocytes hypertrophy, and neovascular invasion (Chen et al. 2017). There are several available treatments that contribute towards temporary relief only (Bannuru et al. 2019). Hence, osteoarthritis can be targeted by TE to develop constructs that can be administered into the body by various surgical methods such as microfracture (MF), autologous chondrocyte implantation (ACI), and osteochondral autologous transplantation (OAT). These tissue-engineered grafts hold clinical potential for the treatment of osteoarthritis (Jiang et al. 2020). This case study focused on investigating several biochemical molecules present in tissue constructs along with their potential for osteoarthritis treatment. The followings are the some of these biochemical molecules.

PLATELET-RICH PLASMA

The platelet concentrate or platelet-rich plasma (PRP) contains a combination of several growth factors like insulin-like growth factor-1 (IGF-1), fibroblast growth factor (FGF), and transforming growth factor beta-3 (TGFβ3), which are required for the differentiation of chondrocytes and preserving the phenotype of hyaline cartilage (Gato-Calvo et al. 2019). PRP also includes definite composition of red blood cells (RBCs), white blood cells (WBCs), and platelet enrichment factors (PEFs). For cartilage regeneration, a composite tissue-engineered construct containing implanted autologous chondrocytes loaded with PRP/alginate-based hydrogel was generated in a 3D chitosan (CH)/chondroitin sulfate (CS)/silk fibroin (SF) scaffold. This hydrogel scaffold helped in better deposition of glycosaminoglycan (GAGs), integration into implantation site, and enhanced collagen type II expression (Singh et al. 2022).

MATRILIN-3

Matrilin-3 (MATN3), a crucial extracellular matrix (ECM) protein for cartilage governs chondrocyte inflammation, proliferation, and ECM synthesis along with TGFβ3 (Muttigi et al. 2016). MATN3/TGFβ3 gelatin microparticles (GMPs) with adipose-derived mesenchymal stem cells (MSCs) spheroids were synthesized to stimulate chondrogenesis in patient with degenerative disk disease. MATN3 bio-molecule was released slowly in patients that integrated MATN3/TGFβ3 GMPs. Chondrogenesis was enhanced at the site of injection when it was paired with MSCs forming a spheroid, thereby decreased the hypertrophy in chondrogenic progenitor cells (Bello et al. 2021).

NARINGIN

Naringin is an active ingredient in traditional Chinese medicine that is extracted from the Drynaria fortunei plant. It has been theorized that naringin can promote cartilage regeneration through the TGFβ superfamily signalling pathway., Naringin was claimed to have demonstrated the highest form of cartilage regeneration when combined with MSCs derived from bone marrow (Ye et al. 2020).

KARTOGENIN

Kartogenin is a tiny, drug-like heterocyclic compound that has been shown to encourage the chondrogenic differentiation of MSCs to form hyaline cartilage (Johnson et al. 2012). Kartogenin allows the decoupling of core-binding factor sub-unit beta (CBFβ) from Filamin A (a protein that interacts with secondary messengers, integrins, and transmembrane receptor complexes for regulating the reorganization of the actin cytoskeleton), thereby empowering CBFβ for interaction with runt-related transcription factor 1 (RUNX1). Additionally, this encourages the expression of vital genes that support chondroprotection and chondrogenesis (Johnson et al. 2012; Fazal-Ur-Rehman, Karen, and Hongsik 2016). Kartogenin encapsulated by poly(lactic-co-glycolic acid) microspheres (PLGAMPs) and MSCs derived from bone marrow were loaded into the cartilage-derived ECM (CECM). CECM was generated from patellar groove and decellularized porcine femoral condyle. The continuous, gradual release of Kartogenin from PLGAMPs-embedded CECM encouraged MSCs proliferation and chondrogenesis (Zhao et al. 2020).

Although there are many factors contributing to the treatment of osteoarthritis, it can be reliably inferred that cell signaling molecules are crucial in regulating the integrity of the tissue microenvironment. Tissue engineering has a lot of promise for osteoarthritic joints, even though techniques like MF and ACI have shown some success in the field. The same is demonstrated by commercial products like Chondrosphere®, Bioseed®-C, NeoCart®, and Hyalograft® C (Jiang et al. 2020). As demonstrated in this case study, promising possibilities for the development of tissue-engineered grafts for the treatment of osteoarthritis include biomolecules and substances like PRP, kartogenin, and others.

TISSUE ENGINEERING APPROACH FOR ARTICULAR CARTILAGE REGENERATION—A CASE STUDY

Clinical trials have used autologous chondrocyte implantation, mosaicplasty, and bone marrow stimulation as treatments for articular cartilage defects. But each one of these methods has certain drawbacks. Some researchers are now fascinated by mesenchymal stem cells from the host's bone marrow (BMSCs), which could multiply without losing their ability to differentiate. When BMSCs was first administered to rabbits with injured articular cartilage, osteochondral tissue was produced successfully. Thereafter, BMSCs have been transfered to humans. According to past research, chondral defects in the knee and elbow joints can be treated with BMSCs to decrease their clinical symptoms.

Researchers investigated the efficacy of BMSCs for osteoarthritic knees treated with a high tibial osteotomy by comparing 12 patients who received BMSCs transplants with 12 cell-free patients. Over a 16-months interval, statistically negligible variations in clinical improvement were seen in both groups; however, the group that received cell transplantation provided better results on arthroscopy and histological grading. Over a period of 10-years follow-up, Hospital for Special Surgery knee scores in the BMSCs transplantation and cell-free therapy groups increased to 76 and 73, respectively, which were higher than the preoperative assessment score obtained for knee. The clinical safety of this treatment was further demonstrated by the absence of hypertrophy in the reconstructed tissue throughout the clinical study and the absence of malignancies or infections in any of the patients. Although histologically calcification over the tidemark was never seen in either humans or the rabbit model, the restored cartilage was not entirely generated from hyaline cartilage (Yamasaki et al. 2014).

Three different forms of TE techniques for articular cartilage are referred to as "cell-scaffold construct", "cell-free construct", and "scaffold-free construct". The "cell-scaffold construct" technique is comprised of the seeding of stem cells or autologous chondrocytes. Some of the commercially accessible "cell-scaffold constructs", such as BioSeed®-C and CaReS®, use autologous chondrocytes as seeding cells. Clinical trials are now being carried out for various products, including NOVOCART® 3D. Most of the stem cells used for the development of constructs come from a variety of sources, which are mesenchymal in origin and pluripotent by nature. TruFit and MaioRegen are the two instances of cell-free techniques that delicately utilize the capacity of stem cells for repairing and regenerating damaged cartilage in clinical contexts. Other relevant technologies, such as NOVOCART® 3D, have led to encouraging short-term repair outcomes. The technology without scaffolds so called "scaffold free construct" is an additional novel development route (Jiang et al. 2020).

Individuals with focal and degenerative articular cartilage abnormalities have significantly lower quality of life. Despite the development of several remedies, especially surgical intervention, a definitive cure has not yet been found. Several cell therapy products are already available in the market. In this study, the development of tissue engineered products created for articular cartilage repair using cell therapy was based on the data acquired from the ClinicalTrial.gov website. Despite not disclosing all of the trial results, this website contains information on prospective clinical trials, including some that are currently ongoing. This makes it easier to study the facts in chronological order. A total 203 studies from ClinicalTrial.gov that focused on cartilage regeneration were selected. A few of them are stated in Table 10.1. Clinical translation was shown to differ between cells employed in the treatment derived from adipose tissue and those derived from cartilage and BMSCs. A fewer clinical studies using bone marrow or fat cells than cartilage cells have been entered to the phase III, indicating that most of the discoveries from adipose tissue, BMSCs and cartilage are not successful. The clinical trials from Phases I to Phase III took more than 100 months to complete, wherein all of them used the same product. ClinicalTrials. gov may provide a worldwide perspective on clinical research trends which were difficult to observe previously (Negoro et al. 2018).

CLINICAL TRIALS

Numerous species of animals, including sheep and rabbit, have been employed in the study of mesenchymal stem cells to better understand their mechanisms and potential clinical uses. In order to demonstrate the present status of clinical MSCs therapy for bone healing, the clinical trials that have been made publicly available were collected from the ClinicalTrials.gov database (June 2019) as listed in Table 10.1.

TABLE 10.1
Clinical Trials for Repair of Bone Fractures Using Mesenchymal Stem Cells

NCT Number	Title	Status	Defect Area	Inferences
NCT02140528	Allogeneic Mesenchymal Stem Cell Transplantation in Tibial Closed Diaphyseal Fractures	Completed	Tibial fracture	Injection of mesenchymal stem cells, Placebo
NCT01788059	The Efficacy of Mesenchymal Stem Cells for Stimulate the Unio in the Treatment of Non-united Tibial and Femoral Fractures in Shahid Kamyab Hospital	Completed	Non-union fracture	Injection of mesenchymal stem cells in non-union site
NCT02755922	Bone Regeneration with Mesenchymal Stem Cells	Completed	Mandibular fractures	Autologous mesenchymal stem cell application
NCT00250302	Autologous Implantation of Mesenchymal Stem Cells for the Treatment of Distal Tibial Fractures	Completed	Tibial fracture	Implantation of autologous mesenchymal stem cells
NCT01206179	Treatment of Non-union of Long Bone Fractures by Autologous Mesenchymal Stem Cell	Completed	Non-union fractures	Injection of cells
NCT03325504	A Comparative Study of 2 Doses of BM Autologous H-MSC+Biomaterial vs. Iliac Crest Auto Graft for Bone Healing in Non-Union	Recruited	Non-union fracture	Use of cultured mesenchymal stem cells, Autologous graft from iliac crest
NCT01532076	Effectiveness of Adipose Tissue Derived Mesenchymal Stem Cells as Osteogenic Component in Composite Grafts	Terminated	Osteoporotic fractures	Augmentation of cellularized composite graft, Augmentation of acellularized composite graft

(continued)

TABLE 10.1 (Continued)
Clinical Trials for Repair of Bone Fractures Using Mesenchymal Stem Cells

NCT Number	Title	Status	Defect Area	Inferences
NCT02177565	Autologous Stem Cell Therapy for Fracture Non-union Healing	Completed	Non-union fractures	Use of carrier and autologous BMSCs expanded
NCT01842477	Evaluation of Efficacy and Safety of Autologous MSCs Combined with Biomaterials to Enhance Bone Healing	Completed	Delayed union after fracture of humerus, tibia or femur	Use of autologous cultured mesenchymal stem cells and implantation of bone substitute
NCT03905824	The Effectiveness of Adding Allogeneic Stem Cells After Traditional Treatment of Osteochondral Lesions of the Talus	Recruiting	Osteochondral fracture of talus	Use of umbilical cord derived allogenic stromal mesenchymal stem cells, debridement and microfracture
NCT01409954	Collecting Bone Graft During Spinal Decompression and Posterolateral Lumbar Fusion to Better Define Bone Making Cells	Enrolling by Invitation	Pseudarthrosis after fusion or arthrodesis	–
NCT01041001	Study to Compare Efficacy and Safety of Cartistem and Microfracture in Patients with Knee Articular Cartilage Injury	Completed	Cartilage injury, osteoarthritis	CARTISTEM, treatment of microfracture
NCT03856021	Microfracture vs. Microfracture and BMAC for Osteochondral Lesions of the Talus	Enrolling by invitaion	Osteochondral lesion of talus	Microfracture, microfracture with bone marrow aspirate concentrate (BMAC)
NCT01747681	Results at 10 to 14 Years after Microfracture in the Knee	Completed	Articular chondral defect	Microfracture

NCT number	Title	Status	Condition	Intervention
NCT02696876	Synovium Brushing to Augment Microfracture for Improved Cartilage Repair	Recruiting	Defect of articular cartilage, cartilage injury, osteoarthritis (knee)	Arthroscopic synovial brushing, microfracture
NCT01626677	Follow-up study of CARTISTEMA Versus Microfracture for the Treatment of Knee Articular Cartilage Injury or Defect	Completed	Degenerative osteoarthritis, defect of articular cartilage	CARTISTEM, Microfracture
NCT00512434	Percutaneous Autologous Bone-marrow Grafting for Open Tibial Shaft Fracture	Completed	Tibial fractures, fractures (open)	Osteosynthesis- the reconstructive surgery
NCT02483364	A Clinical Trial to Assess the Effect of HC-SVT-1001 and HC-SVT-1002 in the Surgical Treatment of Atrophic Pseudarthrosis of Long Bone (Bone Cure)	Recruiting	Pseudoarthrosis	HC-SVT-1001 initial protocol, HC-SVT-1002 protocol amendment
NCT00557635	Osseous Setting Improvement with Co-implantation of Osseous Matrix and Mesenchymal Progenitors Cells from Autologous Bone Marrow	Suspended	Tibia or femur pseudoarthrosis	Surgical procedure

Source: Iaquinta et al. (2019).

It has been reported that some clinical trials involving cartilage engineering, including NCT01041001, NCT03856021, and NCT01747681, are in progress. NCT01041001 is the research to examine the safety and efficacy of microfracture and cartistem in patients having knee articular cartilage injuries which is in its Phase III trials. NCT03856021 involves Osteochondral Talus Lesions: Microfracture vs. Microfracture with BMAC, where the goal of this study is to evaluate the impact of adding BMAC to the usual microfracture method on clinical and radiographic outcomes. Moreover, NCT01747681 intends to look at potential indicators of positive and negative results as well as an extended clinical outcome 10 to 14 years post microfracture of articular cartilage abnormalities in the knee.

Despite the fact that MSCs therapy is an intriguing advancement in the field of TE, further research is required to recommend new MSCs treatments for bone repair caused by a lack of information from the aforementioned completed clinical investigations.

REGULATORY ASPECT

Engineered tissue products are new class of therapeutics providing innovative approach for curing bone and related tissue defects. However, the framing of new and comprehensive regulatory prerequisites by the regulatory authorities is the most important factor for successful clinical translation of these products commercially. The researchers who are the developers of the TEPs and the medical industries who are responsible for commercializing these products must have knowledge and adapt the regulatory criteria to promote the development of TEPs and their marketing approval required by the regulatory agency. Certain regulatory criterias which are crucial to adhere, include organization of human tissue and cells, fabrication in accordance with validated standard operating procedures, in-process controls, the confirmation of quality control, preservation, and storage of cells as well as engineered tissue products. The regulatory framework may vary that depends on the jurisdiction under which the product is to be marketed. In Europe, the corresponding directives and norms guarantee the highest levels of safety standards for donation, quality, testing, procurement, and processing. Whereas, the, adherence to the yearly revised "Current Good Manufacturing Practice" (cGMP) requirements for bioreactor systems for bone tissue engineering is necessary in the United States. In order to make it easier to adopt GMP standards for the growth and development of human embryonic stem cells inside a stirred tank bioreactor, protocols have been established. The development and validation of a sealed, highly automated production process for the expansion of stem cells and progenitor cells when human bone marrow mononuclear cells were present was also described. The GMP standards are met by the ZRP cell and tissue culturing systems (Zellwerk GmbH, Deutschland), and RBBs Medistat RBS (B. Braun Biotech International GmbH) that enable the culture and fabrication of 3D tissue-engineered grafts. A closed perfusion bioreactor system was used for generating two marketable products such as Dermagraft and TransCyte. In order to achieve this, allogenic dermal fibroblasts were seeded onto a scaffold (Biobrane) and grown in a bioreactor system that enables automatic seeding of the cells, change of media, in-process monitoring of storage, growth, development, and delivery at the same

TABLE 10.2
Authorized Bone and Cartilage Tissue-Based Products

Name (marketing authorization Holder)	Therapeutic Indication	Date of Authorization	Clinical Status
SPHEROX (CO. DON AG)	Symptomatic defects of the articular cartilage present in the femoral condyle and patella of the knee. Can be used to treat defects upto sizes of 10 cm².	July 2017	MA under considerable obligations (studies postauthorization)
MACIa (Vericel Denmark ApS.)	Symptomatic, full-thickness cartilage defects of size 3–20 cm² (for adults) present in the knee.	June 2013	MA under obligation MA suspended (Sept. 2014)
MACI[a] (Vericel Denmark ApS)	Symptomatic, full-thickness cartilage defects of the knee that may or may not involve bone in adults.	Dec 2016	In the market
Carticel (Vericel Denmark ApS)	Symptomatic cartilage defects caused by the acute or repetitive trauma of the femoral condyle	August 1997	In the market
JACC (Japan Tissue Engineering Co., Ltd.)	Symptoms of traumatic cartilage defects and osteochondritis dissecans	July 2012	In the market

Source: Oberweis et al. (2C20).

time. However, none of the cell-based, tissue-engineered synthetic bone substitutes grown in a bioreactor system have yet been used in a clinical setting. The adherence of proposed products with the GMP standards will be a fundamental requirement to open the door for bioreactor-stimulated, tissue-engineered scaffolds for regeneration of bone in patients (Petite et al. 2000). GLP guidelines are also important to ensure the safety and efficacy of the TEPs when used in humans. Practically, these guidelines are necessary to produce tissue products that are used in clinical trial. GLP guideline provides information on the quality documentation, non-clinical documentation, and clinical documentation for tissue engineered products under clinical trials.

Many tissue engineering products (TEPs), such as cartilage tissue engineered products (CTEPs), bone tissue engineered products (BTEPs), and their complex derivative like osteochondral, have been developed in the past few decades. These engineered tissue products can be used for repairing, or regenerating the damaged tissue of the patients, if these are produced following the stipulated regulatory norms. The clinical translation of novel products as described in Table 10.2 offers a new and extensive regulatory frameworks to the regulatory authorities. For the researchers and industries, understanding and adjusting to these regulatory issues are crucial since they support the development of TEPs along with their consent and commercialization of the tissue engineered products. Although the European Union (EU) and the United States have established precise and detailed regulatory frameworks for such products, the supervision of these products in other jurisdictions is still difficult due to the absence of platform to regulate and supervise the performance of TEPs (Oberweis et al. 2020).

TEPs are new and leading products, which are in their developing stage and the legislations are reframed based on scientific and technological advances, which are usually complex, and have distinctive regulatory issues due to their innovative attributes (Oberweis et al. 2020). Therefore, it is essential that these TEPs meet with regulatory regulations so that they can maintain high standards of quality, effectiveness, and safety during their production and legal administration. The granting of a marketing authorization (MA) for a TEP's eventual commercialization by the competent authority is a crucial stage in its development and is extremely important throughout the entire register method. Even while CTEPs and BTEPs have advanced quickly, some of the products have approved MA as displayed in (Table 10.2), and the social impact of these goods is very less (Gálvez et al. 2013).

Major international regulatory authorities have developed specific legislative frameworks for TEPs because of their leading character, as their active component like cells or tissues demand a complicated and exclusive process. Therefore, the EU is a pioneer in this field in order to build a specialized regulatory system for synthetic tissue-based therapeutics. This framework may serve as a regulatory guideline for other nations. In addition, Canada, the United States, South Korea, Australia, and Japan have announced their own regulatory policies. In spite of this, the absence of a uniform regulation for TEPs worries the health care regulatory organizations (Guadix et al. 2019).

EXERCISE

1. What are the various clinical treatments used for articular cartilage defect?
2. Explain microfracture surgery. How it is different from other surgical procedures?

3. What is MACI? How does it differ from ACI?
4. What is mosaicplasty? Give one example.
5. Name a few crucial clinical applications for articular cartilage repair. Explain any one of them.
6. Why engineered cartilage tissue products could not reach their clinical trials?
7. What are the parameters those are important for the development of neocartilages?
8. What are the types of cells that were used for cartilage repair? What were their sites of extraction? Mention their advantages and disadvantages.
9. What are the advantages and disadvantages of MSCs for the repairing of articular cartilages?
10. How are hydrogels beneficial for repairing lesions in focal cartilage region?
11. List out the problems related to the use of scaffolds in treating cartilage lesions. How does mechanobiology help to overcome these problems?
12. What are the parameters required for developing cartilage *in vitro*? Explain with case study.
13. What is the current status of cartilage tissue products in the domain of clinical trials?
14. What are the various stages of tissue product formation processes at industrial scale?
15. How is the biofabrication process helpful for development of tissue constructs for clinical application?
16. Mention a few clinical trials conducted for repair of bone fractures using mesenchymal stem cells.
17. What are the regulatory criteria that a engineered bone tissue product needs to fulfil?
18. What is cGMP? How are GMP standards fulfilled? Mention the countries that follow cGMPs.
19. Name a few cartilage-based product along with their therapeutic indication and clinical status.
20. Name the countries who have announced their regulatory policies and framework for tissue engineered products.
21. Mention the first cartilage-based product that was marketized.
22. Explain how regulatory aspects are important for clinical application of tissue products.
23. Give your opinion about future translational strategy for clinical application of the engineered bone and cartilase tissue products.
24. Write about clinical status of osteochondral tissue graft.

REFERENCES

Appelman, T. P., J. Mizrahi, J. H. Elisseeff, and D. Seliktar. 2009. "The differential effect of scaffold composition and architecture on chondrocyte response to mechanical stimulation." *Biomaterials* 30 (4): 518–525.

Bannuru, R. R., M. C. Osani, E. E. Vaysbrot, N. K. Arden, K. Bennell, S. M. A. Bierma-Zeinstra, V. B. Kraus, L. S. Lohmander, J. H. Abbott, and M. Bhandari. 2019. "OARSI guidelines for the non-surgical management of knee, hip, and polyarticular osteoarthritis." *Osteoarthritis and Cartilage* 27 (11): 1578–1589.

Bartha, L., A. Vajda, Z. Duska, H. Rahmeh, and L. Hangody. 2006. "Autologous osteochondral mosaicplasty grafting." *Journal of Orthopaedic & Sports Physical Therapy* 36 (10): 739–750.

Bello, A. B., Y. Kim, S. Park, M. S. Muttigi, J. Kim, H. Park, and S. Lee. 2021. "Matrilin3/TGFβ3 gelatin microparticles promote chondrogenesis, prevent hypertrophy, and induce paracrine release in MSC spheroid for disc regeneration." *NPJ Regenerative Medicine* 6 (1): 1–13.

Benedek, T. G. 2006. "A history of the understanding of cartilage." *Osteoarthritis and Cartilage* 14 (3): 203–209.

Bilgen, B., P. Sucosky, G. P. Neitzel, and G. A. Barabino. 2006. "Flow characterization of a wavy-walled bioreactor for cartilage tissue engineering." *Biotechnology and Bioengineering* 95 (6): 1009–1022.

Butler, D. L., N. Juncosa-Melvin, G. P. Boivin, M. T. Galloway, J. T. Shearn, C. Gooch, and H. Awad. 2008. "Functional tissue engineering for tendon repair: A multidisciplinary strategy using mesenchymal stem cells, bioscaffolds, and mechanical stimulation." *Journal of Orthopaedic Research* 26 (1): 1–9.

Chen, D., J. Shen, W. Zhao, T. Wang, L. Han, J. L. Hamilton, and H.-J. Im. 2017. "Osteoarthritis: toward a comprehensive understanding of pathological mechanism." *Bone Research* 5 (1): 1–13.

Ebert, J. R., M. Fallon, A. Smith, G. C. Janes, and D. J. Wood. 2015. "Prospective clinical and radiologic evaluation of patellofemoral matrix-induced autologous chondrocyte implantation." *American Journal of Sports Medicine* 43 (6): 1362–1372.

Eschen, C., C. Kaps, W. Widuchowski, S. Fickert, W. Zinser, Ph Niemeyer, and G. Roël. 2020. "Clinical outcome is significantly better with spheroid-based autologous chondrocyte implantation manufactured with more stringent cell culture criteria." *Osteoarthritis and Cartilage Open* 2 (1): 100033.

Fahy, N., M. Alini, and M. J. Stoddart. 2018. "Mechanical stimulation of mesenchymal stem cells: Implications for cartilage tissue engineering." *Journal of Orthopaedic Research* 36 (1): 52–63.

Fazal-Ur-Rehman, B., A. H. Karen, and C. Hongsik. 2016. "Kartogenin induced chondrogenesis of stem cells and cartilage repair." *International Journal Stem Cell Research and Therapy* 3: 036.

Frank, E. H., M. Jin, A. M. Loening, M. E. Levenston, and A. J. Grodzinsky. 2000. "A versatile shear and compression apparatus for mechanical stimulation of tissue culture explants." *Journal of Biomechanics* 33 (11): 1523–1527.

Gálvez, P., B. Clares, A. Hmadcha, A. Ruiz, and B. Soria. 2013. "Development of a cell-based medicinal product: Regulatory structures in the European Union." *British Medical Bulletin* 105 (1): 85–105.

Gato-Calvo, L., J. Magalhaes, C. Ruiz-Romero, F. J. Blanco, and E. F. Burguera. 2019. "Platelet-rich plasma in osteoarthritis treatment: Review of current evidence." *Therapeutic Advances in Chronic Disease* 10: 2040622319825567.

Gou, G.-H., F.-J. Tseng, S.-H. Wang, P.-J. Chen, J.-F. Shyu, C.-F. Weng, and R.-Y. Pan. 2020. "Autologous chondrocyte implantation versus microfracture in the knee: a meta-analysis and systematic review." *Arthroscopy: The Journal of Arthroscopic & Related Surgery* 36 (1): 289–303.

Guadix, J. Antonio, J. López-Beas, B. Clares, J. L. Soriano-Ruiz, J. Luis Zugaza, and P. Gálvez-Martín. 2019. "Principal criteria for evaluating the quality, safety and efficacy of hMSC-based products in clinical practice: current approaches and challenges." *Pharmaceutics* 11 (11): 552.

Gudas, R., A. Gudaitė, A. Pocius, A. Gudienė, E. Čekanauskas, E. Monastyreckienė, and A. Basevičius. 2012. "Ten-year follow-up of a prospective, randomized clinical study of mosaic osteochondral autologous transplantation versus microfracture for the treatment of osteochondral defects in the knee joint of athletes." *American Journal of Sports Medicine* 40 (11): 2499–2508.

Hall, A. C. 1999. "Differential effects of hydrostatic pressure on cation transport pathways of isolated articular chondrocytes." *Journal of Cellular Physiology* 178 (2): 197–204.

Hall, A.C. 2019. "The role of chondrocyte morphology and volume in controlling phenotype -- Implications for osteoarthritis, cartilage repair, and cartilage engineering." Curr Rheumatol Rep 21: 38.

Iaquinta, M. R., E. Mazzoni, I. Bononi, J. C. Rotondo, C. Mazziotta, M. Montesi, S. Sprio, A. Tampieri, M. Tognon, and F. Martini. 2019. "Adult stem cells for bone regeneration and repair." *Frontiers in Cell and Developmental Biology* 7: 268.

Jiang, S., W. Guo, G. Tian, X. Luo, L. Peng, S. Liu, X. Sui, Q. Guo, and X. Li. 2020. "Clinical application status of articular cartilage regeneration techniques: tissue-engineered cartilage brings new hope." *Stem Cells International* 2020: 1–16.

Johnson, K., S. Zhu, M. S. Tremblay, J. N. Payette, J. Wang, L. C. Bouchez, S. Meeusen, A. Althage, C. Y. Cho, and X. Wu. 2012. "A stem cell–based approach to cartilage repair." *Science* 336 (6082): 717–721.

Kang, H. W., Lee, S. J., Ko, I. K., Kengla, C., Yoo, J. J., & Atala, A. 2016. "A 3D bioprinting system to produce human-scale tissue constructs with structural integrity." *Nature biotechnology* 34 (3): 312–319.

Kurniawan, N. A. 2019. "The ins and outs of engineering functional tissues and organs: evaluating the in-vitro and in-situ processes." *Current Opinion in Organ Transplantation* 24 (5): 590.

Lee, C. R., A. J. Grodzinsky, and M. Spector. 2003. "Biosynthetic response of passaged chondrocytes in a type II collagen scaffold to mechanical compression." *Journal of Biomedical Materials Research Part A: An Official Journal of the Society for Biomaterials, the Japanese Society for Biomaterials, and the Australian Society for Biomaterials and the Korean Society for Biomaterials* 64 (3): 560–569.

Lee, D. A., and D. L. Bader. 1997. "Compressive strains at physiological frequencies influence the metabolism of chondrocytes seeded in agarose." *Journal of Orthopaedic Research* 15 (2): 181–188.

Li, Z., L. Kupcsik, S.-J. Yao, M. Alini, and M. J. Stoddart. 2010. "Mechanical load modulates chondrogenesis of human mesenchymal stem cells through the TGF-β pathway." *Journal of Cellular and Molecular Medicine* 14 (6a): 1338–1346.

Mauck, R. L., B. A. Byers, X. Yuan, and R. S. Tuan. 2007. "Regulation of cartilaginous ECM gene transcription by chondrocytes and MSCs in 3D culture in response to dynamic loading." *Biomechanics and Modeling in Mechanobiology* 6 (1): 113–125.

Mauck, R. L., M. A. Soltz, C. C. B. Wang, D. D. Wong, P.-H. Grace Chao, W. B. Valhmu, C. T. Hung, and G. A. Ateshian. 2000. "Functional tissue engineering of articular cartilage through dynamic loading of chondrocyte-seeded agarose gels." *Journal of Biomechanical Engineering* 122 (3): 252–260.

McCormick, F, B. J. Cole, B. Nwachukwu, J. D. Harris, H. D. Adkisson IV, and J. Farr. 2013. "Treatment of focal cartilage defects with a juvenile allogeneic 3-dimensional articular cartilage graft." *Operative Techniques in Sports Medicine* 21 (2): 95–99.

Medvedeva, E. V., E. A. Grebenik, S. N. Gornostaeva, V. I. Telpuhov, A. V. Lychagin, P. S. Timashev, and A. S. Chagin. 2018. "Repair of damaged articular cartilage: Current approaches and future directions." *International Journal of Molecular Sciences* 19 (8): 2366.

Meinert, C., K. Schrobback, D. W. Hutmacher, and T. J. Klein. 2017. "A novel bioreactor system for biaxial mechanical loading enhances the properties of tissue-engineered human cartilage." *Scientific Reports* 7 (1): 1–14.

Mirza, M. Z., R. D. Swenson, and S. A. Lynch. 2015. "Knee cartilage defect: Marrow stimulating techniques." *Current Reviews in Musculoskeletal Medicine* 8 (4): 451–456.

Mizuno, S., F. Allemann, and J. Glowacki. 2001. "Effects of medium perfusion on matrix production by bovine chondrocytes in three-dimensional collagen sponges." *Journal of Biomedical Materials Research: An Official Journal of the Society for Biomaterials, the Japanese Society for Biomaterials, and the Australian Society for Biomaterials and the Korean Society for Biomaterials* 56 (3): 368–375.

Mollon, B., R. Kandel, J. Chahal, and J. Theodoropoulos. 2013. "The clinical status of cartilage tissue regeneration in humans." *Osteoarthritis and Cartilage* 21 (12): 1824–1833.

Musumeci, G., C. Loreto, S. Castorina, R. Imbesi, and R. Leonardi. 2013. "Current concepts in the treatment of cartilage damage: A review." *Current Concepts in the Treatment of Cartilage Damage: A Review* 118 (2): 189–203.

Muttigi, M. S., I. Han, H.-K. Park, H. Park, and S.-H. Lee. 2016. "Matrilin-3 role in cartilage development and osteoarthritis." *International Journal of Molecular Sciences* 17 (4): 590.

Negoro, T., Y. Takagaki, H. Okura, and A. Matsuyama. 2018. "Trends in clinical trials for articular cartilage repair by cell therapy." *NPJ Regenerative Medicine* 3 (1): 1–10.

Nicodemus, G. D., and S. J. Bryant. 2010. "Mechanical loading regimes affect the anabolic and catabolic activities by chondrocytes encapsulated in PEG hydrogels." *Osteoarthritis and Cartilage* 18 (1): 126–137.

Niethammer, T. R., M. F. Pietschmann, A. Horng, B. P. Roßbach, A. Ficklscherer, V. Jansson, and P. E. Müller. 2014. "Graft hypertrophy of matrix-based autologous chondrocyte implantation: A two-year follow-up study of NOVOCART 3D implantation in the knee." *Knee Surgery, Sports Traumatology, Arthroscopy* 22 (6): 1329–1336.

Oberweis, C. V., J. A. Marchal, E. López-Ruiz, and P. Gálvez-Martín. 2020. "A worldwide overview of regulatory frameworks for tissue-based products." *Tissue Engineering Part B: Reviews* 26 (2): 181–196.

Palmoski, M. J., and K. D. Brandt. 1984. "Effects of static and cyclic compressive loading on articular cartilage plugs in vitro." *Arthritis & Rheumatism: Official Journal of the American College of Rheumatology* 27 (6): 675–681.

Park, Y.-B., C.-W. Ha, C.-H. Lee, Y. C. Yoon, and Y.-G. Park. 2017. "Cartilage regeneration in osteoarthritic patients by a composite of allogeneic umbilical cord blood-derived mesenchymal stem cells and hyaluronate hydrogel: Results from a clinical trial for safety and proof-of-concept with 7 years of extended follow-up." *Stem Cells Translational Medicine* 6 (2): 613–621.

Pavlovich, M. J., J. Hunsberger, and A. Atala. 2016. "Biofabrication: A secret weapon to advance manufacturing, economies, and healthcare." *Trends in Biotechnology* 34 (9): 679–680.

Petite, H., V. Viateau, W. Bensaid, A. Meunier, C. de Pollak, M. Bourguignon, K. Oudina, L. Sedel, and G. Guillemin. 2000. "Tissue-engineered bone regeneration." *Nature Biotechnology* 18 (9): 959–963.

Salinas, E. Y., J. C. Hu, and K. Athanasiou. 2018. "A guide for using mechanical stimulation to enhance tissue-engineered articular cartilage properties." *Tissue Engineering Part B: Reviews* 24 (5): 345–358.

Salinas, E. Y., A. Aryaei, N. Paschos, E. Berson, H. Kwon, J. C. Hu, and K. A. Athanasiou. 2020. "Shear stress induced by fluid flow produces improvements in tissue-engineered cartilage." *Biofabrication* 12 (4): 045010.

Santoro, R., A. L. Olivares, G. Brans, D. Wirz, C. Longinotti, D. Lacroix, I. Martin, and D. Wendt. 2010. "Bioreactor based engineering of large-scale human cartilage grafts for joint resurfacing." *Biomaterials* 31 (34): 8946–8952.

Savadipour, A., R. J. Nims, D. B. Katz, and F. Guilak. 2022. "Regulation of chondrocyte biosynthetic activity by dynamic hydrostatic pressure: the role of TRP channels." *Connective Tissue Research* 63 (1): 69–81.

Schulz, R. M., N. Wüstneck, C. C. van Donkelaar, J. C. Shelton, and A. Bader. 2008. "Development and validation of a novel bioreactor system for load-and perfusion-controlled tissue engineering of chondrocyte-constructs." *Biotechnology and Bioengineering* 101 (4): 714–728.

Singh, B. N., A. Nallakumarasamy, S. Sinha, A. Rastogi, S. P. Mallick, S. Divakar, and P. Srivastava. 2022. "Generation of hybrid tissue engineered construct through embedding autologous chondrocyte loaded platelet rich plasma/alginate based hydrogel in porous scaffold for cartilage regeneration." *International Journal of Biological Macromolecules* 203: 389–405.

Smith, R. L., S. F. Rusk, B. E. Ellison, P. Wessells, K. Tsuchiya, D. R. Carter, W. E. Caler, L. J. Sandell, and D. J. Schurman. 1996. "In vitro stimulation of articular chondrocyte mRNA and extracellular matrix synthesis by hydrostatic pressure." *Journal of Orthopaedic Research* 14 (1): 53–60.

Wang, Y., et al. 2018. "Bone remodeling induced by mechanical forces is regulated by miRNAs." *Bioscience Reports* 38 (4): BSR20180448.

Wernike, E., Z. Li, M. Alini, and S. Grad. 2008. "Effect of reduced oxygen tension and long-term mechanical stimulation on chondrocyte-polymer constructs." *Cell and Tissue Research* 331 (2): 473–483.

Yamasaki, S., H. Mera, M. Itokazu, Y. Hashimoto, and S. Wakitani. 2014. "Cartilage repair with autologous bone marrow mesenchymal stem cell transplantation: Review of pre-clinical and clinical studies." *Cartilage* 5 (4): 196–202.

Ye, C., J. Chen, Y. Qu, H. Liu, J. Yan, Y. Lu, Z. Yang, F. Wang, and P. Li. 2020. "Naringin and bone marrow mesenchymal stem cells repair articular cartilage defects in rabbit knees through the transforming growth factor-β superfamily signaling pathway." *Experimental and Therapeutic Medicine* 20 (5): 1–1.

Zhao, Y., X Zhao, R. Zhang, Y. Huang, Y. Li, M. Shan, X. Zhong, Y. Xing, M. Wang, and Y. Zhang. 2020. "Cartilage extracellular matrix scaffold with kartogenin-encapsulated PLGA microspheres for cartilage regeneration." *Frontiers in Bioengineering and Biotechnology* 8: 600103.

Index

Note: Figures are indicated by *italics*. Tables are indicated by **bold**.

For Product Safety Concerns and Information please contact our EU
representative GPSR@taylorandfrancis.com
Taylor & Francis Verlag GmbH, Kaufingerstraße 24, 80331 München, Germany

www.ingramcontent.com/pod-product-compliance
Lightning Source LLC
Chambersburg PA
CBHW060804220326
41598CB00022B/2537